CLINICAL PROBLEMS IN VASCULAR SURGERY

CLINICAL PROBLEMS IN VASCULAR SURGERY

EDITED BY

Robert B Galland MD, FRCS
Consultant Surgeon, Royal Berkshire Hospital, Reading, UK

AND

Charles AC Clyne MS, FRCS(Ed), FRCS(Eng)
Formerly Consultant Surgeon, Torbay Hospital, Torquay, UK

Edward Arnold
A member of the Hodder Headline Group
LONDON BOSTON MELBOURNE AUCKLAND

First published in Great Britain 1994

Distributed in the Americas by Little, Brown and Company
35 Beacon Street, Boston, MA 02108

British Library Cataloguing in Publication Data
Available on request

ISBN 0-340-56437-7

Whilst the advice and information in this book is believed to be true and accurate at the date of going to press, neither the author nor the publisher can accept any legal responsibility or liability for any errors or omissions that may be made. In particular (but without limiting the generality of the preceding disclaimer) every effort has been made to check drug dosages; however, it is still possible that errors have been missed. Furthermore, dosage schedules are constantly being revised and new side effects recognised. For these reasons the reader is strongly urged to consult the drug companies' printed instructions before administering any of the drugs recommended in this book.

Typeset in 10/11pt Linotron Century Old Style by
Rowland Phototypesetting Limited, Bury St Edmunds, Suffolk.
Printed and bound in Great Britain for Edward Arnold,
a division of Hodder Headline PLC,
338 Euston Road, London NW1 3BH by
Butler and Tanner Limited, Frome, Somerset.

Preface

This book has been written to provide a background of basic principles in vascular surgery. Common problems have been identified and their management described by clinicians having an interest and expertise in that subject. We have aimed the book primarily at trainees in vascular surgery, particularly those about to undertake postgraduate examinations. However, we hope that it will also be of value and interest to more senior surgeons who encounter vascular problems from time to time but whose main interests lie elsewhere.

Sadly, Charles Clyne died before the project was completed.

Bob Galland
Reading, April 1993

Contents

Contributors

Ali Bakran BSc, FRCS(Ed), FRCS
Consultant Transplant and Vascular Surgeon, The Royal Liverpool University Hospital Trust, Liverpool

Aires AB Barros D'Sa MD, FRCS, FRCS(Ed)
Consultant Vascular Surgeon, Royal Victoria Hospital, Belfast

Jonathan D Beard FRCS, ChM
Consultant Vascular Surgeon, Vascular Surgery Unit, Royal Hallamshire Hospital, Sheffield

Jill JF Belch MD, FRCP
Consultant Physician and Reader, University Department of Medicine, Ninewells Hospital and Medical School, Dundee

Peter RF Bell MD, FRCS, FRCS(Glasg)
Professor of Surgery, University Department of Surgery, Leicester Royal Infirmary, Leicester

Ken Burnand MS, FRCS
Professor of Vascular Surgery, St Thomas' Hospital, London

Kevin G. Callum MS, FRCS
Consultant Surgeon, Derbyshire Royal Infirmary, Derby

W Bruce Campbell MS, MRCP, FRCS
Consultant Surgeon, Royal Devon and Exeter Hospital, Exeter

John Chamberlain FRCS(Ed)
Consultant Vascular Surgeon, Freeman Hospital, Newcastle upon Tyne

Anthony DB Chant BSc, MS, FRCS
Consultant Vascular Surgeon, Royal South Hants Hospital, Southampton

NJW Cheshire FRCS
Research Fellow, Vascular Unit, St Mary's Hospital, London

Jack Collin MA, MD, FRCS
Consultant Surgeon and Reader in Surgery, John Radcliffe Hospital and University of Oxford

RJ Corson FRCS(Ed)
Research Fellow, University Hospital of South Manchester

Simon G Darke MS, FRCS
Consultant Vascular Surgeon, Royal Bournemouth Hospital, Bournemouth

HHG Eastcott MS, FRCS, FRCOG, Hon. FACS, Hon. FRACS
Consulting Surgeon, St Mary's Hospital, London; Emeritus Consultant in Surgery and Vascular Surgery to the Royal Navy

AT Edwards FRCS
Department of Surgery, University Hospital of South Manchester

Robert B Galland MD, FRCS
Consultant Surgeon, Royal Berkshire Hospital, Reading

Anthony AEB Giddings MD, FRCS
Consultant Surgeon, Royal Surrey County Hospital, Guildford

Peter L Harris MD, FRCS
Consultant General and Vascular Surgeon, the Royal Liverpool University Hospital Trust, Liverpool

Stephen M Jones FRCS
Consultant Surgeon, Taunton and Somerset Hospital, Taunton

Nigel C Keddie MA, FRCS, FRCS(Ed)
Consultant Surgeon, West Cumberland Hospital, Whitehaven; Honorary Clinical Lecturer in Surgery, University of Newcastle upon Tyne

Gordon DO Lowe MD, FRCP(Ed, Glasg, Lond)
Professor of Medicine and Consultant Physician, University of Glasgow and Royal Infirmary, Glasgow

CN McCollum MD, FRCS
Department of Surgery, University Hospital of South Manchester

Averil O Mansfield ChM, FRCS
Consultant Surgeon, St Mary's Hospital Vascular Unit, London
Jonathan A Michaels MA, MChir, FRCS(Ed)
Clinical Lecturer, Nuffield Department of Surgery, John Radcliffe Hospital and University of Oxford, Oxford
Mohammed S Quraishy FRCS(Ed)
Research Fellow, Royal Surrey County Hospital, Guildford
Michael R Rees BSc, FRCR, MRCP, FACA
Professor of Radiological sciences and Cardiovascular Interventions Keele University, School of Postgraduate Medicine, Hartshill, Stoke-on-Trent
C Vaughan Ruckley ChM(Ed), FRCS(Ed), FRCP(Ed)
Consultant Surgeon, Vascular Surgery Unit, Edinburgh Royal Infirmary and Professor of Vascular Surgery, University Department of Surgery, Edinburgh
John H Scurr FRCS
Senior Lecturer and Consultant Surgeon, University College and Middlesex School of Medicine, London
Shukri K Shami MS, FRCS(Ed)
Research Fellow, Department of Surgery, University College and Middlesex Hospital School of Medicine, London
JF Thompson MS, FRCS
Consultant Surgeon, Royal Devon & Exeter Hospital, Exeter
Chandy Verghese FRCA
Consultant in Intensive Care and Anaesthesia, Royal Berkshire Hospital, Reading
CS Waldmann MA, FFARCS, EDICM
Director of Intensive Care and Consultant Anaesthetist, Royal Berkshire Hospital, Reading
John HH Webster MA, MChir, FRCS
Consultant Vascular Surgeon, Royal South Hants Hospital, Southampton
John HN Wolfe MS, FRCS
Consultant Vascular Surgeon, Regional Vascular Unit, St Mary's Hospital, London and Honorary Senior Lecturer, Royal Postgraduate Medical School, Hammersmith Hospital, London

1

Historical comment

HHG Eastcott

Ancient learning

The study of vascular disease is much older than most of us realize. 4000 years ago, in *The Yellow Emperor's Classic of Internal Medicine*,[1] Huang Ti wrote:

> 'All the blood in the body is under the control of the heart . . . the blood flows continuously in a circle and never stops.'

This remarkable author went on to a more clinical observation:

> 'When the feet receive blood it strengthens the foot-steps . . . When the blood coagulates within the feet it causes pains and chills.'

The stone-age diet was a healthy one; wild meat, fruit, beans, tubers and roots, brought into the cave mostly after exertion. Those ancestors did not live as long as we do, so atheroma was probably a rarity among them.

Palaeopathological studies by Sir Marc Ruffer[2] on Egyptian mummies dating between 1580 and 527 BC describe calcification in many large and peripheral arteries. One example from the XVIIIth–XXth Dynasty included:

> '. . . the thoracic aorta from a point just above the origin of the left subclavian artery and the whole of the abdominal aorta. The internal coat is studded with small calcareous patches, and the two largest, nearly the size of a shilling, are situated just above the bifurcation. The left subclavian at a point just above its origin is almost blocked by a raised, ragged calcareous excrescence, as large as a threepenny bit (calcified atheromatous ulcer) . . . The common carotid arteries show small patches of atheroma, but the most marked changes are found in the pelvic arteries and in those of the lower limbs.'

Many specimens of the tibial and peroneal arteries showed nodules and calcification. Some were normal, more often in the upper limb arteries. These remnants seem to speak clearly across the centuries. Their message to us is that occlusive atherosclerosis, in the distribution that we know so well, was already a disease of civilization three thousand years ago.

Such aneurysms as survive in the records were nearly all traumatic, often also iatrogenic. Galen was familiar with the false aneurysm that follows unskilful efforts at blood letting from the elbow flexure. Sir William Osler[3] has left us an amusing account of this:

> '. . . a young and inexperienced surgeon had opened an artery instead of a vein and the blood spurted out . . . I took in the situation at once . . . prepared a medicine . . . viscid, conglutinable and obstructive . . . and bound it strongly over the lips of the wound . . . I charged the surgeon not to dress the wound before the fourth day, and not without me. The cure was complete, and Galen remarks that this was the only successful case of the kind, as in all others aneurysm had followed.'

As surgeon to the school of gladiators at Pergamos in Asia Minor, Galen became skilled in the treatment of wounds, and wrote on this[4] and on the related subject of aneurysms. He also distinguished between dry and moist gangrene.[5]

The first ligation for the cure of peripheral aneurysm seems to have been performed by Antyllus, a Greek surgeon practising in Rome during the second century. Osler writes:

> '. . . not a fact of his life is known, yet through the mists of eighteen centuries he looms large as one of the most daring and accomplished surgeons of all time.'

Osler also relates, from the records of Oribasius, court physician to the Emperor Julian, Antyllus's account of the distinctive features of true and false aneurysms, with directions for their cure by ligation.[3] Of this work the great French surgeon and anthropologist, Paul Broca (quoted by Osler), remarked: 'In every line one recognises the author who has seen and done the things of which he speaks.'

During the dark ages after the fall of Rome, when medicine allied itself to the supreme authority of the Church, the practice of surgery fell to the less privileged class of monk and barber surgeon, whose only schooling was a practical apprenticeship. The greatest of these, appearing on the scene just as the Renaissance was beginning, was Ambroise Paré. His treatment of war wounds with dressings of wine, instead of the cautery-iron, foreshadowed the discovery of its scientific basis by his compatriot, Louis Pasteur. Paré knew that syphilis could cause spontaneous aortic aneurysm, with the pounding peripheral pulses of aortic incompetence, and that the enlarging sac would follow an inexorable progress towards a fatal rupture.[4]

The return of medicine as a science stemmed from the great school of Padua,[4] where in the mid-sixteenth century Andreas Vesalius, as the newly appointed professor of anatomy and surgery, showed the true inner form of the human body for the first time. He also recorded the first clinico-pathological description of an abdominal aortic aneurysm. At the same school, early in the seventeenth century, William Harvey was inspired by his famous practical observation of cadaver vein valves and movement of blood in the living forearm to an acceptable and easily proved explanation of the basic working of the circulation.

The birth of vascular surgery

It was in Newcastle in June 1759 that Samuel Hallowell, acting upon the suggestion of his younger associate Richard Lambert, repaired an iatrogenic brachial artery laceration by transfixing it with a pin, and binding this in place with a length of thread wound round it as a figure of eight. This innovation succeeded and the two pioneers reported it to William Hunter,[6] though like most of the other great advances in vascular surgery it was either forgotten or largely ignored for many years.*

William Hunter practised in London as a surgeon, obstetrician and anatomist. Two years before the Newcastle repair case, and in the same journal, he published the first truly scientific account of a traumatic arteriovenous fistula, including its effect in causing dilatation of the draining veins as well as enlargement of the artery, and a clear description of a palpable thrill at the point of injury.[7] His more famous brother John came down from Scotland to work with him for twelve years. John then joined the army as a surgeon to gain experience and improve his finances. During three years' active service in Belle Isle and Portugal he learned much about war wounds. We may still read about this today in one of his few surviving works.[8] On his return to London his practice and professional standing soon increased sufficiently to support his own experimental work in comparative anatomy and surgical science. His pupils included many who went on to fame and success, including Sir Astley Cooper, Edward Jenner, and the Americans, Valentine Mott and Philip Syng Physick.[5] His best known contribution was the Hunterian ligation for popliteal aneurysm,[9] the advantages of which were its safe, indirect surgical approach in the adductor (Hunter's) canal, and a slowing, rather than a complete arrest of the blood flow through the aneurysm, giving time for the establishment of a collateral circulation. He made other advances of comparable importance in transplantation and in dental surgery.[10] His death from myocardial infarction occurred shortly after an acrimonious committee meeting at St George's Hospital.

These were the years of the French Revolution, which brought Napoleon Bonaparte to power. Accompanying him in each and every campaign was his army surgeon, Baron Larrey. Like Ambroise Paré two centuries before him, Larrey, in times of action, was always close to the battle line. He knew, as his helicopter-borne successors do today, the importance of speed in the treatment of war casualties. On the field of Borodino he achieved 200 amputations in a single day. As a clinician, he recognized the pulsating collateral arteries about the knee condyles that develop in favourable cases after popliteal artery ligation or occlusion. Some years later he met Astley Cooper and with him discussed their experiences, methods and results in major arterial ligation.[11]

Such was the state of vascular surgery through most of the nineteenth century. At a time when medical science was at last attaining a more modern form, and anaesthesia and antisepsis had removed much of the suffering from operative surgery, vascular surgery stood still. Yet, there were gleams of the future. Nikolai Eck in 1877 constructed a portacaval fistula in a dog.[12] In 1888 Rudolph Matas conceived and proved the merits of operating inside an aneurysm, though by the end of the century had experience of only three more cases.[13] The advantages of this revolutionary change in surgical tactics were clear to Matas from the outset, but it was to be another 60 years before they became accepted in vascular practice through the separate contributions of Hushang Javid, Oscar Creech and Stanley Crawford (see below[14]).

* For example, arteriography, endoaneurysmorrhaphy, heparin, percutaneous angioplasty, prostaglandins, thrombolysis, vascular ultrasonography and vascular grafting.

Glimpses of the future

Alexis Carrel, visionary and mystic though he may have been, brought the quantum leap in surgical principles that led directly to vascular and transplantation surgery as we know them today.[15] With his associate Charles C. Guthrie[16] he devised and tested most of the methods that we now use in vascular suture; tubular and patch grafting, coronary bypass, renal and limb transplantation. Later, with Charles Lindbergh, he constructed the prototype artificial heart.

Yet almost none of this found surgical acceptance at the time. A few courageous operators tried out the vein grafting method for lower limb aneurysms. The first to succeed was José Luis Goyanes, at that time an assistant on the Surgical Professorial Unit in the General Hospital, Madrid. In 1906, after training himself in the techniques of vascular repair in the experimental laboratory,[17] he turned this experience to clinical use by substituting the popliteal vein as an *in situ* bypass graft across the convexity of a left popliteal aneurysm. The patient was a 40-year-old confectioner, an alcoholic, whose aneurysm may have been syphilitic. While an assistant pressed on the femoral artery in Scarpa's triangle, Goyanes used the medial approach to expose the aneurysm which lay behind and above the knee. Controlling the vessels with rubber-covered haemostats he clamped, divided and ligated the popliteal artery above the sac. The leg went rather blue. Using the triangulation method of Carrel he anastomosed the upper stump of the popliteal, end-to-end to the popliteal vein, and then turned to the lower end of the sac. This anastomosis proved more difficult, owing to the state of the arterial wall, which tore when the first sutures were inserted. He noticed that the aneurysm no longer pulsated, though on release of the clamps the vein graft pulsated well and the blood within it became red. The distal popliteal and the tibial arteries also resumed their pulses; so the wound was closed with the knee immobilized in slight flexion.

This was not Goyanes' only human arterial operation; he also repaired a traumatic false aneurysm of the profunda femoris, and a popliteal arteriovenous fistula. Also reported was an axillary vein graft after excision of malignant lymph nodes from a breast cancer. He showed the safety of arterial puncture and catheterization for regional drug infusion.[18] Goyanes lived until 1964, to see most of his methods become accepted and routine.

Though Carrel's innovations and the principles he established were rewarded with the Nobel Prize in Physiology and Medicine in 1912, his work received very little general attention among surgeons. When he died in Vichy France in 1944 they were still little more than speculative curiosities. Matas ignored vein grafting[13] and Halstead condemned it.[14] All through the two World Wars the vascular wounded received little more than did Larrey's patients a century earlier. There were, it is true, isolated examples of surgical courage and dedication. An army surgeon, Vogislav Soubbotitch, by 1913 had restored vascular continuity in 32 cases during the Serbian wars, and showed his results at a meeting in Oxford in 1914 at which Matas was present.[19] In 1925, in an almost forgotten communication,[20] the Polish surgeon Ramuald Weglowski reported the first large series of venous arterial replacement grafts, in Russian Army casualties from conflicts continuing until 1921.

Heparin and arteriography: the missing ingredients

Several of the essentials for successful vascular repair were lacking. We still needed heparin, safe blood transfusion and arteriography. Though heparin had been discovered in 1916 by Jay McLean, a medical student working in WH Howell's laboratory at Johns Hopkins, from the clinical viewpoint it was virtually shelved until in the late 1930s. Then Gordon Murray and Charles Best in Toronto found that a purified, standardized form could safely be used for the prevention of venous thrombosis, and that it could maintain patency of an arterial segment during the clamping time required for the insertion of a graft.[21]

Within three months of Roëntgen's discovery of X-rays, two Viennese physicists, Haschek and Lindenthal, were injecting the wrist artery of a cadaver with thin barium. The result was a perfect, modern-looking photograph of all the arteries of the hand. Calcification was shown in the living aorta by Huber in Berlin and in the tibial arteries by Hoppe Selyer in Kiel.[22]

Peripheral arteriography owes its existence today to Reynaldo dos Santos of Lisbon.[23] He was a friend of Carrel, Cushing, Leriche and Tuffier; he was also an artist and musician and the father of a famous son, John Cid dos Santos (Fig. 1.1). Their work together was inspired by the remarkable, earlier achievements of their neurologist compatriot, Egaz Moniz, who made the first cerebral angiograms in

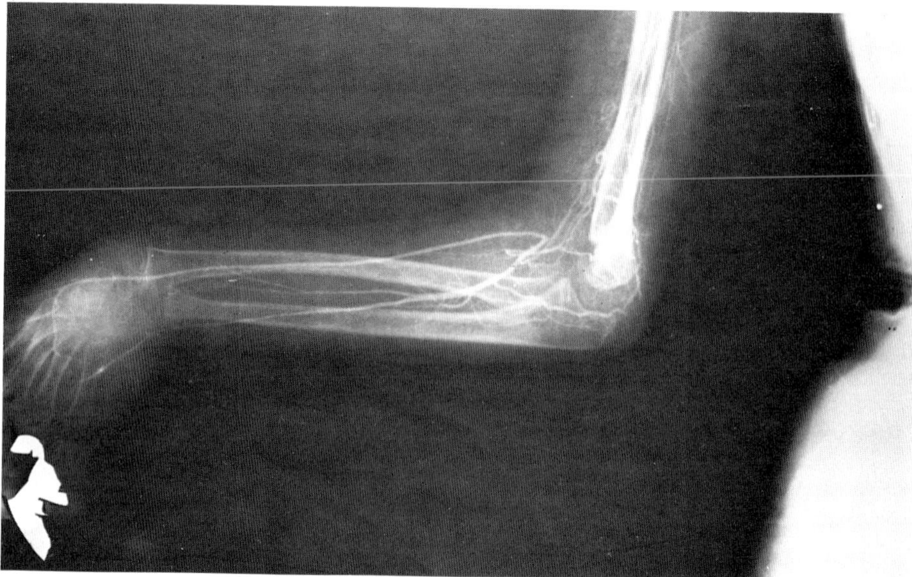

Fig. 1.1 Brachial arteriogram of a 7-year-old boy with Volkmann's contracture, taken in 1937 by John Cid dos Santos, whose note states: 'Fracture of the elbow two months previously. Dissection of the humeral artery at its upper third for arteriography. Artery very thin. Obliteration of the distal humeral artery and rehabilitation of the arteries of the forearm. After the arteriography, liberation of the artery, the median and the radial nerves from the scar tissue which involved them. Patient got better.' (Picture and case details courtesy of the Royal College of Surgeons of Edinburgh.)

1927, and in 1937 showed the association of carotid occlusive disease with cerebral strokes.[24]

The beginnings of success

At that time John Cid dos Santos was a medical student; while helping his father he determined to become a surgeon. Later, on learning of Murray's successes with heparin in venous and aneurysm surgery, he decided to see if it could maintain the patency of surgically 'disobliterated' limb arteries, from which the protective endotheleal layer – so essential, as Carrel and Guthrie had shown, to the fluidity of the blood – must inevitably be removed. The first case, in 1946, was in a young woman of 35, who for three months had suffered severe ischaemia of the right arm and hand from a thrombosis of the right subclavian–axillary artery due to compression by the scalenus. Late patency at two years was confirmed at the time of the report,[25] and again 29 years later in the Leriche Memorial Lecture in Edinburgh[26] in 1975 at which dos Santos made his last public appearance. He died later that year. Another early success cited in the first paper was in a patient aged 40 whose right external iliac and common femoral had occluded.

These and other early thromboendarterectomies by French surgeons were based on the philosophy of René Leriche, now best remembered for his syndrome of aortic bifurcation obstruction with extensive claudication and male sexual impotence. His belief that the affected segment exerted some damaging influence, possibly neurological, was the basis of his policy to excise all such segments and the lumbar sympathetic chain as well.[27] Thus, a local operation for disobliteration was a logical step for the early European and American vascular surgeons trained by Leriche, including John Cid dos Santos himself, his friend Michael DeBakey, a Matas protégé, and EJ Wylie, of San Francisco, who soon reported an extensive experience of thrombo-endarterectomy in the limbs, abdomen and neck.

There was, however, another of Leriche's pupils whose ideas were quite different. Jean Kunlin could see that nature's method in chronic vascular occlusion was less often to recanalize the block than to bypass it with collaterals. He resolved to imitate this, using a venous autograft, with end-to-side anastomoses to the main artery, above and below the diseased segment, at suitable sites near the upper and lower faces of the block. Replacement, he knew, was something that 'had been practised since the opening years of this century . . . but the poor state of the vessel wall in these cases was a good reason to abandon [long, direct-replacement] grafts'. He then describes the case of a man aged 54, whose gangrenous left toes had failed to heal after a lumbar sympathectomy with excision of the occluded superficial femoral artery. A mid-thigh amputation was in prospect:

> 'On the 3rd June 1948 we joined the common femoral to the popliteal by means of a 26 cm saphenous vein graft. The patient's transformation was immediate. The ulcers healed within two weeks. His pain ceased after the operation. The foot which had been cold and purple, with scaly skin, became normal . . . he could walk without pain.'

He then goes on to describe ten more cases with two early graft occlusions. One, in poor condition from his extended suffering, died; but the nine remaining patients did well, and showed the same striking benefits as the first.[28]

The surgery of the aorta

Direct repair of congenital coarctation was achieved in 1945 at almost the same time in Stockholm and Boston. Success in these human cases flowed from the experimental work of Gross and Hufnagel,[29] and stimulated a revival of Carrel's technique for the cold-storage of arterial homografts.[30]

The first successful grafting operations on an abdominal aortic aneurysm were carried out in Paris, using refrigerated human aortic segments.[31,32] Jacques Oudot (a celebrated mountaineer, acclaimed for his part in the first ascent of Annapurna in June 1950) replaced the occluded aorta and its bifurcation, in a woman aged 51 years, using the left oblique retroperitoneal approach. A difficulty occurred over access to the right iliac artery, so to overcome this the resourceful operator made the first known use of the crossover principle. The patient recovered well and soon was able to walk a half mile without difficulty.[31] Tragically, Oudot's promising career was cut short soon afterwards in a road accident.

The first surgical cure of an abdominal aortic aneurysm by grafting was achieved in 1951 (also in Paris) by Charles Dubost,[32] to whom I am indebted for some recollections of his famous case:

> 'I did the operation on a patient in his mid-fifties who presented with claudication in his left leg. His physician examined him and found a huge pulsatile mass in his abdomen and referred the patient for a wrapping or a wiring. When I saw the patient I ordered an aortography which showed a big aneurysm starting immediately below the origin of the renal arteries, associated with a complete obstruction of the primitive iliac artery. In those conditions I thought that any kind of palliative operation would be ineffective, and I estimated that the best chance for the patient was to resect the aneurysm, to remove the whole of the left primitive iliac artery, and to put a graft between the aorta and both iliac vessels. Since 1947 we were familiar at Broussais with preserved human grafts, and we had developed a bank of vessels that we used in peripheral arterial surgery, portal surgery and also in certain cases of the Blalock operation, when the subclavian artery was too short. Unfortunately it was impossible to find a Y-shaped graft whose calibre would be adequate, so I had to prepare a segment of straight thoracic aorta which was preserved by cold storage.
>
> The patient accepted the idea of being submitted to a new operation without anxiety and with great confidence. I had been interested in the surgery of aneurysms for a few years, and had previously had the chance to resect a saccular aneurysm of the ascending aorta which represented the first success since the first attempts of Tuffier in 1903; * so I was thinking that operating and resecting an aneurysm of the below-renal aorta could be less dangerous. Broussais's activity [included] major thoracic and abdominal visceral surgery and we had specially a good experience of oesophageal cancer resection . . . so as I intended to use a combined thoraco-abdominal approach I could anticipate no major problem in this field . . .
>
> After performing an end-to-end aorta-graft anastomosis the straight piece of thoracic aorta was sutured in end-to-end fashion to the right primitive iliac artery. Then the left one was resected to remove the block and an end-to-side anastomosis was performed between the artery and the graft, [thus] a Y-shaped aortic bifurcation was reconstructed. The most difficult part of the operation was the removal of the sac, due to lumbar vessels and to adhesions of the sac to the inferior vena cava. Several small pieces of it were left in place. We had trouble in controlling a spermatic vein and we had (if my memory is good) to reoperate the patient on the same evening. Then the postoperative course was uneventful and the patient was discharged from the hospital after 15 days.
>
> He survived eight years; his death was sudden, at home . . . (?myocardial infarction).

* Tuffier of Paris, a pioneer in thoracic and vascular surgery (who also introduced contrast radiology for study of the kidney), advocated resection of these saccular aneurysms with local repair of the defect in the aortic wall after an apparent success, marred by disruption and secondary haemorrhage after two weeks.[33] Forty years later Bahnson used this method successfully in six cases involving the proximal aorta, syphilis having been confirmed as the cause in most of them.[34]

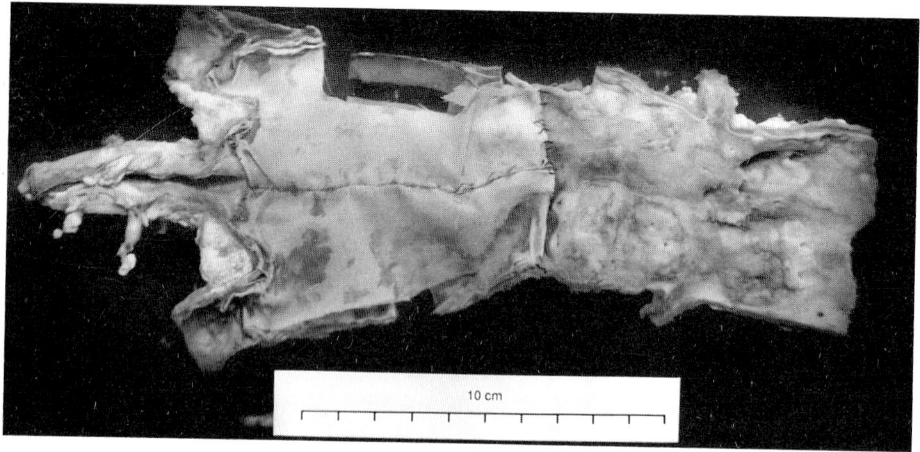

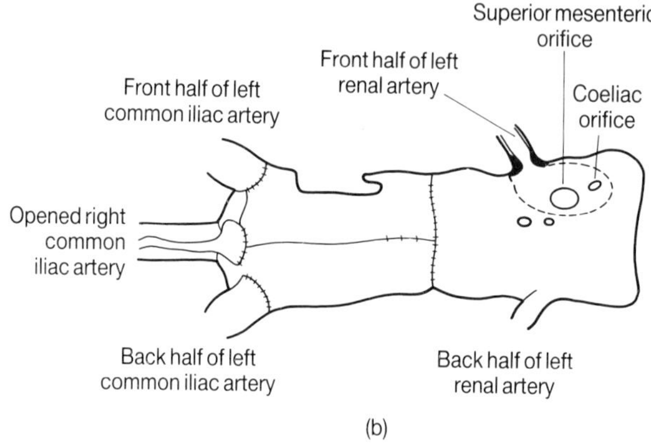

Fig. 1.2 An early fabric prosthesis, inserted at the author's district general hospital in February 1955, in a man aged 64, after favourable experience of a similar case at St Mary's Hospital in November 1954. Both these grafts were made from a piece of Orlon woven cloth, supplied by Charles Hufnagel, and made up with the front and back panels sewn together with a French seam, by the author's wife, as instructed by Hufnagel. The patient made a good recovery, only to die two and a half years later from pulmonary tuberculosis, for he was intolerant to antituberculous chemotherapy. The specimen is sliced open along its left border, though the left renal and left common iliac arteries, and gives much the kind of view that we now see during Stanley Crawford's endoaneurysmal repair of a thoracoabdominal aneurysm,[54] with grouping together of the coeliac, superior mesenteric and right renal orifices (dotted line in diagram).

I would never have thought that so many cases would have been operated in the years following. The coming of prosthetic material and the technique of "graft inclusion" make things rather simple today [just] a simple major surgical procedure.'

As Dubost observed, the greatest impetus towards a safe, simple and relatively cheap method for the replacement of large arteries up to the size of the aorta itself came soon after the two French cases. Voorhees and his colleagues in New York discovered in 1952 that plastic cloth tubes would be accepted by the dog aorta.[35] By 1954 they were able to report clinical results in 17 patients in whom these seamed, home-made segments had been implanted after resection of an abdominal aortic aneurysm.[36] Fig. 1.2 shows such a graft in its third year. The specimen is from one of two cloth-grafted cases of the author's, operated upon during the winter of 1954–55. Both of these patients suffered from tuberculosis, which was still common in the UK at that time.* These two, and three others, did well for two

* During those early post-war years in the UK tuberculosis and syphilis were still common causes of advanced surgical disease. Of our first ten patients grafted at St Mary's Hospital for abdominal aortic aneurysm between 1954 and 1955, one was syphilitic, two were tuberculous and one sac was mycotic. Sir William Osler, in his famous 1905 paper on 16 cases of abdominal aortic aneurysm, reported that nine had syphilis, and ten were alcoholics.[37]

years or more, though one developed a dehiscence of the French seam at 6½ years.

At Christmas time that same winter, Frank Gerbode of San Francisco (who like Charles Dubost was also a cardiac surgeon) rescued one of his old patients. This was a Japanese gentleman whose aneurysm, until then treated conservatively, ruptured while the patient was out fishing. The leak was of the partly 'contained' type, so there was time for Gerbode to place the proximal clamp above the renals and swiftly insert a frozen aortic homograft.[38,39]

The golden age of arterial surgery

The flexible, seamless arterial prosthesis as we know it today began with a chance observation. Sterling Edwards and his medical engineering associate JS Tapp found that when removing a woven, nylon cloth tube from a glass mandril after chemical treatment with formic acid, the tube assumed a permanently crimped or corrugated form which allowed it to be bent and looped without obstructing the lumen.[40] Bifurcations were soon available, in Dacron and Teflon, both of which proved better than nylon. Soon, almost all the major peripheral arteries had been either grafted or bypassed, notably by Michael DeBakey and his associates in Houston, Texas.[41] The golden age of arterial surgery had arrived.

Meanwhile, a revolutionary development was under way. Thomas J Fogarty, at that time in a junior post in Cincinnati, was assisting his chief, John J Cranley, with an embolectomy at which there was difficulty in extracting all the distal thrombus. Fogarty modified a ureteric catheter by fixing a small inflatable rubber balloon to its end. The device was an immediate success;[42] hundreds of limbs were saved and new directions and incentives were opened up for percutaneous, endovascular procedures of numerous kinds. These developments are much in evidence today under the heading of 'minimal access' surgery. More than by anyone, the initiative was taken by Charles Dotter, of Portland, Oregon.[43] He introduced transluminal angioplasty, thrombolysis and supporting stents, and showed that it was possible to cure an arteriovenous fistula and some previously intractable malformations by catheter-introduced emboli, free balloons and glue. He was also largely responsible for the introduction of coronary angiography.

Ultrasound as a medical diagnostic tool began to be used in the 1960s, first for imaging. Though interest then concentrated on its obstetric applications, Ian Donald, the leader in this research, included an examination of an abdominal aortic aneurysm in his classic paper in 1961.[44,†] Flow velocity estimations using the Doppler effect soon followed, with Rushmer and Strandness applying basic physics to common clinical situations.[45]

A new dimension in radiography presented itself in 1973, with the arrival of computed tomography (CT).[46] Such was the importance of this advance that Sir Godfrey Hounsfield (who led the research) received the Nobel Prize in 1979. Early systems were limited to the examination of the head. Even so, new prospects in neurodiagnosis immediately presented themselves and vascular surgeons soon adopted CT for the assessment of patients with possible carotid-derived stroke symptoms. When body-sized units became available, the anatomy and pathology of aortic aneurysms and dissections could be studied from a viewpoint that complemented that of arteriography.[47]

Noninvasive vascular investigations have since burgeoned; even angiography has distanced itself from the formerly universal arterial puncture since the arrival of computerized intravenous arteriography[48] which has virtually eliminated the discomforts and morbidity of arterial puncture. Carotid arteriography, in particular, benefited from the change, for in cerebrovascular occlusive disease there has always been a small but apparently unavoidable mortality to this investigation (which, since most carotid surgery aims at prevention, must mean that the price of benefit to some patients is paid for by complications in others).

Carotid surgery for stenosis with repeated, transient hemisphere ischaemia began in 1954 at St Mary's Hospital, London.[49] Though adopted with enthusiasm in the USA it was never as widely practised in the UK.[50] Controlled trials, one of which virtually ended the practice of intra-extracranial anastomosis for complete carotid occlusion,[51] have examined the outcome of carotid endarterectomy versus the best medical treatment and have lately shown a highly significant benefit from the operation when the narrowing is severe.[52,53] This would clearly only apply to operations under optimum conditions and best surgical skill.

† Both Dotter and Donald later became cardiac surgical patients, and both suffered a long and distressing illness.

Into the future

The risk–benefit ratio in vascular surgery has always varied between hospitals and between countries. When Stanley Crawford in 1965 first applied the endoaneurysmorrhaphy principle to the seemingly insoluble problem of an expanding, recurrent thoracoabdominal aneurysm,[54] it remained a lonely and unattainable surgical summit for nearly a quarter of a century. Now it is within the capacity of most vascular centres and, in emergency, some district hospitals.

History is a continuing process; moreover, as Sir Winston Churchill observed, as we look back it teaches us to look into the future. For vascular surgeons and their patients this seems likely to bring more accurate diagnosis by less invasive methods, safer support services, the monitoring scrutiny of the audit, and a growing use of intraluminal techniques.

References

1. Veith I. *Huang Ti Nei Ching Su Wen; The Yellow Emperor's Classic of Internal Medicine.* Berkeley and Los Angeles: University of California Press, 1966.
2. Ruffer MA. On arterial lesions found in Egyptian mummies. *J Path Bact* 1911; **15:** 453–61.
3. Osler W. Remarks on arterio-venous aneurysm. *Lancet* 1915; **i:** 949–55.
4. Guthrie D. *A History of Medicine.* Edinburgh: Nelson, new edition 1985.
5. Zimmerman LM, Veith I. *Great Ideas in the History of Surgery.* Baltimore: Williams & Wilkins, 1961.
6. Lambert R. Account of a new method of treating an aneurysm. Medical Observations and Enquiries by a Society of Physicians in London. London: Wm Johnston, 1764; **2:** 360–4.
7. Hunter W. Further observations on a particular species of aneurysm. *Ibid.* 1757; **1:** 323–57.
8. Hunter J. A treatise on the blood, inflammation and gun-shot wounds. London: Sherwood, Giblert & Piper, 1828.
9. Schechter DC, Bergan JJ. Popliteal aneurysm: a celebration of the bicentennial of John Hunter's operation. *Ann Vasc Surg* 1986; **1:** 116–26.
10. Qvist G. *John Hunter, 1728–1793.* London: Wm Heinemann Medical Books, 1981.
11. Dible JH. *Napoleon's Surgeon.* London: Wm Heinemann Medical Books, 1970.
12. Child CG. Eck's fistula. *Surg Gynec Obstet* 1953; **96:** 375–6.
13. Matas R. An operation for the radical cure of aneurism based upon arteriorrhaphy. *Ann Surg* 1903; **37:** 161–95.
14. Schumacker HB. Evolution of an operation. *J Cardiovasc Surg* 1981; **22:** 60–7.
15. Edwards P, Edwards WS. *Alexis Carrel: Visionary Surgeon.* Springfield: CC Thomas, 1974.
16. Guthrie CC. Blood vessel surgery and its applications (a reprint). Harbison SP, Fisher B (eds). Pittsburgh: University of Pittsburgh Press, 1959.
17. Goyanes J. Nuevos trabajos de chirurgia vascular: sustitucion plastica de las arterias por las venas, o arterioplastica venosa, como nuevo metodo al tratimiento de las aneurismas. *Siglo Medico* 1906; **53:** 546–8, 561–4.
18. Barros JL. Investigaciones sobre los trabajos vasculares del Dr Jose Goyanes Capdevila. *Cirurgia, Genecologia y Urologia* 1965; **19:** 1–26.
19. Soubbotitch V. Military experiences of traumatic aneurysms. *Lancet* 1913; **ii:** 720–1.
20. Shumacker HB. Weglowski and what might have been. *Aust NZ J Surg* 1990; **60:** 219–24.
21. Murray GDW. Heparin in thrombosis and embolism (Hunterian Lecture at the Royal College of Surgeons of England, June 1939). *Br J Surg* 1939; **27:** 567–78.
22. Doty T. *Development of Angiography and Cardiovascular Catheterisation.* Littleton, Mass: Publishing Sciences Group, 1976.
23. dos Santos R, Lamas A, Caldas J. L'artériographie des membres, de l'aorte et de ses branches abdominales. *Bull Mem Soc Medchir* 1929; **55:** 587–601.
24. Moniz E, Lima A, de Lacerda R. Hémiplégies par thrombose de las carotide interne. *Presse Méd* 1937; **52:** 977–8.
25. dos Santos JC. Note sur la désobstruction des anciennes thromboses artérielles. *Presse Méd* 1949; **39:** 544–5.
26. dos Santos JC. From embolectomy to endarterectomy or the fall of a myth (Leriche Memorial Lecture). *J Cardiovasc Surg* 1976; **17:** 113–28.
27. Leriche R. De la résection du carrefour aortic–iliaque avec double sympathectomie pour thrombose artéritique de l'aorte; le syndrome de l'obliteration termino-aortique par artérite. *Presse Méd* 1940; **48:** 601–4.
28. Kunlin J. Le traitement de l'artérite oblitérante par la greffe veineuse longue. *Arch Mal du Coeur* 1949; **42:** 371–2.
29. Gross RE, Hufnagel CA. Coarctation of the aorta. Experimental studies regarding its correction. *N Engl J Med* 1945; **233:** 287–93.
30. Hufnagel CA. Rapid freezing technique for preserved homologous arterial transplants. *Bull Am Coll Surg* 1947; **32:** 321 (abstract).
31. Oudot J. La greffe vasculaire dans les thromboses du carrefour aortique. *Presse Méd* 1951; **59:** 234–6.
32. Dubost C. A propos du traitement des anévrismes de l'aorte. Ablation de l'anévrisme. Rétablissement de la continuité par greffe d'aorte humaine conservée. *Mem Acad Chir* (Paris) 1951; **77:** 381–3.
33. Tuffier T. A propos du traitement chirurgicale des

anévrismes de l'aorte. *Bull Mèm Soc Chir Paris* 1911; **37:** 843–8.
34. Bahnson HT. Considerations in the exclusion of aortic aneurysms. *Ann Surg* 1953; **138:** 377–86.
35. Voorhees AB, Jaretski A, Blakemore AH. The use of tubes constructed of Vinyon 'N' cloth in bridging arterial defects: a preliminary report. *Ann Surg* 1952; **135:** 332–6.
36. Blakemore AH, Voorhees AB. The use of tubes constructed from Vinyon 'N' cloth in bridging arterial defects. Experimental and clinical. *Ann Surg* 1954; **140:** 324–34.
37. Osler W. Aneurysms of the abdominal aorta. *Lancet* 1905; **ii:** 1089–96
38. Gerbode F. Ruptured aortic aneurysm: a surgical emergency. *Surg Gynec Obstet* 1954; **98:** 759 (editorial).
39. Gerbode F. Personal communication, 1983.
40. Edwards WS, Tapp JS. Chemically treated nylon tubes as arterial grafts. *Surgery* 1955; **38:** 61–70.
41. DeBakey ME. The development of vascular surgery. *Am J Surg* 1979; **137:** 697–738.
42. Fogarty TJ, Cranley JJ, Krause RJ, *et al.* A method for the extraction of arterial emboli and thrombi. *Surg Gynec Obstet* 1963; **116:** 241–4.
43. Dotter CT, Ruble EJ. Transluminal treatment of arteriosclerotic obstruction: description of a new technique and a preliminary report of its application. *Circulation* 1964; **30:** 654–70.
44. Donald I, Brown TG. Demonstration of tissue interfaces within the body by ultrasonic echo sounding. *Br J Radiol* 1961; **35:** 539–46.
45. Strandness DE, McCutcheon EP, Rushmer RF. Application of a transcutaneous Doppler flowmeter in the evaluation of occlusive arterial disease. *Surg Gynec Obstet* 1966; **122:** 1039–45.
46. Hounsfield GN. Computerized transverse axial scanning (tomography). *Br J Radiol* 1973; **46:** 1016–22.
47. Williams LR, Flinn WR, Yao JST, *et al.* Extended use of computer tomography in the management of complex aortic problems: a learning experience. *J Vasc Surg* 1986; **4:** 264–71.
48. Crummy AB, Mistretta CA, Strother CM, *et al.* Computerized fluoroscopy: digital subtraction for intravenous angiocardiography. *Am J Radiol* 1980; **135:** 1131–40.
49. Eastcott HHG, Pickering GW, Rob CG. Reconstruction of internal carotid artery in a patient with intermittent attacks of hemiplegia. *Lancet* 1954; **ii:** 994–6.
50. Murie JA, Morris PJ. Carotid endarterectomy in Great Britain and Ireland. *Br J Surg* 1986; **73:** 867–70.
51. The EC/IC Bypass Study Group. Failure of extracranial–intracranial arterial bypass to reduce the risk of ischemic stroke. *N Engl J Med* 1985; **313:** 1191–200.
52. European Carotid Surgery Trialists' Collaborative Group. European Carotid Surgery Trial: interim results for symptomatic patients with severe (70–99%) carotid stenosis and with mild (90–29%) carotid stenosis. *Lancet* 1991; **337:** 1325–43.
53. North American Symptomatic Carotid Endarterectomy Trial Collaborators. Beneficial effect of carotid endarterectomy in symptomatic patients with high-grade carotid stenosis. *N Engl J Med* 1991; **325:** 445–53.
54. Crawford ES. Thoraco-abdominal and abdominal aortic aneurysms involving the renal, superior mesenteric and celiac arteries. *Ann Surg* 1974; **179:** 763–72.

2

Vascular audit

Stephen M Jones

> 'The attainment of surgical progress is best secured by planting a high standard before the mind, with the determination of approaching as near to it as one has strength to do.'
>
> (John Hilton, FRS, FRCS, late president of the Royal College of Surgeons of England[1])

Regular review of the quality of patient care in the UK has become an integral part of the work of every surgeon, indeed of every doctor. This activity has been stimulated by increased patient expectations, promoted by professional bodies such as the Royal Colleges and the World Health Organization,[2,3] and formalized in the NHS White Paper, *Working for Patients*.[4]

The difference between what is now called 'surgical audit' and the traditional practice of case review, mortality and morbidity meetings, etc., is that the new audit should be a systematic review of the whole of clinical practice, not just a selective review of interesting cases. It is meant to be an educational exercise aimed at increasing the quality of patient care and is not intended to identify and punish the wrongdoer. John Hilton's exhortation to surgeons to set high standards and then to attempt to achieve them is particularly relevant in the current climate.

Auditing in vascular surgery is already producing benefits. For example, the Lothian operative surgery audit and the Confidential Enquiry into Perioperative Deaths (CEPOD) demonstrated reduced mortality for ruptured abdominal aortic aneurysm when patients were operated upon by experienced vascular surgeons.[5,6]

It is now important to integrate auditing into everyday clinical practice.

Principles of surgical audit

Definition

Surgical audit is the process by which medical staff collectively review, evaluate and improve their practice.[2] As defined in *Working for Patients*, (medical) audit is 'the systematic, critical analysis of the quality of medical care, including the procedures used for diagnosis and treatment, the use of resources and the resulting outcome and quality of life for the patient.' Expressed more simply it is:

- *What do we do?*
- *How well do we do it?*
- *How can we improve?*
- *Have we improved?*

This process has been called the 'audit cycle', a useful term because it stresses the need to complete the process and discover the answer to the final question, 'Have we improved?' To answer these questions effectively, the surgical audit requires an explicit definition of the standard of patient care to which surgeons and patients aspire. By establishing clear objectives it becomes possible to assess their achievement and monitor improvements.

Scope of surgical audit

From the above definition, it is clear that the audit should encompass the broad range of activity involved in treating patients and should include the availability of the service in question (access), the problems encountered in treating patients (process) and the outcome of treatment, not only in terms of technical success of surgical procedures, but also the functional result and degree of satisfaction of the patient with the treatment given (outcome audit).[2,7]

Selection of subjects for audit

The range of possible subjects for such review is shown in Table 2.1. While many of these topics can be covered by information obtained from hospital information systems or from personal computer audit data, some require specific prospective study involving extra time and cost. These are the studies increasingly being undertaken by medical audit ana-

Table 2.1 Subjects for vascular audit

	Data available on hospital systems	Requires specialty data collection	Requires targeted 'topic' audit
Access	Waiting time for outpatient appt Waiting time for admission Cancellation: by hospital by patient Special facilities	Non-medical delay in: investigation operation	Waiting time in clinic Appropriateness of referral: consultation admission
Process	Caseload: outpatients admissions: day cases % inpatients % emergency %	Work load: consultations investigations operations case-mix complexity emergency % trainee supervision	Case-note quality Communications: referral letters discharge letters
Outcome	Crude mortality figures	Unplanned events: mortality readmission return to theatre transfer to ITU complications: specific general	Patient satisfaction: return to work social activity Effectiveness: relief of symptoms
Resource utilization	Theatres: allocation used % duration of lists Beds: length of stay Staffing levels: actual ideal	Non-medical delay in: discharge	Case-mix costing

Modified from reference 7.

lysts, appointed to clinical departments as a result of central Department of Health funding for medical auditing. The subjects of most value are likely to be those of relevance to local problem areas (e.g. the 'occasional' vascular surgeon), high-volume activities (e.g. varicose veins, referrals for claudication), or high-cost activities (e.g. major arterial reconstructions).

If the audit is to be truly systematic, an indication of total work-load and case-mix, including changes over time, is essential. To achieve this, data collection systems are required which provide basic information on all patients who are seen. This should include not only patients who undergo a surgical procedure but also those seen just for consultation and patients admitted to hospital without an operation being performed. Where possible, the information should also be viewed against the background of disease in the community (Fig. 2.1).

Collection of data

Existing hospital systems for collection of such data are insufficient at present to allow the required systematic audit and will need to be developed to include this information. A number of pioneering starts in developing tailor-made computer systems have been made by some enthusiasts,[8–10] but comprehensive, low-cost, integrated data collection is still only available to a few. Useful guidance on the main require-

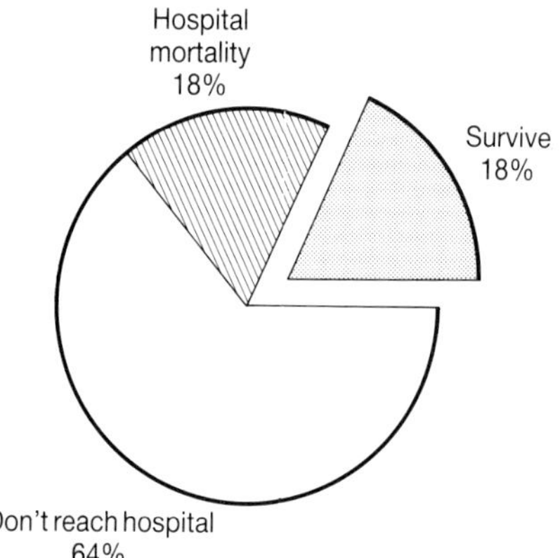

Fig. 2.1 Survival after aortic aneurysm rupture. By including deaths outside hospital and patients admitted but not offered operation for ruptured abdominal aortic aneurysm, the true mortality is seen to be considerably in excess of the impression gained by looking only at operative mortality. (See also Chapter 27.)

ments of such integrated computer systems is available in a publication by the Department of Health.[11] A basic list of essential information required for each surgical patient (minimum data set) has been published by the Royal College of Surgeons of England.[12] However, even in well organized studies experience shows that completeness of data is difficult to achieve; for example, the Vascular Registry in Southern Sweden[13] experienced problems in obtaining complete follow-up data on such basic items as pre- and postoperative Doppler pressure measurements and graft patency.

It should be remembered that the Data Protection Act (1984) requires that all computer systems holding data identifiable to a living individual should be registered with the Data Protection Registrar, and that patients have a right to check that data held about them on computer are accurate. In a similar way, the Access to Health Records Act (1990) allows patients access to the information held about them in manual records like hospital case-notes, and the Access to Medical Reports Act (1990) allows the patient to see the contents of medical reports written about them to a third party before they are released.

A word on data definitions

Locally developed audit systems have tended to create their own nomenclature of diseases and operative procedures. This has benefits in fitting local needs, avoiding ambiguity to the users and making data collection easier. But to allow comparison with other centres, all systems should be capable of mapping to the current UK standards of ICD9 diagnostic coding (International Classification of Disease, ninth revision) and OPCS4 procedure coding (Office of Population Censuses and Surveys, fourth revision). While not themselves ideal (ICD9 in particular allows little detailed coding of vascular disease) they are currently the only ones available for national comparisons. The Read classification offers some promise for improvement in the future.

Another difficulty in making interdistrict, interregional, national and international comparisons is the lack of consensus on terminology and definitions used. There are, as yet, few publications on audit of vascular case-mix, but those that are available have used different groupings of procedures which prevents direct comparison.[14–20] There is an urgent need for agreement on such operative procedure groupings, perhaps via specialist associations (Table 2.2).

Table 2.2 Suggested surgical procedure groups for audit

Abdominal aortic aneurysm:
elective
emergency
Aorto-femoral bypass
Extra-anatomic bypass
Femoro-popliteal bypass
Femoro-infrapopliteal bypass
Thoraco-abdominal aneurysm
Carotid artery reconstruction
Upper-limb revascularization
Thoracic outlet decompression
Major amputation
Embolectomy
Balloon angioplasty
Thrombolytic therapy
Sympathectomy
Varicose veins operation

From a questionnaire circulated by the Vascular Surgical Society of Great Britain and Ireland.

Auditing a vascular surgical service

Access to the service

Although waiting times for outpatient consultation and waiting lists for operations are properly the concern of managers, surgeons need to be aware of the state of their own waiting lists and the changes that occur over time. It is also necessary for surgeons to be involved in maintaining the accuracy of operation waiting lists as this can only be accomplished with any accuracy by an experienced member of the surgical team. In such a validation exercise, in which patients waiting for varicose veins operation were re-examined, Brewster *et al.* 'reduced' their waiting list to a remarkable 42% of the original number, and only 7% required surgery as an inpatient.[21]

In the same way, an evaluation of the appropriateness of use of a vascular service by referring clinicians can only be done by surgeons. Vascular audit should therefore include, for example, the number of inappropriate 'nonarterial' referrals for an outpatient opinion (Table 2.3) and the mode of referral for vascular emergencies which have such a disruptive effect on the cold surgery undertaken by a department.[18]

Table 2.3 New outpatient referrals for arterial assessment (vascular clinic 1990–91)

	n	(%)
Claudication	71	(41)
Critical ischaemia	37	(21)
Aneurysm	20	(12)
Diabetic	9	(5)
Cerebrovascular	1	(1)
Vasospasm	2	(1)
NOT arterial cause	32	(19)
	172	

NB: Varicose veins excluded

The process of investigation and treatment

Case-mix

Vascular surgery is time-consuming and expensive and any assessment of the efficiency of a service can only be undertaken against a background knowledge of the mix of cases treated in a department. For example, in planning an outpatient vascular service the case-mix needs to be known since the time taken to see an arterial referral (estimated by Stoodley[22] to average 23 minutes) is significantly longer than that for a patient with varicose veins (7 minutes). The case-mix for a one-consultant DGH service receiving referrals of patients with suspected arterial disease is shown in Table 2.3.

Similarly, vascular surgical operations consume a disproportionate amount of theatre time, and much vascular surgery is undertaken by general surgeons with an interest in vascular surgery. The mix of general and vascular operative procedures will therefore be relevant in service planning.[15] Resource planning in vascular surgery is further complicated by the high proportion of emergency admissions (about one-third of vascular admissions) and this information should be available when making comparisons between departments.

Work-load

Nationally, information on vascular work-load has been collected by the Vascular Surgical Society of Great Britain and Ireland[17] and further studies are under way. All surgical work-load is conventionally estimated by a simple count of the number of operations performed, regardless of the complexity of the operation or the time taken to perform it. The relative complexity of many vascular operations makes it necessary to weight the work-load in vascular surgery to give a more realistic assessment of surgical 'work' done. One way of achieving this is to use the 'Intermediate Equivalent' (IE) weighting, which gives such an assessment by comparing the surgical work involved in a given procedure with that required for a 'standard' intermediate operation (e.g. inguinal hernia repair) (Table 2.4). By calculating the work of a vascular surgeon and that of nonvascular colleagues using the IE, the contribution by the vascular surgeon was seen to be equal to that of his colleagues.[23] A further refinement, described by Collins, enables calculation of the work-load contribution of trainee surgeons relative to the consultant, by determining the Service Equivalent Value (SEV) of each grade.[24]

Documentation

Audits of case-notes and discharge summaries will

Table 2.4 Intermediate Equivalent (IE) values

Group	Example	IE
Minor	Circumcision OGD	0.5
Intermediate	Inguinal herniorrhaphy Breast lump excision	1.0
Major	Mastectomy Partial thyroidectomy	1.75
Major plus	Partial gastrectomy Hemicolectomy	2.2
Complex major operation	Aortic aneurysm repair AP resection	4.0

prove particularly illuminating. The regular assessment of the quality of case-notes, against published standards,[25] is effective in raising the standards of note-keeping and has become popular as an audit activity. It is accomplished without extensive data collection, and indeed just the knowledge that case-notes are under review can result in improvement. This activity has been given fresh impetus by the Access to Health Records Act (1991) which gives patients a right of access to the information contained in their case-notes.

Two-way communication between general practitioners and consultants is also a fruitful field for audit, because both parties at present feel that correspondence leaves much to be desired. Consultants identify legibility (13%) and information about current treatment (70%) as defects in referral letters.[26] General practitioners identify the delay in receiving summaries, review intentions (62%) and information given to patients (90%)[27] as defects in hospital discharge summaries.

Trainee experience

Accurate recording of the experience gained by surgical trainees is necessary not only so that a 'log book' of surgical experience can be presented at the FRCS examination and for Higher Surgical Training accreditation, but also to permit the assessment of the training value of a particular post. In this respect it is important to record the cases at which the trainee (a) was the assistant, (b) was the surgeon, assisted by a senior, and (c) was the surgeon unassisted. Such information will in time become essential for accreditation of surgical training in the UK, as it already has elsewhere (e.g. in Australia).[17]

Assessing the value of investigations, including the value of high-volume or high-cost investigations (e.g. arteriography, computed tomography, magnetic resonance imaging) has relevance to the safety of the patient, the efficient arrival at a diagnosis and the effective use of limited resources. Similarly, the effectiveness of prophylaxis of deep vein thrombosis and pulmonary embolus and the use of antibiotics to prevent postoperative infection are quality indicators for a surgical service.

Auditing outcomes

General outcome measures

The outcome of treatment is both the most relevant indicator of the quality of a surgical service and the most difficult to assess. All surgeons have an interest in the outcome of the surgical procedures they perform on patients, yet to follow up every patient to assess this accurately would bring the outpatient service to a halt. Harris has proposed a scheme of follow-up for patients undergoing vascular reconstructions[28] and, although this is based on the clinical needs of the patient rather than an audit, it provides a minimum requirement which would also allow an opportunity for outcome assessment.

Little has been written on the overall estimation of outcome for vascular patients. General outcomes based on a simple scoring system can give an overall impression of outcome (Fig. 2.2). They are very easy to collect but give only an overview of the general performance of the service.

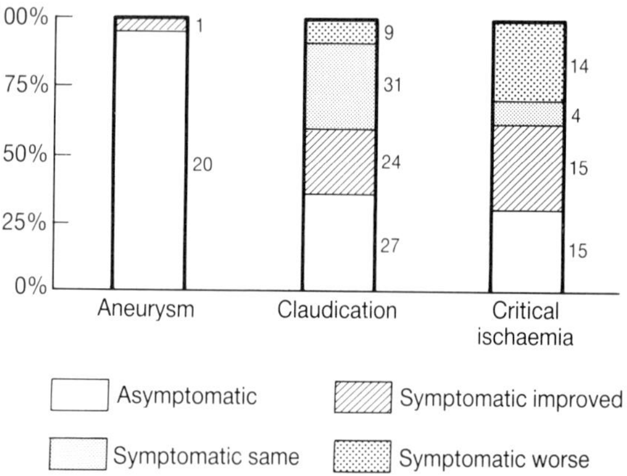

Fig. 2.2 General vascular outcomes in the clinic 1990–91. Results of 170 consecutive vascular outpatient follow-up assessments using the general outcome groups: asymptomatic, symptomatic improved, symptomatic same, symptomatic worse.

Specific outcome measures

Therapeutic procedures in vascular surgery (e.g. vascular reconstructions and percutaneous transluminal angioplasty) offer reasonably discrete short-term end-points that are easy to record. Graft or vessel patency, limb salvage and the associated secondary amputation rate, and unplanned return to theatre or admission to ITU, give a useful indication of the technical quality of the surgery performed, provided that the indications for these procedures are taken into account.

Postoperative complications, if accurately recorded, provide an indirect measure of quality (Table 2.5). Experience of information about complications collected systematically shows a generally higher

Table 2.5 Postoperative complications

Specific	General
Graft thrombosis	Wound infection
Haemorrhage	Wound haematoma
Distal embolization	Deep vein thrombosis
Lymph leak	Pulmonary embolism
Lymph collection	Chest infection
Graft infection	Septicaemia
False aneurysm	Urinary retention
	Urinary infection
	Renal failure
	Cardiac failure
	Myocardial infarction
	CVA
	Pressure sore
	Anaesthetic complication
	Return to theatre

complication rate than clinical impression might give. This is probably due, in part, to the natural tendency of the surgeon to forget his mistakes, but also to the enthusiastic recording of every minor problem by those who currently collect this information systematically. To interpret complication rates meaningfully it is necessary to establish which are the important complications; i.e. the ones that significantly affect the patient. Therefore, as well as recording the complication, it is also necessary to note whether it is major or minor. In this context, major complications are those that are fatal, endanger the life of the patient, or that prolong their stay in hospital. Minor complications cause significant morbidity (and may incur extra cost).

Patient perspective

Perhaps the most important outcome measure of all is the degree to which the patient's expectation of the outcome of treatment has been realized. As far as the patient is concerned the outcome is rather ill-defined and is measured in terms of symptom relief, subsequent dependancy, and economic or social capability. Satisfaction will depend on how these parameters measure up to preoperative expectations, whether realistic or not. The importance of preoperative counselling by surgeons is becoming increasingly apparent, making information about procedures and likely outcomes, in the form of patient information sheets, a priority.

Numerous attempts have been made to design objective measures of 'health status', but those currently available tend to be complex, time-consuming and expensive to collect, making them inappropriate for routine use. As research tools these are, however, useful and include the Nottingham Health Profile,[29] QALYS (quality-adjusted life years)[30] and, perhaps to have been expected, the EuroQol.[31]

Patient satisfaction questionnaires are notoriously difficult to assess because most studies show that 80% of patients are satisfied with their treatment overall, almost regardless of what questions were asked. Specific questions regarding known problem areas are likely to provide more useful replies, but even then patients' views are likely to be coloured by other factors such as the politeness and friendliness of the doctor – the 'halo effect'.[32]

The outcome as judged by the patient may not accord with the views of the surgeon. In assessing the outcome of treatment for varicose veins, for example, there is often a discrepancy between the views of the surgeon about the outcome and those of the patient. Outcomes of varicose vein operations are notoriously difficult to assess. Robbins *et al.* discussed the advantages and disadvantages of the following indicators: clinical signs, subjective symptoms, peripheral venous physiology and iatrogenic effects.[33] It is not possible to collect such information routinely, and for the present it is best to concentrate on the more easily measured general outcomes already described.

Monitoring the use of resources

As those who are primarily responsible for committing health care resources, doctors have an obligation to ensure the efficient use of the limited funds available and should show a willingness to achieve competent resource husbandry.

The avoidance of waste is an obvious example; but the degree to which use of operating theatres (as recommended in the Bevan report[36]) and the value of a daytime emergency operating theatre (as advocated in the CEPOD report[6]) can be accurately assessed is limited at present by the sparse information available. Better provision of such information will make this task easier. In addition, the demonstration of inadequate staffing as a possible cause of postoperative complications will only be of significance if there is a possibility of change resulting from identifying such defects.

Holding an audit meeting

Who should attend?

In short, everyone. Peer review is best achieved in a forum comprising all medical staff within the unit. It is particularly important that trainees attend as well as consultants, since the meeting is an educational opportunity in which they must play an active part.

Most vascular surgery in the UK is performed within departments of general surgery; a local vascular audit is therefore usually undertaken within the general surgery framework. This has certain advantages: a chance to compare techniques and results with surgeons having a special interest in vascular surgery, to view the management of vascular emergencies against management by 'experts', and to offer advice to colleagues on best practice in vascular surgery.

There is also a need to compare performance with other vascular units within regions and nationally as well as internationally. Regional projects like the Lothian audit provide information which enables individuals to compare their practice more widely, and nationally the Confidential Comparative Audit Service of the Royal College of Surgeons provides individual ranking, in confidence, for surgeons who provide data from their own personal surgical practice. Although the service is aimed at general surgery, 1992 data include case-load, complications and mortality for abdominal aortic aneurysm.

Confidentiality

It is quite clear that, for a medical audit to achieve its stated aim of improving the quality of care for patients, the profession must have complete confidence in the security of any information produced as a result of the audit endeavour. The Department of Health stresses the importance of this issue in its guidance on the conduct of a medical audit and on the use of computer systems:

> 'For medical audit to be effective it must be conducted in an atmosphere of trust; confidentiality of data must be guaranteed.'[11]

> 'It is important that doctors should not feel that they are under a greater threat of litigation because of their involvement in medical audit.'[34]

A record of the audit meeting is necessary for future reference, for training approval and as a demonstration that audit is taking place, but it is important to avoid naming individual patients or doctors.

Methods of presentation

Using graphical presentation where possible, an overview of the work of a department is an essential first step to promoting interest in a more detailed analysis of selected items. The following should be shown initially:

- the case-load for the month for each department
- deaths and complications recorded for the month.

This should be followed by a detailed presentation of a topic which was previously selected as suitable for study.

The method of criterion-based audit described by Shaw[35] is most useful. After deciding on a necessary study, a number of standards (criteria) are agreed in advance. A number of records chosen at random are then scrutinized for these criteria. The results are presented, conclusions are reached and a decision about the need for change is then made. The crucial final step is to revisit the subject after an interval and assess the same criteria to discover whether improvement has occurred and been maintained.

Using the results of an audit

To be of lasting value, an audit must result in beneficial change and improve the quality of patient care. Good intentions often result from an audit study, but the passage of time allows the reappearance of the problem if it is not kept alive by repetition. It is well worth reviewing the particular activity after an interval to see whether the initial good intentions have become permanent changes for the better, or have lapsed and been forgotten. To maintain the initial improvement, agreed changes can be encapsulated in a locally agreed protocol of patient management which can be disseminated widely and given to new staff as they arrive. Experience with surgical audits to date has shown a readiness to agree protocols for investigation, patient management, surgical treatment, etc. The additional benefits of such protocols are that they can eliminate idiosyncratic preferences of different consultants, allowing trainees to feel confident that what they are doing is accepted by the whole department. There is also the benefit that protocols make the understanding and learning of surgical care more ordered and rational for the trainee.

The danger is that having protocols for just about every clinical eventuality can mean that each department becomes rigid in its management of patients. This can stifle original thought and innovation, and the newly arrived trainee can be faced with what amounts to a local texbook on patient management which must be learned and from which he/she fears to divert, for fear of reprimand or even litigation. Protocols, then, should be used with caution.

It is sometimes argued that there is little point in a medical audit since there is no extra funding to pay for the necessary changes. While this may sometimes be the case, there are many situations in which an audit can result in financial savings, which in turn can be diverted to other areas within a department. But if the outcome of an audit is that more funding is required to put right a problem, then the careful, critical evaluation resulting from a well conducted audit will provide excellent data on which to base an argument for an increase in resources.

Auditing has now been accepted by the profession and there is no turning back from the recent developments. However, if surgical auditing is to succeed there must be adequate information, adequate resources to support the process, a willingness to change practice and a determination to ensure that the changes are permanent.

Recommended further reading

1. Royal College of Surgeons of England. *Guidelines to Clinical Audit in Surgical Practice.* London: 1989.
2. Standing Medical Advisory Committee of the DoH, *The Quality of Medical Care.* London: HMSO, 1990.
3. Shaw C. *Medical Audit – A Hospital Handbook.* London: King's Fund Centre, 1989.
4. Devlin HB. Audit and the quality of clinical care. *Ann Roy Coll Surg Eng* 1990; **72** (Suppl): 3–4.

References

1. Hilton J. *On Rest and Pain: A Course of Lectures.* London: Bell & Sons, 1877.
2. Royal College of Surgeons of England. *Guidelines to Clinical Audit in Surgical Practice.* London: 1989.
3. World Health Organization Regional Office for Europe. *Targets for Health for All.* Copenhagen: WHO, 1985.
4. Department of Health. *NHS Review 'Working for Patients'. Working Paper 6: Medical Audit.* London: HMSO, 1989.
5. Gruer R, Gordon DS, Gunn AA, Ruckley CV. Audit of surgical audit. *Lancet* 1986; **1:** 23–6.
6. Buck N, Devlin HB, Lunn JN. *Report of the Confidential Enquiry into Perioperative Deaths.* London: Nuffield Provincial Hospital Trust and the King's Fund for Hospitals, 1987.
7. Jones SM. Clinical audit experience in the South West region. *Postgrad Med J* 1990; **66:** S8–10.
8. Dunn DC. Audit of a surgical firm by microcomputer: five years' experience. *Br Med J* 1988; **296:** 687–91.
9. Ellis WB. How to set up an audit. *Br Med J* 1989; **298:** 1635–7.
10. McCollum PT, Gupta SK, Mantese VA, Joseph M, Karplus TE, Gray-Weale AC, Shanik GD, Lippey ER, de Burgh MM, Lusby RJ. Microcomputer database and system of audit for the vascular surgeon. *Aust NZ J Surg* 1990; **60:** 519–23.
11. Department of Health. *Working for Patients. Medical Audit: Guidance for Hospital Clinicians on the Use of Computers.* London: HMSO, 1990.
12. Royal College of Surgeons of England. *Guidelines for Surgical Audit by Computer.* London: 1991.
13. Vascular surgery in southern Sweden – the first year's experience of a vascular registry. *Eur J Vasc Surg* 1989; **3:** 563–9.
14. Sladen JG. Morbidity Audit, 1984, Canadian Society for Vascular Surgery. *Can J Surg* 1987; **30:** 3–4.
15. Roberts JP, Smallwood JA, Chant AC, Webster JH. Local audit in vascular surgery. *Ann Roy Coll Surg Eng* 1990; **72:** 287–90.
16. Holdsworth JD. Five year vascular audit from a district hospital. *Br J Surg* 1991; **78:** 601–6.
17. Thompson JF, Fergus ME, Royle GT, Webster JH, Chant AD. The Southampton Teaching Triad: an audit of operative surgical instruction. *Ann Roy Coll Surg Eng* 1990; **72:** 243–6.
18. Michaels JA, Galland RB. Prospective audit of vascular surgical emergencies in a district general hospital. *Br J Surg* 1991; **78:** 1271–2.
19. Campbell WB, Souter RG, Collins J, Wood RF, Kidson IG, Morris PJ. Auditing the vascular surgical audit. *Br J Surg* 1987; **74:** 98–100.
20. Lyons C. An interdistrict audit of vascular surgery. *Qual Assur Hlth Care* 1991; **3:** 293–302.
21. Brewster SF, Nicholson S, Farndon J. The varicose vein waiting list: results of a validation exercise. *Ann Roy Coll Surg Eng* 1991; **73:** 223–6.
22. Stoodley BJ. Correspondence. *Ann Roy Coll Surg Eng* 1989; Suppl: 33.
23. Jones SM, Collins CD. Caseload or workload? Complexity scoring of operative procedures. *Br Med J* 1990; **301:** 324–5.
24. Collins CD. Model Workload Agreement for DGH General Surgeon: Discussion Paper. *Ann Roy Coll Surg Eng* 1990; **72** (Suppl): 48–50.
25. Royal College of Surgeons of England. *Guidelines for Clinicians on Medical Records and Notes.* London: 1990.
26. Cybulska E, Rucinski J. Communication between doctors. *Br J Hosp Med* 1989; **41:** 266–8.

27. Fair JF. Hospital discharge and death communications. *Br J Hosp Med* 1989; **42:** 59–61.
28. Harris PL. Follow-up after reconstructive vascular surgery. *Eur J Vasc Surg* 1991; **5:** 369–73.
29. Hunt SM, McWeen J, McKenna SP. The Nottingham Health Profile: subjective health status and medical consultations. *Soc Sci Med* 1981; **15:** 221–9.
30. Office of Health Economics. *Measurement and Management in the NHS.* London: 1989.
31. The EuroQol Group. EuroQol – a new facility for the measurement of health-related quality of life. *Hlth Policy* 1990; **16:** 199–208.
32. Fitzpatrick R. Surveys of patients' satisfaction. 1: Important general considerations. *Br Med J* 1991; **302,** 887–9.
33. Robbins MA, Frankel SJ, Nanchahal K, Caost J. Williams MH. *Epidemiologically Based Needs Assessment of Varicose Vein Treatment.* Bristol: Health Care Evaluation Unit/NHS Management Executive, 1992.
34. Standing Medical Advisory Committee of the DoH. *The Quality of Medical Care.* London: HMSO, 1990.
35. Shaw C. *Medical Audit – A Hospital Handbook.* London: King's Fund Centre, 1989.
36. NHS Management Executive. *The management and utilisation of operating departments* (Chairman: PG Bevan). HMSO, 1989.

3

Management of the acutely ischaemic limb

AEB Giddings and MS Quraishy

Acute ischaemia is more common in the leg than the arm. It threatens an increasing number of the elderly, who may lose a limb, if not their life, when treatment is delayed or unsatisfactory. Rheumatic heart disease with systemic embolism, which was the cause of most of these emergencies several decades ago, is now less frequent than arterial thrombosis. Patients with embolism have a high mortality owing to their underlying cardiac disease. By contrast, those with thrombosis of their limb arteries are at increased risk of amputation.[1] The majority of elderly amputees remain socially and physically crippled, at great cost to both the community and themselves. The successful management of acute limb ischaemia can increase the number of patients who will retain their limb until death. Modern management requires the combined skills of a vascular surgeon and interventional radiologist.

In a district of 200 000 people, about 25 present each year with an acutely threatened limb, roughly equal to the number presenting with an abdominal aortic aneurysm. Originally, the combination of heparin and surgical embolectomy was the standard treatment, and it remains so for acute arterial embolism with a severe motor and sensory defect. However, the main cause of acute limb ischaemia is now arterial thrombosis, and so thrombolytic therapy has become popular and more appropriate.[2] Modern methods of low-dose intra-arterial thrombolysis provide a safe and effective method for the dissolution of obstructing propagation clot, allowing the underlying cause of the thrombosis to be unmasked and surgical or radiological correction undertaken.

Diagnosis

The major causes of acute limb ischaemia are summarized in Table 3.1.

Table 3.1 Common causes of acute limb ischaemia

Embolism:	Cardiac arrhythmia Mural thrombus Valve vegetations Atrial myxoma Arterial atheroma
Thrombosis:	Atheromatous native vessel Arterial graft Aneurysm Cardiac failure Thrombotic states
Dissecting aneurysm	
Trauma:	Penetrating Blunt Iatrogenic Traction
Small vessel disease:	Arteritis

Patients with arterial thrombosis are generally elderly, with diffuse arterial disease, which may be suspected from associated angina, claudication or stroke. Those with embolism may be slightly younger and usually give a history of cardiac disease, such as arrhythmia, valvular disorder or infarction. Rarely, a local arterial abnormality – such as aneurysm, arteritis, arterial entrapment or cystic adventitial disease – will affect young adults or, exceptionally, children. Cardiovascular events, interventions (such as angioplasty and vascular reconstruction), and conditions of medical risk (such as smoking, diabetes mellitus and hypertension) should be noted. Factors influencing thrombosis (such as respiratory disease, immobility, dehydration, infection and malignancy) must also be borne in mind.

The pain of acute ischaemia is usually severe and resists analgesia. It may be less dramatic when preceded by claudication or slowly progressive occlusion. Tissues with the highest metabolic demand are muscle and nerve. Ischaemic muscle is suggested by painful spasm and paralysis, ischaemic nerve by pain and paraesthesiae. Sudden arterial occlusion induces a deathly pallor which is constant, not developing with elevation and changing to the brick-red hue of dependancy, as in the positive Buerger's sign of more chronic, critical ischaemia. After a few hours, the intense vascular spasm relaxes and vessels fill with stagnant deoxygenated blood and propagation clot. Skin blanching on pressure then gives way to a fixed blue and black staining as tissues die, with blistering and liquifaction. If associated dry gangrene is seen, pre-existing and more gradual mortification is likely. The limb will feel cold, often showing a steep temperature gradient. By contrast, the blue and swollen limb of an acute and extensive venous thrombosis will be warm with detectable pulses. Abdominal, limb and carotid pulses should be recorded, not forgetting the popliteal. Irregular rhythm suggests embolism, variable volume suggests severe cardiac disease or incomplete obstruction, while arterial dilatation raises the possibility of an aneurysm with thrombosis or distal embolism. A strong pulse does not necessarily indicate flow and the most prominent pulse may be felt just above a complete occlusion: here, the hand-held Doppler probe will clearly identify little or no flow. The Doppler probe is also of great value in the detection of flow where pulses are difficult to feel because the patient is obese, the arteries are rigid, or proximal occlusion has resulted in a dampened wave due to flow through collateral vessels. Systolic pressures should be recorded if possible, as they are useful to monitor change; but, in significant ischaemia, they are commonly too low to be accurate. Comparison with the contralateral limb is vital to distinguish central from peripheral causes and may help to differentiate unilateral embolism from arterial thrombosis.

The timing of presentation of an ischaemic limb will depend on the speed and severity of onset and the extent to which a collateral circulation develops. When there are adequate collateral vessels, some days may elapse before presentation. Symptoms and signs are then rather subtle but the prognosis is reasonable. Motor and sensory defects in a warm limb should lead to a detailed neurological assessment.

Classical complete obstruction, with a motor and sensory defect, is a dramatic emergency demanding immediate surgical relief.

Initial management

While the ischaemic limb is an urgent problem, assessment of the patient's general medical condition is the first priority. Recent medical deterioration may present with its effects on the peripheral circulation and it is important to detect cardiac failure, which may precipitate thrombosis and renal failure. Sepsis may expose a reduced cardiac reserve, and uncontrolled diabetes may cause dehydration. Pain and toxaemia due to necrosis of muscle may lead to serious problems in medical management. Dealing with the risks of acute renal failure and cardiac arrhythmia is a serious challenge in a patient who may be confused and unable to cooperate.

As soon as haemorrhage or dissection of a major artery has been excluded, anticoagulation with an infusion of 10 000 u of heparin 6-hourly should be given, with isotonic crystalloid and colloid solutions to maintain optimal circulation. In some patients, this will be sufficient to save the limb.[3] Analgesia and sedation in small but frequent intravenous doses is both necessary and humane. The assessment is completed by a full blood count, urea or creatinine, electrolytes, and glucose measurements. An electrocardiogram and chest X-ray are also required.

A series of crucial decisions now follows (Fig. 3.1). First, is this acute limb ischaemia rather than an acute venous thrombosis or a neurological emergency? Secondly, is the most urgent problem the patient's general medical state or is it the limb itself? Thirdly, is the ischaemia of the limb reversible or is primary amputation required? Fourthly, if reversible, is there a severe motor and sensory defect, making immediate embolectomy and fasciotomy the only chance, or is this a more gradual thrombosis, allowing time for arteriography and thrombolysis? Factors which generally distinguish embolism from thrombosis and the differences in prognosis for life and limb are given in Table 3.2.

Embolism and embolectomy

Although surgical embolectomy was first described in 1908, it was not until the development of the balloon embolectomy catheter by Fogarty in 1963 that the technique became well established.[4] The distribution of arterial emboli is shown in Table 3.3. Embolectomy is not an operation for a surgeon with limited vascular experience, since it may require intraoperative arteriography and may lead on to

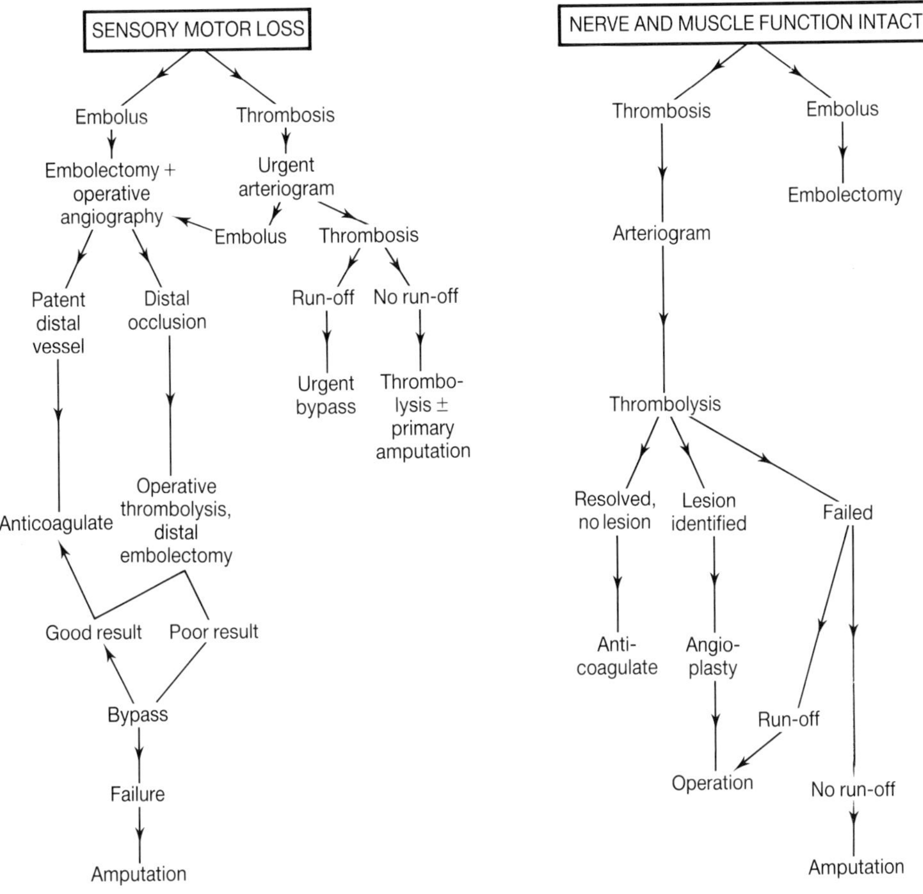

Fig. 3.1 Flow charts for management of acute ischaemia.

Table 3.2 Differences between embolism and thrombosis

	Embolism	**Thrombosis**
Incidence[5]	41%	59%
Onset	Sudden cardiac arrhythmia	Gradual preceding claudication
Examination	Pulse proximal to occlusion	No distal pulses. Contralateral limb pulses may be absent
Arteriography	Seldom required	Mandatory
Arteriography appearances	Filling defect in normal vessel with poor collaterals	General atheroma. Established collaterals
Treatment	Embolectomy	Thrombolysis, angioplasty, surgery
Amputation rate[10]	28%	13%
Mortality	9%	17%

Table 3.3 Incidence and distribution of peripheral emboli

Incidence (%)	
Post mortem series	0.23
Following myocardial infarction	< 1.0
Site of embolization (%)	
Aorta, saddle	15.5
Iliac	17.6
Femoral	43.4
Popliteal	15.0
Upper limb	8.5

Source: reference 5.

further procedures, such as intraoperative thrombolysis and immediate arterial reconstruction. Balloon catheter embolectomy alone is frequently incomplete.

Exposure of the artery under general or local anaesthesia may be used. Local anaesthesia may be preferred in a slim cooperative patient with an enhanced cardiac risk, such as embolism from recent myocardial infarction. An anaesthetist should be always in attendance because additional sedation is helpful and the smooth induction of general anaesthesia may be required in the event of difficulty. Obesity and confusion are strong indicators for general anaesthesia, as is the need to explore arteries at several sites.

The limb should be draped to allow operative arteriography and exposure of the standard sites (femoral, popliteal, brachial, antecubital), and the foot or hand enclosed in a sterile transparent bag for inspection of vascularity. Full intravenous heparin should be continued and a solution of dilute heparin and papaverine available for intra-arterial irrigation.

Aortic saddle emboli require access to both common femoral arteries and vessels should be opened just above their division, since it is there that impaction of clot occurs and access to branches is best. Exposure of the artery should be generous, long enough for safe control and manipulation without trauma. Arterial clamps and slings must be atraumatic. Arteriotomies in soft vessels over obvious emboli should be transverse and closed with fine interrupted sutures of Prolene. Where the vessel is diseased or if an anastomosis could be required at that site, a vertical incision is preferred, but closure must then be made with a vein patch, preferably taken from the long saphenous vein at the ankle.

Local clot may be removed by forceps and gently milking the artery and the limb. Remote clot is removed by passing the smallest embolectomy catheter which will do the job and inflating the balloon with a saline-filled syringe of narrow bore and long stroke (such as a tuberculin syringe) to give the best feel. The balloon should be inflated only when it is moving and extreme gentleness is required, particularly in atheromatous vessels which may be irregular and friable; even normal endothelium is easily injured or stripped by a balloon catheter.

When embolectomy is thought to be complete, an irrigation catheter (such as a fine umbilical catheter) should be passed and the vessels irrigated with 100 ml of a solution of heparinized saline and papaverine. Operative arteriography can then be carried out. This will require approximately 20 ml of nonionic contrast, films being taken with an arrested arterial circulation. Profuse back-bleeding and the easy outflow of irrigating solutions is an encouraging sign, but operative arteriography may show that both are due to patency of the more proximal vessels alone and that a distal obstruction persists. Clot or debris beyond the reach of a femoral or brachial arteriotomy may be removed by distal arteriotomies, but meticulous technique is necessary to avoid intimal damage and snow-ploughing of debris into collateral vessels which can occur when the catheter is drawn distally with the balloon inflated.

When the operative arteriogram shows extensive distal occlusion, intraoperative thrombolysis by the instillation of 100 000 u of streptokinase into an arrested distal circulation over 30 minutes may produce clearance.[6] Lysis of propagation clot may then be sufficient, but undissolved mature emboli or atheromatous debris will require further attempts at physical removal using catheter suction or well targeted arteriotomies closed with vein patches. If all else fails, immediate bypass to a patent distal vessel will be required. Success must be confirmed by observing reactive hyperaemia in the foot or hand, feeling good pulses and/or a satisfactory completion arteriogram. Residual stenoses or loose debris must not be accepted, even if distal pulses return, since rethrombosis is likely.

Postoperatively, anticoagulation with heparin should be converted to warfarin, since this reduces recurrent emboli by two-thirds. Intensive management of cardiac, respiratory and renal function should be continued, since the reperfusion of ischaemic tissues may produce postoperative cardiac depression, arrhythmia and renal failure in at least 10% of patients. In addition, swelling of reperfused muscle may require fasciotomy in at least one patient in 10. This swelling and its effects may not be obvious during the first hour after reperfusion but is the inevitable consequence of severe ischaemia and should be anticipated by fasciotomy before revascularization. All muscle compartments should be opened through full-length skin incisions at the time of embolectomy, or as soon as tender swelling of muscle with a restriction of movement is detected postoperatively. Measurements of compartment pressure to indicate the need for decompression have been recommended, but avoiding the syndrome by prophylactic fasciotomy is to be preferred.

Fasciotomy and inspection of muscles is wise before embolectomy when viability is in doubt. Excision of necrotic muscle or primary amputation can then be performed to avoid the serious risk from reperfusion of dead tissues. Severe but reversible ischaemic injury may be reduced in the future by the development of pharmacological blockade of the lipid mediators of cell injury.

The potential for percutaneous extraction of emboli is being evaluated at present but does require an expert radiologist and large (8–12Fr) catheters.

Thrombosis and thrombolysis

Thrombosis is the most frequent cause of acute limb ischaemia, acting through the principles defined in Virchow's triad which affect the vessel wall, the blood and flow. The patient may give a history suggesting intermittent claudication, cardiorespiratory disease or other medical disorder. Not only is attention to the underlying cause a priority, but the slower onset of thrombotic ischaemia may allow time for a more precise diagnosis by arteriography. Definition of the cause usually makes the choice of correct treatment more obvious and, in particular, should avoid the risks of inappropriate and fruitless surgical thrombectomy.

The modern management of arterial thrombosis requires high-quality and complete arteriography. Useful preliminary information may be gained from arterial mapping, using the Doppler probe or duplex scanning techniques; but contrast examinations by digital subtraction (DSA) or conventional arteriography are more precise. For intra-arterial studies of the lower limbs, puncture of the contralateral groin is to be preferred (Table 3.4). Intravenous DSA studies are convenient, particularly if they have to be repeated: arterial puncture is avoided, but the quality of the information is reduced. Intra-arterial contrast yields excellent films, but arterial puncture – particularly in the aorta, axillary or brachial vessels – may be hazardous in itself and may preclude subsequent thrombolysis at that site. The femoral approach, using small catheters (5Fr), is best to obtain comprehensive pictures of the upper limb or contralateral lower limb with minimal morbidity. Arteriography may show unsuspected emboli, such as aortic saddle emboli, incompletely obstructing the aorto-iliac bifurcation. The patient may then be prepared for surgical embolectomy from both groins, since low-dose intra-arterial thrombolysis is ineffective and impractical in a flowing bloodstream. In most cases, arteriography will demonstrate occlusive thrombus. Lysis of propagation clot, to unmask the underlying cause, would be the next step. Thrombolysis for upper-limb occlusions is, however, more difficult technically and pericatheter thrombosis could lead to cerebral embolization. Embolectomy or bypass should be preferred.

Table 3.4 Advantages of the contralateral approach for lower-limb arteriography

For infusion
The only approach for iliac and common femoral arteries
Easier: fewer puncture and profunda problems
Catheter more stable with less bleeding
Full diagnostic arteriogram
Proximal clot more accessible
For operation
Operation easier since no puncture (and possible haematoma) in affected limb
Catheter well placed for intra-operative arteriogram
Ideal for infusing heparin or lytic drugs postangioplasty or postoperatively

Thrombolysis has been available for more than 30 years, but new drugs, better arterial catheters and (especially) new techniques of administration have improved safety and effectiveness. Originally, large doses of intravenous streptokinase were used, often with dramatic effect. Although large amounts of arterial and venous clot could be removed, systemic fibrinolysis gave rise to serious or fatal bleeding, particularly affecting the intracerebral and retroperitoneal vessels. Intravenous thrombolysis has little application for the acutely ischaemic limb.

The delivery through a fine catheter of low-dose streptokinase into stagnant clot was pioneered by Dotter in 1974,[7] using a continuous infusion for several days, and refined with improved efficacy and safety by Katzen and van Breda.[8] The method depends on achieving a high local concentration of the drug for several hours, while minimizing the systemic effects of lysis. Effectiveness is improved by mechanical disruption of the clot by a guidewire or hydraulic forces. Thrombolysis by infusion and single-film arteriography every 6–12 hours is best managed in an intensive care unit or a high-dependancy unit, where the patient's condition and the conduct of the infusion are under close supervision (though it can be managed satisfactorily on a general surgical ward). Our technique is outlined in Table 3.5.

An alternative technique, using intermittent high-dose bolus injections of thrombolytic agents, was described in 1982 by Hess *et al.*[9] This is carried out under direct radiological screening, with repeated injections every 10 or 15 minutes. Rapid lysis may be achieved and ineffective infusion avoided, but there is a greater time commitment for the radiologist. Infusion alone is slower but less demanding in this respect.

Of the many agents suggested for thrombolysis, streptokinase, urokinase and recombinant tissue plasminogen activator (rtPA) are of practical importance now.[10] All are equally effective and, in large doses, risk haemorrhage, which is probably an inevitable side-effect of potency. Streptokinase is relatively cheap but a foreign protein which may cause allergic reaction, particularly on repeated exposure within six months. Urokinase is a direct plasminogen activator and useful in a patient sensitized to streptokinase, but is very expensive. Tissue plasminogen activator is an expensive product of recombinant DNA technology, although its price is falling with more widespread use. It is an effective lytic drug which can be given without provoking an allergic response. Early claims of clot 'specificity' and a reduced risk of systemic lysis have not been substantiated by clinical experience, and so there is little to choose between the three drugs in terms of effectiveness and safety when equivalent doses are compared (Table 3.6). Some authors recommend the concurrent infusion of heparin to minimize pericatheter thrombosis, but this may increase bleeding and is unnecessary with small catheters which allow brisk pericatheter bloodflow. Any proximal strictures should be dilated first, once they have been cleared of thrombus. Large catheters (8–12Fr) are required for clot suction and may be used with pericatheter heparin. Anticoagulation after thrombolysis does reduce the risk of rethrombosis.

Thrombolysis by infusion should be completed within 24–36 hours. Prolonged ineffective attempts at thrombolysis are associated with an increased risk of serious bleeding, so treatment should be discontinued if there is little progress after 12 hours of infusion or three doses by the bolus technique followed by a similar period of infusion. During infusion, arteriography repeated every 6–12 hours offers an opportunity to consider improving the flow by angioplasty, disruption of clot by guidewires or aspiration through large-bore catheters. As propagation thrombus is removed, the cause is unmasked and should be corrected without delay to avoid rethrombosis. Strictures should be dilated by standard angioplasty techniques and dilatation followed by intra-arterial infusion of heparin.

Up to a third of patients undergoing thrombolysis will require angioplasty. Some lesions may also need arterial stenting to maintain the lumen after dilatation, but this procedure should be reserved for large-calibre arteries, such as the iliac vessels, rather than in the infrainguinal region. For strictures which resist balloon dilatation, or for clot and atheromatous debris which persists despite successful removal of surrounding propagation thrombus, operation will be required. The techniques of balloon

Table 3.5 The authors' technique of thrombolysis

Arteriography:	Contralateral approach 5Fr end-hole catheter Catheter embedded 1 cm into clot
Infusion:	Streptokinase 6000 u/h or rtPA 5 mg in 3 doses, then 0.5 mg/h
Monitoring:	Arteriography every 6–12 hours Catheter advanced if lysis Clot disrupted with guidewire If no lysis, stop infusion If complications, stop infusion
Catheter removal:	When complete lysis has occurred After angioplasty If no improvement If complications occur
After thrombolysis:	IV heparin for 48 hours Then anticoagulation or aspirin

Table 3.6 Comparison of thrombolytic drugs

Drug	Dose	Allergy	Cost
Streptokinase	5000–10 000u/h × 12 h	Yes	Low
Urokinase	250 000u/h once 40 000–60 000u/h × 12 h	No	High
rtPA	5 mg × 3, 0.5–1.0 mg/h	No	High
(± heparin	400–1000u/h)		

embolectomy with direct or vein patch closure are sufficient to treat a further third of patients, but a minority of those requiring operations can be improved only by a more extensive arterial reconstruction. This may involve endarterectomy and interposition grafting for shorter obstructions and standard bypass procedures for longer ones. Occasionally, thrombosis will occur without obvious arterial pathology and a normal patent arterial tree is revealed. Anticoagulation alone is then appropriate.

In approximately one-third of patients undergoing attempted thrombolysis there will be no effect. This is not surprising if the obstruction is due to insoluble and calcified atheromatous debris or the white, platelet and fibrin mesh of old emboli or flow thrombus. It is, however, difficult to understand why fresh red propagation clot should resist thrombolysis by all drugs in a small proportion of patients. Higher doses may marginally improve effectiveness but increase the risk of haemorrhagic complications, of which stroke is the most feared (Table 3.7). Surgical removal of obstructing clot and debris which does not respond to safe thrombolysis is much better. Equally difficult to explain is the ability of fibrinolytic drugs to lyse the mature clot and neo-intima in synthetic grafts which have apparently been well incorporated for months. Though lysis in retroperitoneally implanted grafts can be effective, there is a risk of concealed haemorrhage through the graft wall; angioplasty balloon control of bleeding may be required in an emergency. Surgical clearance may be more rapid and safer in such groups.

Despite the measures outlined above, about 10% of patients will not be relieved by the usual combinations of thrombolysis, angioplasty and surgery. If arteriography demonstrates a patent outflow beyond the obstruction, urgent surgical bypass is required; but in an ischaemic limb, proximal obstruction may prevent even the most expert radiologist from showing patent distal vessels suitable for anastomosis. Intraoperative arteriography, using large volumes of contrast and an arrested circulation, may help, but venous filling can mask the arterial anatomy. Careful preoperative Doppler mapping of all vessels, with the limb dependent,[11] or by pulse-generated runoff technique,[12] may identify a suitable site for a distal anastomosis. Exploration of such vessels must then confirm patency and a suitable runoff. The crude assessment of resistance to a hand injection of irrigating fluid may be refined by impedance analysis, and the results of the reconstruction may be checked by operative arteriography and flow measurements. Satisfactory results make early postoperative failure unlikely.

Table 3.7 Results and complications of thrombolysis

Data from collected series[10]	
Lysis	62%
Major haemorrhage	4%
Mortality	3%
Stroke	1%
Data from Guildford series	
Diagnosis	
Arterial thrombosis	64%
Embolus	16%
Thrombosed femoral-popliteal grafts	10%
Thrombosed aorto-femoral grafts	3%
Unknown	7%
Long-term results	
(52 patients followed for minimum of 3 years)	
Effective lysis	73%
Significant benefit	67%
Sustained benefit	57%

Managing thrombosis at particular sites

Aortoiliac thrombosis

A severely stenotic aorta or aortoiliac bifurcation may occlude slowly, but when occlusion occurs suddenly it carries a grave prognosis. Severe ischaemia should be treated surgically by embolectomy and/or bypass grafting. Less critical patients may be treated by thrombolysis from an axillary approach. Thrombosis of a single iliac artery can frequently be managed by thrombolysis and angioplasty from the contralateral groin. In the event of distal embolism, the catheter is advanced and lysis continued. If lysis is not successful, reconstruction by bifemoral, aortobifemoral, femorofemoral or axillofemoral grafting may be effective, the method chosen depending on the state of the patent aortoiliac segment and the fitness of the patient to undergo an intra-abdominal operation. Similar considerations apply to the treatment of aortoiliac saddle emboli, where impaction in strictured vessels makes extraction difficult, and to the relatively uncommon catastrophe of acute thrombosis of an aortic aneurysm.

Peripheral aneurysm thrombosis

Peripheral aneurysms cause ischaemia by complete thrombosis or by acting as a source of distal emboli.

Such emboli are often multiple and small. Initially, there may be few symptoms or signs, but digital discoloration (the blue toes or finger syndrome) is a serious sign of clots which are usually beyond the reach of embolectomy catheters and resistant to thrombolysis. Reduced outflow may eventually lead to occlusion of the aneurysm itself. Common sites include the subclavian and axillary artery in the upper limb, where thoracic outlet compression or repeated trauma may be implicated. Collateral flow here is usually good and distal embolization is the critical feature. Surgical reconstruction is usually satisfactory in treating the aneurysmal segment. In the leg, the main sites are the femoral arteries and that sinister harbinger of doom, the popliteal aneurysm.

Popliteal aneurysm thrombosis

In the popliteal artery, aneurysm is the commonest cause of acute ischaemia, although thrombosis due to arterial entrapment or cystic adventitial disease may occur. Estimates suggest that popliteal aneurysm presents clinically for every 25 abdominal aortic aneurysms, but this may understate the problem. The condition illustrates a complex of vascular pathologies and management options.

The aneurysms often occur in vessels that are generally ectatic. As dilatation increases, so does intraluminal flow thrombus, turbulence, microembolism and distortion of the outflow. Venous compression may further reduce arterial inflow until there is complete thrombosis.

Popliteal aneurysms are usually obvious on clinical examination. However, the diagnosis is often missed even when the limb is symptomatic, and the greater use of thrombolysis for the treatment of acute lower-limb ischaemia has revealed the thrombosed popliteal aneurysm as an unsuspected cause in up to 20% of cases.[13] Ultrasound examination demonstrates the aneurysm and shows intraluminal clot.

Simple thrombectomy is of little benefit, but thrombolysis is often successful in reopening recently occluded aneurysms and more importantly their outflow,[14] allowing replacement of the aneurysm by a graft, preferably of autogenous vein. Thrombolysis is less effective in restoring patency to vessels that are chronically occluded by old, distal emboli. The risk of thrombosis is increased when the aneurysm contains a large amount of clot and the fate of the limb correlates closely with the patency of the tibial vessels at the time of presentation. The threat of limb loss has led to an aggressive policy of reconstruction for all symptomless popliteal aneurysms over 2 cm in diameter in some centres, but few symptomless patients are improved by surgery. The availability of safe thrombolysis may justify conservative management of the small and symptomless popliteal aneurysm containing little clot. Should thrombosis occur, successful thrombolysis may be followed by reconstruction or, if the patient is very unfit, by anticoagulation alone.

Graft thrombosis

In this condition the diagnosis is usually obvious from the history and sudden change in signs. Symptoms familiar to the patient, and which preceded the reconstruction, may recur. All patients with grafts should be briefed to return to hospital at once if this is the case. Occlusion of grafts within the first postoperative month is almost invariably due to inappropriate selection or a technical defect. Graft compression, kinking or narrowing at the anastomoses is best managed by immediate re-exploration with thrombectomy, intraoperative arteriography and surgical correction, as required. Thrombolysis is more dangerous in the early postoperative period due to bleeding from wounds and suture lines, but intraoperative thrombolysis with an arrested circulation may be helpful for the clearance of distal vessels.

Late graft occlusion should be investigated by arteriography, particularly to detect progression of proximal and distal disease, which requires attention in its own right.

Occlusion of large-calibre synthetic grafts in the aortofemoral position may occur due to progressive neo-intimal hyperplasia, particularly at bifurcations and anastomoses. Mechanical clearance, using embolectomy catheters aided by instrumental stripping of the obstructing material, is often successful and can be carried out from an inguinal approach. Aortic graft thrombosis has been successfully treated by peraxillary thrombolysis, and single iliac occlusion by lysis from the contralateral groin, but there is a significant risk of haemorrhage through the graft wall. More accessible subcutaneous grafts in the axillofemoral, axilloaxillary, femorofemoral or femoropopliteal positions can be safely treated by thrombolysis, since there is little risk of concealed haemorrhage.

If cannulation of these grafts from a contralateral arterial puncture is difficult (perhaps due to stenosis of the graft origin), direct puncture may be successful; thrombolysis by bolus or infusion techniques *under antibiotic cover* may then be employed. Direct puncture is more difficult to achieve in deeply placed grafts or those constructed from autogenous vein; but, if possible, successful lysis is usual in the majority of cases, the closed conduit of the graft being ideal for the development of a high concentration of lytic drug.

Stenoses in the body of synthetic and vein grafts may be dilated by angioplasty balloon, but the late results are disappointing, since neo-intimal hyperplasia does not dilate like atheromatous plaque in native vessels, and surgical revision is generally required. Stenosis of the origin (which is difficult to show), or distal anastomosis, is best managed by additional jump grafting to a new site, since surgical revision – particularly if the original anastomosis is of vein or was patched by vein – requires a difficult dissection with a high risk of technical problems. Thrombosis of vein grafts may cause permanent intimal damage, in contrast to synthetic conduits. Long-term patency is no better for reopened synthetic grafts than autogenous vein. Lysis of an occluded graft will sometimes reveal a normally patent reconstruction with good inflow and outflow vessels. If so, long-term anticoagulation is recommended to reduce the risks of further occlusion.

Other causes of acute limb ischaemia

Aortic dissection

This is an unusual cause of acute limb ischaemia which is most common in men. Hypertension, coarctation, Marfan's syndrome and pregnancy are known risk factors. Severe thoracoabdominal pain is classical, but some patients present with painless loss of peripheral pulses and the diagnosis requires CT or MR scanning and arteriography to demonstrate the characteristic true and false lumens. The induction of hypotension should be followed by surgical correction if possible. Dissection should be suspected if the easy retrograde passage of an embolectomy balloon is not followed by forward flow.

Trauma

The principles of management of trauma are discussed more fully in Chapter 18. In the upper limb, penetrating injuries (including iatrogenic injuries due to cardiac catheterization, arteriography or other invasive procedures) are increasing in incidence. Immediate repair should yield excellent results.

In small children microvascular techniques are required. Arterial occlusion from self-injection of home-made and street-purchased drugs causes severe microvascular chemical injury, as does the inadvertent intra-arterial injection of anaesthetic agents. Such injuries are difficult to treat, but the combination of heparin, intravenous dextran, steroids and thrombolytic agents has been recommended.[16]

Traction injuries in the upper limb may produce intimal arterial fracture and occlusion which may be associated with brachial plexus damage (classically in motorcycle injuries). Skeletal fractures and dislocations permit distraction and occlusion, especially where the vessel is fixed by its branches, such as at the circumflex humeral arteries. A precise angiographic diagnosis is required, particularly when the skeletal injury is remote from the arterial occlusion[17]. Direct repair of localized injury, using vein patches or interposition grafts, will be required.

In the lower limb, the femoral arteries are the most commonly involved in both penetrating and blunt injuries. Disruption of the femoral or popliteal arteries is likely to involve critical damage to the accompanying veins. The repair of both structures is important in limb salvage.

Thoracic outlet syndrome

Arterial compression and friction injury at the thoracic outlet may produce aneurysm, occlusion or local ulceration and microembolization. Complete arteriography is important to deal with both cause and effect.

Surgical microembolism (Trash foot)

This is usually seen following aortoiliac manipulation. Pain, discoloration and forefoot gangrene may occur with bounding ankle pulses. There is no specific treatment, but prevention by careful dissection and early distal control of atheromatous vessels is required.

Arteritis

Arteritis of the larger vessels supplying the limbs may present as a segmental stenosis or occlusion. Treatment with steroids is often effective, but surgical reconstruction may be required in unresponsive patients. Arteritis affecting the small vessels in the hands or feet should also be managed by steroids or immunosuppressive therapy. Vasodilatation by sympathetic blockade and drugs, such as guanethidine, reserpine and intravenous dextran, may all be helpful in a crisis.

Buerger's disease

This obliterative condition of the small vessels in young male smokers may present as an acute gangrene of the toes or, rarely, the fingers. Medium and small arteries are affected and there may be a superficial thrombophlebitis. The primary requirement is for the patient to stop smoking, but vasodilating drugs or sympathectomy may assist in the management of the acute phase.

The diabetic foot

The combination of arterial insufficiency, neuropathic ulceration and infection may lead to fulminating ischaemia as the increased demands of sepsis outstrip the blood supply. Necrosis may be accompanied by nonclostridial gas gangrene. Tissue gas due to clostridial infection is very rare indeed. Control of the infection by surgical debridement and appropriate systemic antibiotic therapy should be the first priority while any potential for arterial reconstruction is assessed.

Venous gangrene

This is a rare cause of acute peripheral ischaemia, secondary to massive venous occlusion. In the early stages there may also be acute arterial spasm. Elevation of the limb and anticoagulation remain the most important management principles.

Conclusions

In the United Kingdom, more than 5000 patients present with acute limb ischaemia annually. Many are elderly and only 70% will leave hospital with an intact limb. Of the remainder, half die in hospital and half require major amputation. Of the amputees, only 20% will maintain mobility with a prosthesis. Early diagnosis and correct management has the potential to save life and limb. The use of heparin and crystalloid alone has been reported to double rates of limb salvage to 87%, with a 12% mortality. Successful embolectomy together with heparin and reconstruction may yield limb salvage rates of up to 92% and a mortality of 10.2%. These excellent results are, however, exceptional. Thrombolytic therapy, followed by angioplasty and surgery, benefits at least 70% of patients with arterial thrombosis, and 57% will have a sustained improvement for at least three years. These elderly and frail patients are more likely to retain their limbs until death from another cardiovascular cause if the diagnosis is made without delay and if they are managed from the outset by an integrated team which includes an interventional radiologist and a vascular surgeon.

Recommended further reading

1. Bell PRF. The management of acute ischaemia of the limbs. In: *Surgical Management of Vascular Disease*, Bell PRF, Jamieson CW, Ruckley CV (eds). WB Saunders, 1992: 409.
2. Parent FN, Bernhard VM. Techniques of embolectomy, fasciotomy and fibulectomy. In: *Surgical Management of Vascular Disease*, Bell PRF, Jamieson CW, Ruckley CV (eds). WB Saunders, 1992: 423.

References

1. Cambria RP, Abbott WM. Acute arterial thrombosis of the lower extremity. Its natural history contrasted with arterial embolism. *Arch Surg* 1984; **119:** 784–7.
2. Walker WJ, Giddings AEB. A protocol for the safe treatment of acute lower limb ischaemia with intra-arterial streptokinase and surgery. *Br J Surg* 1988; **75:** 1189–92.
3. Jivegard LE, Arfvidsson B, Holm J, Schersten T. Selective conservative and routine early operative treatment in acute limb ischaemia. *Br J Surg* 1987; **74:** 798–801.
4. Fogarty TJ, Cranley JJ, Krause RJ, Strasser ES, Hafner CD. A method for extracting arterial emboli and thrombi. *Surg Gynae Obst* 1963; **116:** 241–4.
5. Mills JL, Porter JM. Basic data related to clinical decision-making in acute limb ischaemia. *Ann Vasc Surg* 1991; **5:** 96–8.
6. Quinones-Baldrich WJ, Baker JD, Busuttil RW, *et al.* Intraoperative infusion of lytic drugs for thrombotic complications of revascularization. *J Vasc Surg* 1989; **10:** 408–17.
7. Dotter CT, Rosch J, Seaman AJ. Selective clot lysis with low dose streptokinase. *Radiology* 1974; **111:** 31–7.
8. Katzen BT, van Breda A. Low dose streptokinase in the treatment of arterial occlusions. *Am J Roentgenol* 1981; **136:** 1171–8.
9. Hess H, Ingrisch H, Mietaschk A, Rath H. Local low dose thrombolytic therapy of peripheral arterial occlusions. *N Engl J Med* 1982; **307:** 1627–30.
10. Earnshaw JJ. Thrombolytic therapy in the management of acute limb ischaemia. *Br J Surg* 1991; **78:** 261–9.
11. Bell PRF. Femoro-distal grafts – can the results be improved *Eur J Vasc Surg* 1991; **5:** 607–9.
12. Scott DJA, Vowden P, Beard JD, Horrocks M. Non-invasive estimation of peripheral resistance using Pulse Generated Runoff before femorodistal bypass. *Br J Surg* 1990; **77:** 391–5.
13. Lancashire MJR, Torrie EPH, Galland RB. Popliteal aneurysms identified by intra-arterial streptokinase: a changing pattern of presentation. *Br J Surg* 1990; **77:** 1388–90.

14. Bowyer RC, Cawthorn SJ, Walker WJ, Giddings AEB. Conservative management of asymptomatic popliteal aneurysm. *Br J Surg* 1990; **77:** 1132–5.
15. Parent FN, Piotrowski JJ, Bernhard VM, *et al.* Outcome of intra-arterial urokinase for acute vascular occlusion. *J Cardiovasc Surg* 1991; **32:** 680–90.
16. Silverman SH, Turner WW. Intra-arterial drug abuse: new treatment options. *J Vasc Surg* 1991; **14:** 111–16.
17. Yanni, D, Wetzig NR, Giddings AEB. Remote arterial injury. Another cause of spurious arterial spasm. *J Cardiovasc Surg* 1989; **30:** 948–50.

4

Investigation of chronic occlusive disease

Jonathan D Beard

This chapter deals with the noninvasive and invasive investigation of chronic lower-limb ischaemia. Investigations complement, but do not replace, a careful history and examination. When establishing a diagnosis of vascular insufficiency it is always important to remember that the definition of terms like 'intermittent claudication' and 'rest pain' are symptom-based. Impalpable pulses do not mean that the patient's symptoms are necessarily vascular in origin, and the clue to the precise diagnosis usually lies in the history. Examination of the leg, including a neurological assessment, will usually then confirm or refute a vascular diagnosis. Arterial investigations are most useful when the diagnosis is uncertain, or to evaluate the degree of ischaemia and the location of disease.

Assessment of the general health of the patient is also important. There is little point in requesting expensive investigations for a claudicant if walking is also limited by angina. Detection of risk factors such as smoking, obesity, hyperlipidaemia, diabetes, hypertension and polycythaemia is also essential. Correction of these may produce significant improvements in the patient's symptoms and general health (see Chapter 5).

There are two distinct facets to arterial investigation: function and structure. Functional assessment has been revolutionized by the introduction of Doppler ultrasound. Conventional arteriography remains the standard investigation for providing structural information but is being challenged by newer modalities such as digital subtraction angiography and duplex ultrasound scanning. The sequence of investigations will depend upon the severity of symptoms, progressing from simple, noninvasive methods to time-consuming, invasive techniques. Two questions need to be asked:

1. What is the severity of the ischaemia?
2. Where is the arterial disease located?

Severity of ischaemia

This is the easier of the two questions to answer. It helps to establish that reduced blood flow is responsible for the symptoms, thereby differentiating, for example, true intermittent claudication from pain due to spinal stenosis (cauda equina syndrome).

Doppler ankle pressures

Doppler ultrasound enables blood flow to be monitored in impalpable arteries and, in conjunction with a sphygmomanometer, allows measurement of the systolic blood pressure (Fig. 4.1). Doppler ultrasound relies on the principle that the frequency of sound reflected by a moving object (red blood cells) is shifted in proportion to its velocity.[1] This frequency shift is in the audible range if the probe frequency is 1–10 MHz, giving a characteristic 'whooshing' noise during systole.

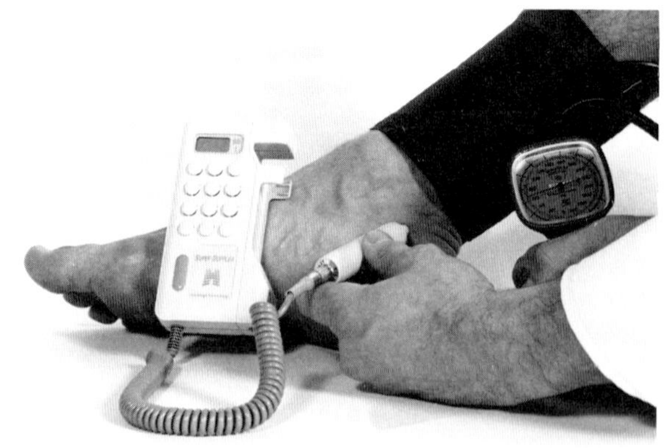

Fig. 4.1 Systolic ankle pressure measured with a Doppler ultrasound probe and a sphygmomanometer cuff. The pressure is normally expressed as an index of the brachial pressure (ABPI).

To measure the Doppler ankle pressure a standard sphygmomanometer cuff is placed around the ankle. The cuff is inflated to a suprasystolic level and then slowly deflated. The onset of blood flow detected by the Doppler probe equals the systolic blood pressure. Both the posterior tibial and dorsalis pedis arteries should be listened to and the highest pressure noted. If neither can be heard, a search should be made for the peroneal artery behind the fibula with the patient prone, or around the lateral malleolus. Very faint signals may be missed if the probe is pressed too hard against the skin. These signals can be improved by placing the feet in a dependent position.

Doppler ankle pressures are often expressed as a ratio of the brachial systolic pressure. This ratio is called the 'ankle brachial pressure index' (ABPI).[2] The index allows comparisons to be made between patients and from day-to-day in the same patient: a change of 0.15 being significant.[3] Normal subjects should have an ABPI of 1.0 or more, whilst in claudicants it is usually less than 0.9 and in those patients with critical ischaemia less than 0.5. Critical ischaemia has been defined by the European Working Group[4] as persistent rest pain for more than two weeks and/or ulceration or gangrene, plus an ankle systolic pressure of less than 50 mmHg. Arterial calcification, common in diabetes, may lead to falsely elevated pressures due to incompressible arteries. However, an experienced operator will be alerted by the damped flow signals if proximal disease is present. This can be confirmed by elevating the leg, which will abolish the Doppler signal. A measure of the pressure can be obtained by recording the height at which the signal disappears. Toe pressures are less likely to be affected by calcification but require small cuffs and are more difficult to measure routinely.

The value of foot X-rays to detect osteomyelitis beneath an ulcer should not be forgotten, especially in diabetics (see Chapter 17).

Exercise testing

If the level of the Doppler ankle pressure is equivocal, it should be repeated after exercise which increases the sensitivity of the test.[5] The increased muscle blood flow required by exercise will result in a fall in the ankle pressure if there is significant arterial disease (Fig. 4.2). Conversely, if there is no fall, the patient can be reassured that arterial disease is not the cause of the symptoms. Unfortunately, the problem of the patient with evidence of both

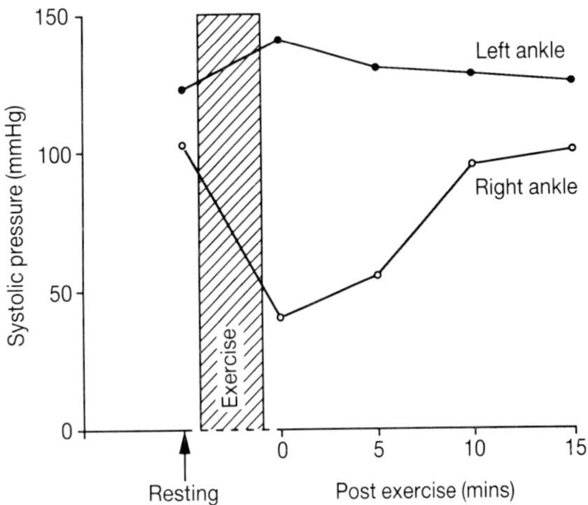

Fig. 4.2 Exercise test of a patient with right calf claudication. After exercise, the pressure falls dramatically, indicating haemodynamically significant disease.

arterial occlusive disease and nerve-root irritation remains. There is currently no reliable method of determining objectively which is the more symptomatic condition, although magnetic resonance imaging, combined with a stress test, may provide the answer in the future. Empirical treatment such as angioplasty may be the best option but patients should be warned that their pain might not be improved.

Most exercise testing is now performed on a treadmill. The speed of the treadmill is usually set at 4 km/h with a gradient of 10 degrees. The duration of exercise may be standardized to one minute,[6] or continued until the patient is stopped by pain. The former may be more reproducible but the latter has the advantage of measuring how far the patient can actually walk.

Some patients may be unable to tolerate a treadmill due to unfamiliarity, shortness of breath, angina or arthritis. These patients can be assessed by a timed walk, at their own pace, down a hospital corridor. Alternatively, Doppler ankle pressures may be measured after hyperaemia induced by ankle flexion/extension, or after release of an occlusive thigh cuff.

Plethysmography

Plethysmography relies on the principle that short-term changes in limb volume are largely due to changes in the amount of blood present.[7] Accurate measurement of the volume changes requires cumbersome equipment, because the leg must be enclosed in a rigid container with an effective seal and the displacement of air or water measured.

Qualitative information is more simply obtained. The change in volume of a segment of the leg under a cuff may be measured by a pulse volume recorder[8] (Fig. 4.3), or the diameter by a mercury strain gauge.[9] The amount of blood in the skin may be measured by infrared photoplethysmography[10] or the flux of blood in the skin by laser Doppler.[11] All of these instruments may be used in an AC (arterial) mode or in a DC (venous) mode. In AC mode they can record pulsation in the leg and in DC mode they can estimate limb blood flow, if combined with a venous tourniquet.

It is difficult to justify the use of plethysmography for the routine assessment of the severity of leg ischaemia. Any plethysmographic technique, in conjunction with a sphygmomanometer, can be used to measure systolic pressures, but they are more complex and expensive than Doppler pressures. They may be of more use in locating the site of arterial disease but their main role is in the noninvasive investigation of venous disease[12] and as research tools. However, automatic digital photoplethysmographic sphygmomanometers have recently become available. These are cheaper and require less expertise than Doppler pressures, and may be useful in the preliminary evaluation of patients with suspected lower-limb ischaemia.

Transcutaneous oximetry

Transcutaneous measurement of the oxygen tension in the skin ($TcPO_2$) depends on the notion that, at equilibrium, the partial pressure of oxygen which diffuses through to the surface of the skin will reflect the oxygen tension of the underlying tissues.[13] The probe consists of a Clark-type oxygen electrode together with a heating element and a temperature sensor. The probe is clipped on to a ring attached to the skin, and filled with an electrolyte solution. Resting $TcPO_2$ measurements are of little value but, in combination with a stress test, can determine the severity of limb ischaemia. However, this is only the case if the skin is not hyperkeratotic and is heated to 43–44°C. It is a time-consuming technique that requires care to achieve reproducible results. It may be of more use in the selection of amputation sites as it has been shown to correlate well with subsequent stump healing.[14] Photoplethysmography,[15] laser Doppler,[16] thermography[17] and isotope clearance[18] have also been shown to be superior to Doppler ankle pressures in this respect,[19] but none has become established for routine use.[20]

Isotope blood flow

Radioisotopes have been used to study blood flow by measuring clearance rates of 99m-technetium pertechnate following intramuscular injection,[21] by first-pass radionuclide arteriography,[22] and by intravenous ^{99m}Tc-labelled human serum albumin combined with hyperaemia, following release of a thigh

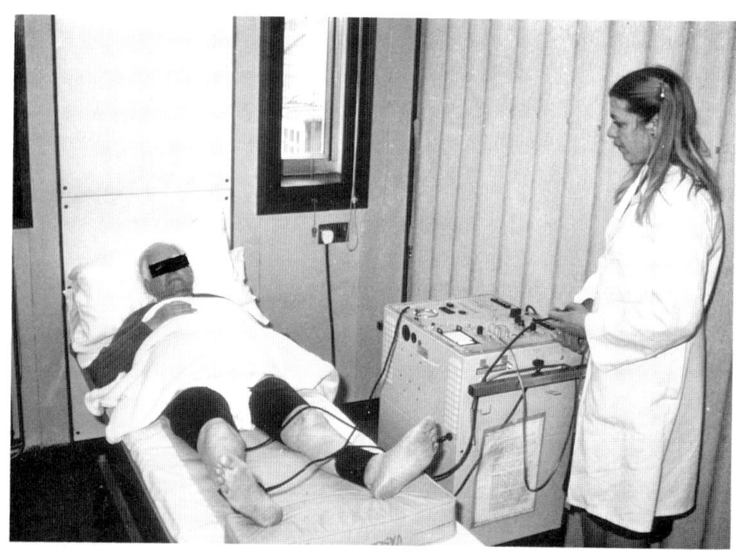

Fig. 4.3 Pulse volume recorder. This is an air plethysmograph that detects pulsatile pressure changes within the thigh and calf cuffs. Proximal arterial disease results in a damped waveform with a reduced amplitude and a slower upstroke time.

tourniquet.[23] These methods are very sensitive in detecting arterial disease and can provide qualitative and quantitative information about limb blood flow. However, this information is of little practical value in terms of patient management. The tests are invasive and more suited to research.

Location of disease

Once the severity of the ischaemia has been established, it is necessary to locate the site of disease if intervention in the form of transluminal angioplasty or reconstructive surgery is contemplated. Atherosclerosis commonly affects the arteries supplying the leg in a segmental fashion. These arterial segments are classified clinically into aortoiliac, femoropopliteal (profunda and superficial femoral arteries), and distal (popliteal trifurcation and calf/foot arteries). To plan treatment effectively, the severity of disease in each segment needs to be assessed. The difficulty arises in determining the most significant lesion when there is multilevel disease. As a general principle, proximal disease is dealt with first, because the results are generally better and the effectiveness of a lower reconstruction might be otherwise limited by poor inflow. However, estimation of the outflow capacity (runoff) is also important as this will determine graft function and patency. There are two main areas of difficulty:

1. the diagnosis of significant aortoiliac disease in the presence of femoropoliteal disease (i.e. is there an inflow problem?) (Fig. 4.4);
2. the detection of patent distal calf arteries in the presence of severe proximal disease (i.e. is there a runoff problem?).

Palpation of the femoral pulse is notoriously unreliable at detecting mild-to-moderate aortoiliac disease that might well be haemodynamically significant.[24] The pulse may be normal at rest and will also be affected by obesity, scarring from previous operation or angioplasty, and vessel calcification. The presence of a bruit may help to confirm the clinical impression of a weak femoral pulse, but this is flow-dependent and may be absent if there is low flow due to coexisting femoropopliteal disease. Palpation of pedal pulses or Doppler ankle pressures are clearly going to be of little use in determining the amount of distal calf artery disease when there is severe femoropopliteal disease.

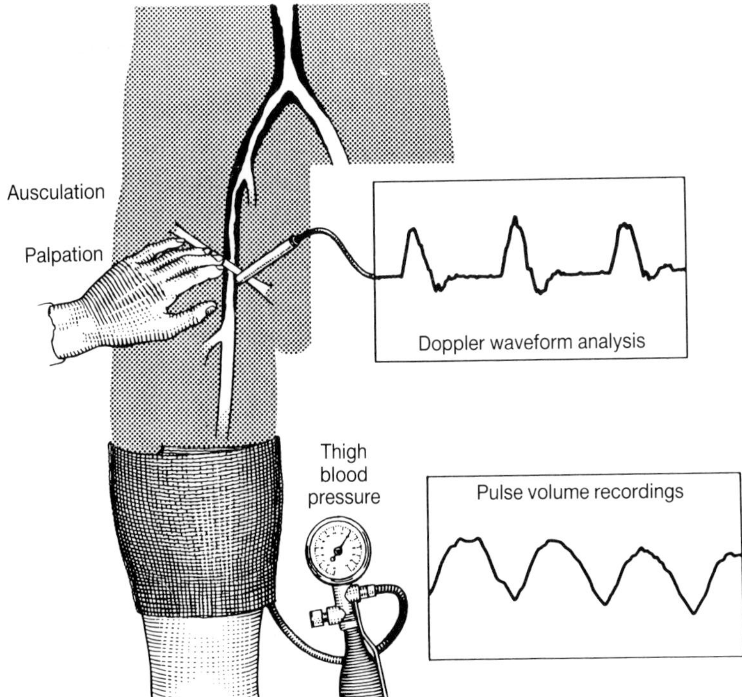

Fig. 4.4 Noninvasive methods of diagnosing aortoiliac disease. However, the 'gold-standard' remains femoral artery pressure measurements.

Segmental arterial pressures

This approach relies on the simple idea that the pressure in arteries in any point in the leg will be reduced if there is significant disease proximal to it. Four cuffs are applied: as high as possible on the thigh, above the knee, below the knee and above the ankle. Each cuff is inflated in turn and the returning signal detected by a Doppler probe placed over an ankle artery, or by a plethysmograph cuff around the hallux. In normal subjects the gradient between adjacent cuffs will be less than 20–30 mmHg and the difference between the same sites on opposite legs not more than 20 mmHg.[25] The technique has the advantage that it is noninvasive but it suffers from two major problems:

1. the remoteness of the detection from the cuff, which may result in a falsely low reading if there is arterial disease below the cuff;
2. the size of the high-thigh cuff, which means that the pressure recorded will be falsely elevated.

As a result, the diagnosis of aortoiliac stenosis is unsatisfactory particularly if femoropopliteal disease is present. However, a 'normal' thigh pressure at rest makes aortoiliac disease unlikely.

Waveform analysis

A bidirectional Doppler recorder is able to distinguish between blood flow towards and away from the probe and can produce a waveform representing the mean blood flow velocity in the vessel.[1] In most peripheral arteries, including the common femoral artery, the flow profile has three phases: powerful forward flow in systole, transient reversed flow, followed by weak forward in diastole. A marked stenosis or occlusion of the aortoiliac segment will give a damped, monophasic waveform. More accurate flow information may be obtained by spectrum analysis of the Doppler signals. A visual display is obtained of all the different blood velocities in the vessel at any one time. A stenosis causes an increase in the peak blood velocity through it and turbulence beyond it (see Fig. 4.11). Turbulence produces a wider range of velocities, termed 'spectral broadening'.

A grossly damped waveform is easy to detect but it is of little diagnostic value as the femoral pulse will be palpably weak or absent. Many methods have been used to analyse femoral artery waveforms in an attempt to detect clinically less obvious, but haemodynamically significant, aortoiliac disease. These include the pulsatility index (Fig. 4.5), derived from dividing the peak height of the waveform by the mean;[26] Laplace transform damping analysis which is a complex mathematical method of fitting a curve to the waveform;[27] and principal component analysis which compares the waveform with that obtained from a sample population.[28]

These methods of analysis are all better than palpation at detecting a significant aortoiliac stenosis. However, they all suffer from the same disadvantage as segmental arterial pressures, in that results may be misleading if femoropopliteal disease is present.[29]

Direct pressure measurement

This is currently the 'gold standard' for functional assessment of the aortoiliac segment. The common femoral artery is punctured, under local anaesthetic, by a needle or cannula connected to a pressure transducer. The brachial or radial artery is also cannulated and the femoral/brachial pressure ratio measured (Fig. 4.6). Papaverine 30 mg is injected into the femoral artery and the percentage fall in the ratio measured. A fall of 20% after papaverine indicates significant proximal disease.[29] The test is relatively unaffected by distal disease unless it is so severe that papaverine, which is a potent vasodilator, does not cause any increase in flow. Similar measurements of the pressure drop across the aortoiliac segment may be made at the time of arteriography.[30]

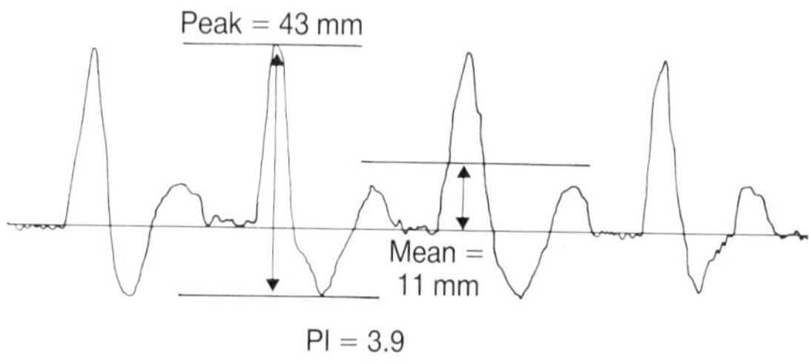

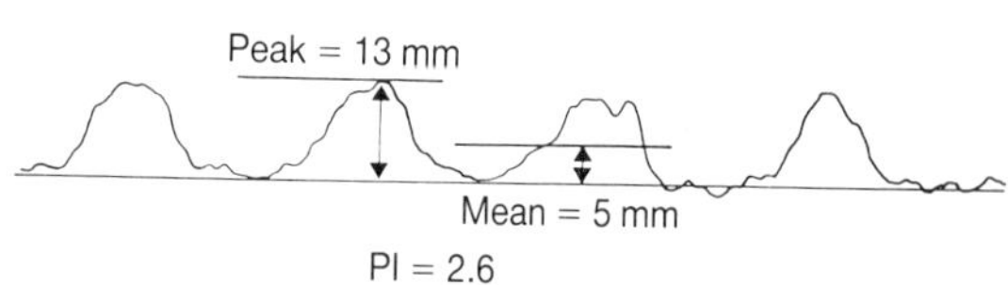

Fig. 4.5 Pulsatility index (PI) calculated from the bidirectional femoral artery Doppler waveform of a normal (top) compared to a patient with aortoiliac disease. Proximal stenosis results in a reduction in the ratio of the peak-to-peak amplitude to the mean.

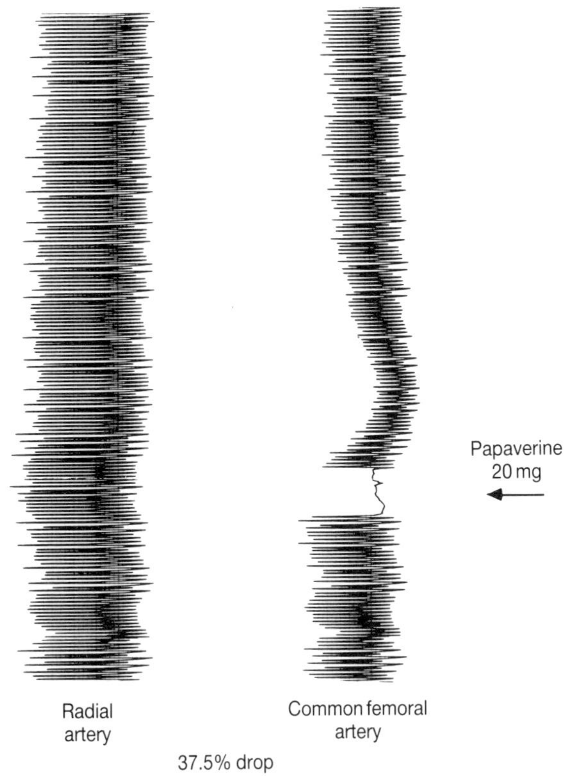

Fig. 4.6 Intra-arterial pressure measurement of the radial and femoral arteries of a patient with haemodynamically significant aortoiliac disease. Although there is little difference at rest, there is a drop of 37.5% after papaverine.

Arteriography

Arteriography remains the best method of providing structural information about the arterial tree upon which decisions regarding the technical aspects of proposed treatment are made. It also has the advantage that percutaneous transluminal angioplasty may be performed at the same time. However, it is an invasive technique with a small but definite risk of complications such as anaphylaxis, thrombosis, embolization and haematoma.[31] Therefore, arteriography should not be performed unless it has been decided that an operation or angioplasty will be carried out if a suitable lesion is demonstrated.

The most common technique is that described by Seldinger.[32] An artery (usually the common femoral) is punctured with a needle, under local anaesthetic, and a guidewire passed up into the abdominal aorta. The needle is withdrawn and a catheter passed over the guidewire which is also removed. Contrast is then injected rapidly by a high-pressure pump. A timed sequence of exposures is taken to demonstrate the entire arterial tree from the aorta to the feet, as contrast flows distally. If there is no femoral access then an alternative approach is required. Intravenous DSA (see later) may provide sufficient detail of the aortoiliac segment but is unlikely to visualize the distal arterial tree very well. The aorta can be punctured directly by a needle passed through the left lumbar muscles (translumbar aortography), but it is uncomfortable for the patient and large retroperitoneal haematomas can occur because pressure cannot be applied to the aorta when the needle is withdrawn. In modern practice, a more popular alternative is catheterization of the brachial or axillary arteries.

Conventional uniplanar arteriography suffers from several limitations. No functional information is obtained; the severity of a stenosis, particularly in the aortoiliac segment, may be under- or overestimated; and patent calf and foot vessels may not be demonstrated.[33] The significance of aortoiliac and femoral stenoses should be further assessed by biplanar views[34] (Fig. 4.7), intra-arterial pressure measurements[30] or duplex scanning (see later). Demonstration of the calf and foot arteries usually requires additional measures, such as injection of contrast into the common femoral artery or producing hyperaemia by an occlusive cuff or vasodilators.[35]

Pulse-generated runoff

It is essential to demonstrate patent calf or foot arteries as these form the runoff upon which a successful femorodistal bypass graft depends. If these arteries are not demonstrated the patient may be condemned to an unnecessary amputation. One way to avoid this is to perform a peroperative arteriogram by direct puncture of the exposed popliteal artery,[36] but this makes preoperative planning difficult (Fig. 4.8).

A better method is to augment the weak Doppler ultrasound signals at the ankle by means of a pneumatic cuff around the calf.[37] The cuff is inflated 60 times a minute by compressed air, and this generates pulsatile flow in patent calf arteries. This 'pulse-generated runoff' (PGR) system has been shown to detect more patent calf arteries than conventional arteriography in severely ischaemic legs and is non-invasive (Fig. 4.9). PGR can also determine whether there is continuity with the pedal arch, and correlates well with operative peripheral resistance measurements and the subsequent outcome of femorodistal bypass.[38]

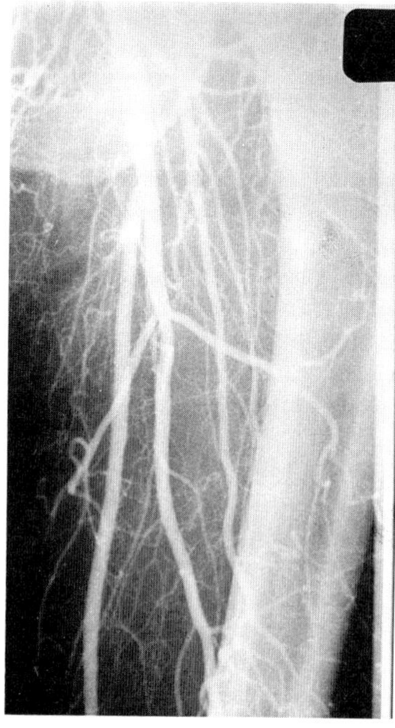

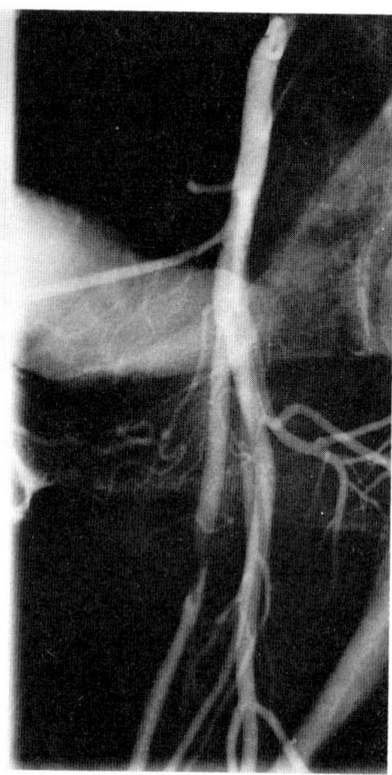

Fig. 4.7 Arteriogram of the common femoral artery bifurcation showing the value of biplanar views. The tight stenosis of the proximal superficial femoral artery can be clearly seen on the oblique view (right), but would have been missed on the AP view (left).

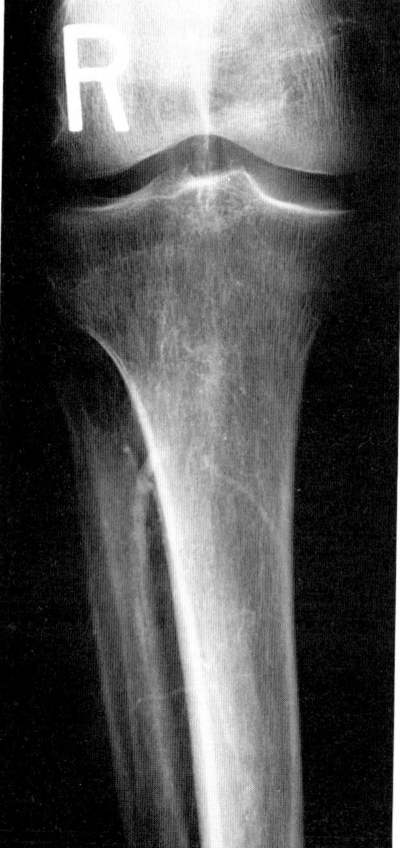

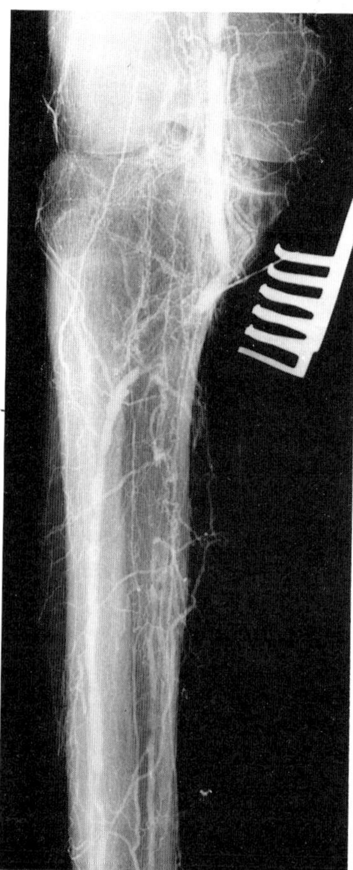

Fig. 4.8 Operative arteriogram performed by direct puncture of the exposed popliteal artery (right) compared with the preoperative arteriogram (left) which only demonstrated the proximal anterior tibial artery because of severe proximal disease. On the operative film, this is shown to be occluded in the mid-calf with distal runoff via the peroneal artery.

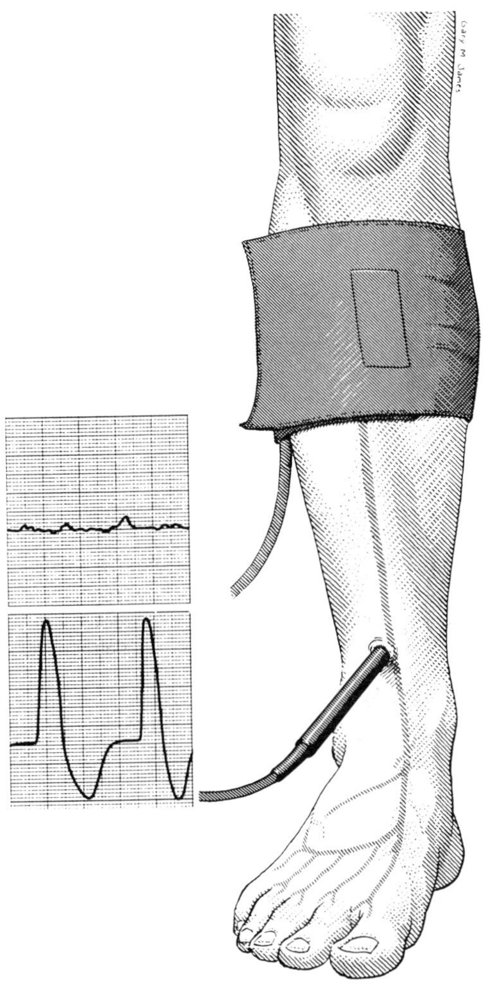

Fig. 4.9 The pulse-generated runoff system (PGR). The pulsatile cuff around the calf augments the existing weak or inaudible Doppler signal at the ankle if the artery is patent.

Digital subtraction angiography

Digital subtraction angiography (DSA) images are obtained by using a computer to digitize an image of the background (bone and soft tissues) and then subtracting this from the image acquired following injection of contrast. The resultant image then shows arterial detail without any overlying structures. Subsequent manipulation of the information is possible to improve the quality of the picture and to replace a certain amount of background detail, if required. Whilst the spatial resolution is not as good as with conventional angiography, this is outweighed by the improvement in arterial visualization and the potential for post-processing and digital storage.

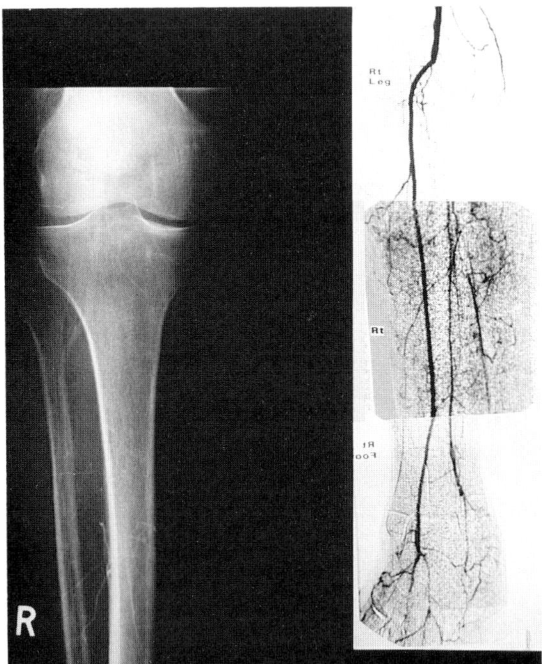

Fig. 4.10 Intra-arterial digital subtraction arteriogram (right) of the lower leg in a patient with severe proximal disease. The conventional arteriogram (left) had failed to demonstrate adequately a patent anterior tibial artery to the foot.

Images obtained over an extended time can demonstrate patent distal vessels that have filled late due to poor flow, and so the problem of incorrect timing associated with conventional techniques is avoided (Fig. 4.10).

The high sensitivity to intra-arterial contrast (IADSA) also means that a smaller volume of contrast is required, permitting the use of narrower 3 or 4F catheters and improving safety.[39] Whilst there was a vogue for the intravenous delivery of contrast agents into the vena cava or right atrium (IVDSA), this requires a relatively large volume of contrast which is unsafe in patients with myocardial insufficiency and it yields pictures of inferior quality.[40] Most equipment now allows an overlay of the arterial tree on the monitor whilst manipulating a guidewire, catheter or balloon. This is invaluable for superselective arteriography, angioplasty or embolization, resulting in a marked reduction in procedure time.

Duplex scanning

The duplex ultrasound scanner combines real-time, B-mode imaging and a pulsed Doppler into one instrument.[41] The former uses the reflections of ultrasound from tissue interfaces, rather than from blood movement as in the Doppler technique. A high-resolution image of the vessel can be obtained together with spectral analysis of the blood flow within it (Fig. 4.11). The latest generation of colour duplex scanners also provide real-time colour-coded mapping of the blood flow velocities in the arteries, but they are expensive. Theoretically, it is also possible to calculate blood flow with a duplex scanner because the probe to vessel angle and the vessel diameter can be measured. In practice, there are many sources of error, such as estimation of the true mean blood velocity, which make such measurements unreliable in diseased arteries.[42]

The combination of simultaneous structural and functional information obtained noninvasively is unique and has resulted in duplex scanning becoming the definitive investigation for carotid artery disease[43] (see Chapter 19). However, the same cannot be said for the lower-limb arteries. Duplex scanning of the aortoiliac segment has been shown to be as good as arteriography in detecting significant disease, but visualization may be difficult in obese patients and bowel gas may also obscure the image.[44] This is less of a problem with the more distal arteries, but the length of time and technical expertise required to obtain a complete assessment does not justify its routine use at present. The duplex scanner may be of use in assessing the suitability of arterial stenoses or occlusions for angioplasty as it can provide information about the composition of the lesion. It can also be used as a screening test before proceeding to arteriography in claudicants with clinical evidence of SFA occlusion, and symptoms sufficient to warrant angioplasty but not reconstructive surgery. Duplex scanning can easily determine whether the origin of the SFA is patent, which is a prerequisite for angioplasty. It is also of value in the preoperative evaluation of the long saphenous vein prior to femoropopliteal bypass grafts[45] and in monitoring these grafts postoperatively to detect stenoses[46] (see Chapter 8).

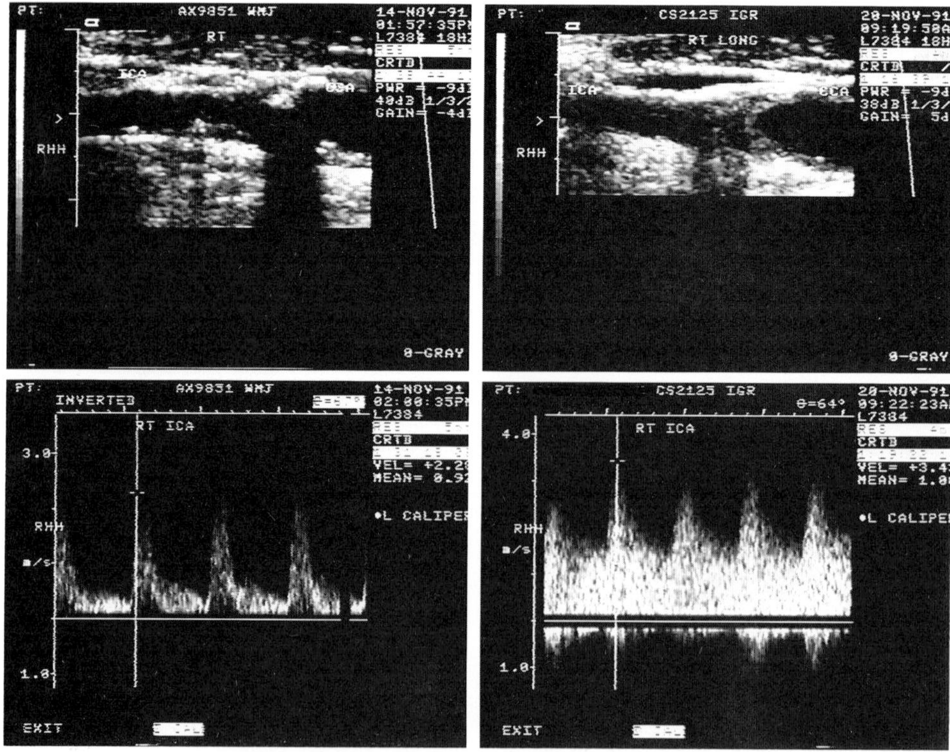

Fig. 4.11 Duplex ultrasound scan of a 60% arterial stenosis (top left) and an 80% stenosis (top right). The images give a fair impression of the severity of the stenoses, and further information about this can be obtained from spectral analysis of the waveform. Flow through the 60% stenosis (bottom left) shows an increased peak velocity and spectral broadening, indicating turbulence. Flow through the 80% stenosis (bottom right) shows severe turbulence with a very high peak velocity.

Magnetic resonance imaging

Magnetic resonance imaging (MRI) offers exciting possibilities for the future.[47] Like duplex scanning it can also provide structural and functional information noninvasively. Magnetic resonance angiography (MRA) offers the potential to examine the peripheral vessels noninvasively, without the complications of iodinated contrast or exposure to ionizing radiation. Images are normally acquired in the coronal plane using a large field of view to cover the region of interest, although demonstration of small vessels can be facilitated by using a surface coil to improve the signal quality. The data may then be processed to produce either sequential 2-dimensional images or a 3-dimensional model.

Major disadvantages at present are the high cost, poor resolution and time taken to scan each patient. Undesirable flow phenomena (such as turbulence) cause signal loss and overestimation of the severity of stenoses. This problem may be ameliorated in the future by better imaging and processing techniques, and by the use of paramagnetic contrast agents.

Conclusions

Many sophisticated techniques are now available for the investigation of lower-limb ischaemia. However, the simplest test remains the best: namely Doppler ankle pressures, combined with an exercise test if necessary. If further assessment is required, conventional arteriography usually provides adequate structural information but is being challenged by DSA and duplex scanning. Direct pressure measurements give superior functional information about the aortoiliac segment and remain the 'gold-standard'. MRI offers exciting prospects for the noninvasive investigation of both vascular structure and function in the future.

References

1. Atkinson P, Woodcock JP. *Doppler Ultrasound and its Uses in Clinical Measurements*. London: Academic Press, 1982.
2. Yao JST, Hobbs JT, Irvine WT. Ankle systolic pressure measurements in arterial disease affecting the lower extremities. *Br J Surg* 1969; **56:** 676–9.
3. Baker JD, DeEtle Dix PAC. Variability of Doppler ankle pressures with arterial occlusive disease: an evaluation of ankle index and brachial ankle pressure gradient. *Surgery* 1980; **89:** 134–7.
4. Dormandy J. *European Consensus Document on Critical Limb Ischaemia*. Berlin: Springer-Verlag, 1989.
5. Berglund B, Eklund B. Reproducibility of treadmill exercise in patients with intermittent claudication. *Clin Physiol* 1981; **1:** 253–6.
6. Laing SP, Greenhalgh RM. Standard exercise test to assess peripheral arterial disease. *Br Med J* 1980; **280:** 13–16.
7. Brodie TG, Russell AE. On the determination of the rate of blood flow through an organ. *J Physiol* 1905: 32–47.
8. Raines JK, Darling RC, Buth J, *et al.* Vascular laboratory criteria for the management of peripheral vascular disease of the lower extremities. *Surgery* 1976; **79:** 21–9.
9. Holling HE, Boland HC, Russ E. Investigation of arterial obstruction using a mercury-in-rubber strain gauge. *Am Heart J* 1961; **62:** 194–203.
10. Lee BY, Trainor FS, Kavner D, Crisologo JA, Shaw WW, Madden JL. Assessment of the healing potentials of ulcers of the skin by photoplethysmography. *Surg Gynae Obst* 1979; **147:** 232–9.
11. Allan PIM, Goldman M. Laser Doppler assessment of skin blood flow in arteriopathic limbs. *Clin Phys Physiol Meas* 1987; **8:** 1779–82.
12. Ruckley CV. *Surgical Management of Venous Disease*. London: Wolfe Medical, 1988: 18–31.
13. Franzeck UK, Talke P, Bernstein EF, Golbranson FL, Fronek A. Transcutaneous pO_2 measurements in health and peripheral vascular disease. *Surgery* 1982; **91:** 156–63.
14. Ratcliffe DA, Clyne CAC, Chant ADB, Webster JHH. Prediction of amputation wound healing: the role of transcutaneous pO_2 assessment. *Br J Surg* 1984; **71:** 219–22.
15. Van Den Broek TAA, Dwars BJ, Rauwerda JA, Bakker FC. Photoplethysmographic selection of amputation level in peripheral vascular disease. *J Vasc Surg* 1988; **8:** 10–13.
16. Karanfilian RG, Lynch TG, Zirul VT, *et al.* The value of laser Doppler velocimetry and transcutaneous oxygen tension determination in predicting healing of ischaemic forefoot ulceration and amputation in diabetic and nondiabetic patients. *J Vasc Surg* 1986; **4,** 511–16.
17. Stoner HB, Taylor L, Marcuson RW. The value of skin temperature measurements in forecasting the healing of below-knee amputation for end-stage ischaemia of the leg in peripheral vascular disease. *Eur J Vasc Surg* 1989; **3:** 355–61.
18. Moore WS, Henry RE, Malone JM, Daly MJ, Patton D, Childers SJ. Prospective use of Xenon Xe-133 clearance for amputation level selection. *Arch Surg* 1981; **116:** 86–8.
19. Welch GH, Leiberman DP, Pollock JG, Angerson W. Failure of Doppler ankle pressure to predict healing of conservative forefoot amputations. *Br J Surg* 1985; **72:** 888–91.

20. Savin S, Sharni S, Shields DA, Scurr JH, Coleridge-Smith PD. Selection of amputation level: a review. *Eur J Vasc Surg* 1991; **5:** 611–20.
21. Cutajar CL, Brown NJG, Marston A. Muscle blood flow studies by the technetium ($^{99}Tc^{m}$) clearance technique in normal subjects and in patients with intermittent claudication. *Br J Surg* 1971; **58:** 532–7.
22. Oshima M, Ijima H, Kohda Y, *et al.* Peripheral arterial disease diagnosed with high count rate radionuclide arteriography. *Radiology* 1984; **152:** 161–6.
23. Wilkinson D, Vowden P, Parkin A, Wiggins PA, Robinson PJ, Kester RC. A reliable and readily available method of measuring limb blood flow in intermittent claudication. *Br J Surg* 1987; **74:** 516–19.
24. Green IL, Greenhalgh RM. Objective evaluation of the femoral pulse. In: *Diagnostic Techniques and Assessment Procedures in Vascular Surgery*, Greenhalgh RM (ed). Orlando: Grune & Stratton, 1986: 241–50.
25. Walker WF, Spence VA, McCollum PT. Systolic pressure measurements in the ischaemic lower limb. *Hosp Update* 1986; **12:** 343–58.
26. Gosling RG, Dunbar G, King DH, *et al.* The quantitative analysis of occlusive peripheral arterial disease by a non-intrusive ultrasonic technique. *Angiology* 1971; **22:** 52–5.
27. Baird RN, Bird DR, Clifford PC, Lusby RJ, Skidmore R, Woodcock JP. Upstream stenosis: its diagnosis by Doppler signals from the femoral artery. *Arch Surg* 1980; **115:** 1316–22.
28. Prytherch DR, Evans DH, Smith MJ, Macpherson DS. On-line classification of arterial stenosis using principal component analysis applied to Doppler ultrasound signals. *Clin Phys Physiol Meas* 1982; **3:** 191–200.
29. Macpherson DS, Evans DH, Bell PRF. Common femoral artery Doppler waveforms: a comparison of these methods of objective analysis with direct pressure measurements. *Br J Surg* 1984; **71:** 46–9.
30. Udoff EJ, Barth KH, Harrington DP, Kaufman SL, White RI. Haemodynamic significance of iliac artery stenosis: pressure measurements during angiography. *Radiology* 1979; **132:** 289–93.
31. Hessel SJ, Adams DF, Abrams HL. Complications of angiography. *Radiology* 1981; **138:** 273–83.
32. Doby T. A tribute to Seldinger. *AJR* 1984; **142:** 1–11.
33. Campbell WB, Fletcher EL, Hands LJ. Assessment of the distal lower limb arteries: a comparison of arteriography and Doppler ultrasound. *Ann Roy Coll Surg Eng* 1986; **18:** 37–9.
34. Sethi GK, Scott SM, Takaro T. Multiplane angiography for more precise evaluation of aortoiliac disease. *Surgery* 1975; **8:** 154–9.
35. Feins RH, Roedersheimer LR, Baumstark AE, Green RM. Predicted hyperaemic angiography: a technique of distal arteriography in the severely ischaemic limb. *Surgery* 1981; **89:** 202–5.
36. Flannigan DP, Williams LR, Keifer T, Schuler JJ, Berend AJ. Pre-bypass operative arteriography. *Surgery* 1982; **92:** 627–33.
37. Beard JD, Scott DJA, Evans JM, Skidmore R, Horrocks M. Pulse generated runoff: a new method of determining calf vessel patency. *Br J Surg* 1988; **75:** 361–3.
38. Scott DJA, Hunt G, Beard JD, Hartnell GG, Horrocks M. Arteriogram scoring systems and pulse-generated runoff in the assessment of patients with critical ischaemia for femorodistal bypass. *Br J Surg* 1989; **76:** 1202–6.
39. Kaufman SL, Chang R, Kadir S, Mitchell SE, White PI. Intra-arterial digital subtraction angiography in diagnostic arteriography. *Radiology* 1984; **151:** 323–7.
40. Sumner DS, Porter DJ, Moore DJ, Windes RE. Digital subtraction angiography: intravenous and intra-arterial techniques. *J Vasc Surg* 1985; **2:** 344–53.
41. Evans DH, McDicken WN, Skidmore R, Woodcock JP. *Doppler Ultrasound: Physics, Instrumentation and Clinical Applications.* Chichester: John Wiley, 1989: 47–63.
42. Gill RW. Measurement of blood flow by ultrasound: accuracy and sources of error. *Ultrasound Med Biol* 1985; **11:** 625–41.
43. Flanigan M, Schuler JJ, Vogel M, Borozan PG, Gray B, Sobinsky KR. The role of carotid duplex scanning in surgical decision making. *J Vasc Surg* 1985; **2:** 15–25.
44. Legemate DA, Teeuwen C, Hoeneveld H, Eikelboom BC. Value of duplex scanning compared with angiography and pressure measurement in the assessment of aortoiliac arterial lesions. *Br J Surg* 1991; **78:** 1003–8.
45. Leopold PW. Shandall A, Kupinski AM, *et al.* Role of B-mode venous mapping in infra-inguinal *in situ* vein arterial bypasses. *Br J Surg* 1989; **76:** 305–7.
46. Grigg NJ, Nicolaides AN, Wolfe JHN. Femorodistal vein bypass graft stenoses. *Br J Surg* 1988; **75:** 737–40.
47. Bydder GM. Magnetic resonance imaging: present status and future perspectives. *Br J Radiol* 1988; **61:** 889–97.

5

Conservative management of chronic occlusive arterial disease

Gordon DO Lowe

Epidemiology and pathology

Intermittent claudication is the commonest clinical presentation of chronic arterial disease of the lower limbs. It is common in developed countries: questionnaire surveys have shown a prevalence of about 5% in the population aged over 50 years.[1–3] The prevalence of *asymptomatic* arterial disease is much higher. For example, in a survey of the Edinburgh population aged 55–74 years, 8% had a severely abnormal ankle brachial pressure index (ABPI) and/or reactive hyperaemia test; while another 17% had moderate abnormalities in these two tests.[2,3] In total, therefore, about a quarter of the older population have some detectable manifestation of chronic occlusive disease, even though only one in five is symptomatic. This high prevalence of disease is in keeping with necropsy studies.[4] It is quite likely that many patients with asymptomatic disease do not complain of claudication because they never exercise enough to experience pain!

While many people who do exercise enough to experience claudication worry about progression of their claudication to critical leg ischaemia, the good news for claudicants is that the natural history of limb symptoms is usually benign. Less than 50% experience continued deterioration in symptoms and/or consult a doctor; and less than 5% ever require a major amputation.[1,2,5] The probable pathological basis of stepwise deterioration and spontaneous symptomatic improvement in chronic peripheral occlusive disease is outlined in Fig 5.1. The main predictor of local progression is the ABPI followed by male sex, smoking and diabetes, age has only a weak effect[5] (Table 5.1). These predictive variables can be assessed at the clinic in a few minutes.

The bad news for claudicants is that their claudication is a symptom of generalized atherosclerosis and arterial thrombosis, which affects also the aorta, coronary and cranial arteries and results in a high risk of cardiovascular death.[1,2] Men with chronic leg ischaemia have a 5-year mortality 2–3 times higher than men of similar age without such symptoms: 50% die of ischaemic heart disease, 15% of stroke, 10% of abdominal vascular disease, and only 25% die non-cardiovascular deaths.[1] Hence the major risk in claudication is to life rather than limb. Risk predictors for early cardiovascular events and death include low ABPI (presumably as an index of the severity of generalized atherosclerosis), history of coronary artery disease, diabetes, hypertension and a high white blood cell count.[5] Again, these predictors can easily be assessed at a clinic visit.

The major population risk associations for chronic occlusive arterial disease are similar to those for ischaemic heart disease and cerebrovascular disease: age, male sex, cigarette smoking, hyperten-

Table 5.1 Predictive value of various risk factors for all-cause mortality and for deterioration of leg ischaemia in 1969 claudicants (control group of the PACK study); univariate analysis showing relative risk and 95% confidence intervals in brackets

	All-cause mortality	Deterioration of leg ischaemia
Age (per 10 years)	2.1 (1.6–2.7)	1.2 (1.0–1.4)
ABPI (≤ 0.5)	2.0 (1.3–3.2)	2.3 (1.6–3.4)
Coronary artery disease	2.0 (1.3–3.1)	1.3 (0.9–1.9)
Hypertension	1.8 (1.1–2.8)	1.0 (0.7–1.4)
Diabetes	1.7 (1.0–2.8)	1.3 (0.8–2.1)
Male sex	1.3 (0.7–2.3)	1.7 (1.0–2.8)
Stroke	1.1 (0.5–2.2)	1.8 (1.1–3.0)
Smoking (past 6 months)	0.8 (0.5–1.3)	1.4 (0.9–2.2)
Previous vascular surgery	0.6 (0.3–0.9)	1.7 (1.2–2.4)

Source: reference 5

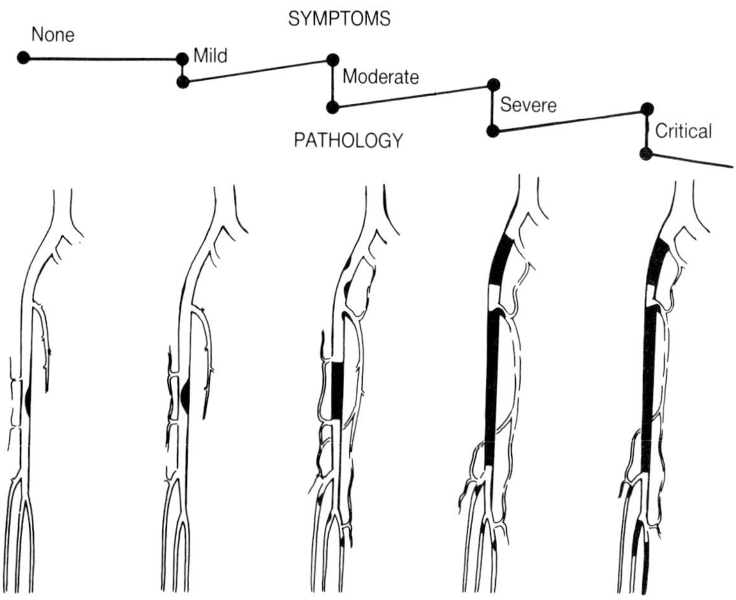

Fig. 5.1 Diagram relating progression of the pathological changes in chronic occlusive arterial disease of the lower limb to the symptoms. Each deterioration is followed by a period of spontaneous symptomatic improvement due to collateral circulation and other factors. (Reproduced with permission from Ruckley CV, Symptomatic and asymptomatic disease; in reference 2.)

sion, hyperlipidaemia, diabetes, obesity and lack of exercise.[2,6] Cigarette smoking is of particular importance to risk of peripheral arterial disease.[2,6] Diabetes is of particular importance as a risk factor for critical leg ischaemia and amputation, possibly due to increased frequency of distal disease, peripheral neuropathy, and predisposition to foot infection.[7] There is increasing epidemiological evidence that many of these risk predictors may operate in part through alterations in haemostatic factors (endothelial disturbance; activation of platelets and coagulation; fibrinogen and fibrin deposition) and in haemorheological factors which affect blood flow (blood and plasma viscosity; haematocrit; fibrinogen and white cell count).[2,7–9] For example, plasma fibrinogen and blood viscosity levels are related to the extent of peripheral arterial disease in the population,[8] and to deterioration in claudication;[10] fibrinogen level is also related to occlusion of femoropopliteal vein grafts.[11] In the Edinburgh Artery Study, plasma viscosity was an independent determinant of the risk of claudication for a given degree of arterial resistance (ABPI), consistent with a role for viscosity as well as for arterial occlusion in the pathogenesis of symptomatic leg ischaemia.[8]

Assessment of symptomatic disease

A careful history and examination should be performed in patients with lower-limb pain, to answer the following questions:

1. Are the symptoms due to arterial occlusion, or to other disease?
2. If yes, is the occlusion atherosclerotic, thrombotic, or caused by other pathology?
3. Do the symptoms merit investigation with a view to operation or other invasive procedures?
4. What risk-factor modification and/or medication is indicated, to reduce the risk of ischaemic heart disease and cerebrovascular disease, as well as to reduce the risk of progression of leg ischaemia?

Symptoms due to arterial occlusion?

This is usually apparent after a careful history and examination, but may require investigations such as measurement of ABPI, before and after treadmill exercise, to confirm or refute the diagnosis (see Chapter 4.) *Venous claudication* is suggested by the absence of arterial occlusive disease, a history of deep vein thrombosis, and signs of venous insufficiency. *Orthopaedic causes of leg pain* (spinal stenosis, sciatica, arthritis) are suggested by the history and by skeletal and neurological examination.

Pathology of the occlusion?

The typical patient with claudication is aged over 50 years, has cardiovascular risk factors (especially a history of smoking), and often a history of other arterial occlusive disease (angina, myocardial infarction, stroke, transient ischaemic attacks). The onset of exercise-limiting symptoms is often sudden with stepwise progression (due to recurrent thrombosis on atherosclerotic stenoses) and gradual improvement (due to collateral formation) (Fig. 5.1). In younger patients (age under 50 years) the clinician should consider rarer causes of arterial occlusion, as well as primary prothrombotic states.[12]

Cardiac thromboembolism usually presents with acute critical ischaemia, but occasionally presents with acute onset of claudication without limb threat. The diagnosis is suggested by a history of heart valve disease, atrial fibrillation, or heart murmurs. Ultrasound examination may reveal a potential source of embolism and sometimes intracardiac thrombus.

Buerger's disease is rare in the United Kingdom. It is suggested by heavy smoking, critical limb ischaemia, and thrombophlebitis.

Arteritis is suggested by other features of systemic lupus erythematosus, polyarteritis nodosa, giant cell arteritis or syphilis. A markedly raised plasma viscosity or erythrocyte sedimentation rate (ESR) is suggestive.

Fibrosis is suggested by a history of radiotherapy, or features of retroperitoneal fibrosis (including raised plasma viscosity or ESR).

Developmental abnormalities include coarctation of the aorta (suggested by hypertension, absent or delayed femoral pulses, and visible collaterals on the chest wall); and popliteal aneurysm (suggested by careful palpation of the popliteal fossa, and confirmed by ultrasound – which also confirms cystic adventitial disease of the popliteal artery).[12]

Prothrombotic states should be excluded in all patients with lower-limb ischaemia by measurement of a full blood count (to exclude polycythaemia, thrombocythaemia and hyperleucocytic leukaemia) and plasma viscosity or ESR (to exclude plasma hyperviscosity syndrome, as well as to screen for arteritis and fibrosis).[13] In patients aged under 50 years a 'thrombophilia screen' should also be considered: measurement of the coagulation inhibitors, antithrombin III, protein C and protein S, to exclude congenital thrombophilias; and screening for a lupus anticoagulant and antiphospholipid antibodies.[12,13] Interpretation of results can be difficult and referral to a haematologist is often appropriate. Homocystinaemia is a rare cause of premature arterial disease; however there is recent interest in the milder, heterozygous form which may be relatively common in premature arterial disease: diagnosis requires a methionine tolerance test.

Do the symptoms merit invasive procedures?

The complications and costs of invasive investigations, catheter procedures and operation are justified if ischaemia is either limb-threatening[7] or (in some cases) lifestyle-limiting. Assessment of lifestyle limitation requires a careful history, noting occupation, social habits, and other disease (especially exercise limitation by angina, heart failure, chronic lung disease or arthritis: all conditions which frequently coexist with claudication). Because the natural history of claudication tends towards spontaneous improvement (Fig. 5.1), a trial of conservative treatment should be given before invasive procedures are considered in patients whose symptoms are limited to claudication.[14] The features of critical limb ischaemia and its management have been reviewed elsewhere.[7]

Risk-factor modification and/or medication?

Assessment of risk factors and contributory diseases has already been discussed. Their modification and the place of medication are discussed in the next section.

Management of symptomatic disease

Education

Following confirmation of the diagnosis of chronic occlusive arterial disease and assessment of the whole patient as discussed above, the patient should be given a simple explanation of the nature of the arterial disease and of the basis of intermittent claudication.[15] This can be reinforced by giving an explanatory leaflet.[16] He or she should be reassured that (in the absence of critical limb ischaemia) the prognosis for the limb is usually good; that the claudication will tend to improve (especially if of recent onset); and that the risk of critical limb ischaemia and amputation is small, especially if they comply with advice to avoid smoking and to take exercise and aspirin (see below). They should, however, be warned to avoid trauma to their feet (for example, from ill-fitting shoes, inexpert cutting of toenails, or hot water bottles) and to report promptly any foot injury, rest pain, or marked change in skin colour or temperature. Such advice is especially important in patients with neuropathy (e.g. due to diabetes or alcohol).[7]

Enquiry about work and lifestyle will reveal the circumstances under which claudication usually occurs, and will guide advice to minimise its occurrence. Walking more slowly to keep below the patient's 'claudication threshold' can help, as can adjustments in work patterns and leisure activities (including use of public transport, a car, or even a mobile golf caddy as appropriate).

Patients should be encouraged to 'stop smoking and keep walking'[17] for two reasons. First, these measures are likely to slow down progression of peripheral arterial disease, and to increase walking distance. Second, both measures are likely to reduce the patient's overall risk of cardiovascular events (see below). Losing weight should also be recommended in obese patients (for similar reasons); however if an increase in weight is the price of stopping smoking, stopping smoking should have priority. Attention to other cardiovascular risk factors (hypertension, hyperlipidaemia) is also appropriate (to reduce the risk of stroke and heart disease) and is best approached as a multifactorial exercise, using a combined risk-factor score.[18] Diet and exercise may be sufficient to reduce high blood pressure and hyperlipidaemia in many patients.

Smoking

Because smoking is the strongest risk factor for peripheral arterial disease;[2,6,19] progression to critical leg ischaemia;[7,20,21] occlusion of femoropopliteal grafts;[11] ischaemic heart disease;[22] and stroke;[23] all patients with chronic occlusive arterial disease should receive strong and continuing advice and help to stop smoking, and not restart.

In canine experiments, cigarette smoking increased the permeability of the arterial wall to fibrinogen, and the carbon monoxide component appeared responsible.[24] Smoking is also the most important cause of raised plasma fibrinogen levels in the population.[2] An epidemiological study has shown that peripheral arterial disease (measured by the ABPI) is associated with both cigarette smoking and with plasma fibrinogen levels, which have an interactive effect in decreasing the ABPI;[8] possibly due to smoking-induced vascular endothelial damage combined with fibrinogen infiltration of the arterial wall[24] in proportion to its plasma concentration. Smoking and fibrinogen level also have an interactive effect on the risk of femoropopliteal graft occlusion.[11] Smoking and occlusive arterial disease are associated with increased plasma levels of activation markers of endothelial cells, platelets, leucocytes and blood coagulation; as well as increased blood viscosity which is partly due to increased haematocrit, and partly to increased fibrinogen levels which increase plasma viscosity and red cell aggregation.[2,8,9]

Stopping smoking is associated with decrease in risk of ischaemic heart disease;[22,25] and stroke;[26] as well as risk of graft occlusion.[11,19] Stopping smoking is also associated with reduction in blood viscosity and haematocrit[27,28] as well as a fall in fibrinogen levels.[28,29] The fall in viscosity may be relevant to improvement in thrombotic risk in claudicants.

About 25% of smokers are untruthful when asked about current smoking habits at peripheral vascular clinics, as shown by measurement of objective smoking markers such as carboxyhaemoglobin, thiocyanate or cotinine levels. These markers may therefore be useful in patient monitoring.[19] The experience of one London clinic was that about 50% of patients with peripheral arterial disease can be persuaded to stop, especially if they have had vascular surgery, a stroke or a myocardial infarction.[19] Whether or not specialized smoking classes add to the efficacy of clinic advice remains to be seen.

Exercise

Like cigarette smoking, lack of regular exercise has now been shown to be a risk factor for ischaemic heart disease;[30] stroke;[31] and peripheral arterial disease;[30] as well as associated with increased levels of blood viscosity and fibrinogen.[32]

Exercise has been suggested as a treatment for intermittent claudication for about 100 years.[33] Four controlled studies of exercise training in claudicants have been reported, as well as several uncontrolled studies. The total results suggest that exercise training doubles the walking distance in patients with claudication by 3 months, with a further slight improvement by 6 months.[33] This compares with a mean 300% increase in walking distance after surgical reconstruction, which improves to a mean 500% increase if surgical reconstruction and exercise training are combined.[34] Guidelines for training programmes have been suggested.[33] Possible mechanisms for the beneficial effects of exercise training on walking distance include increased blood flow to exercising muscles (due to either collateral development or to reduced blood viscosity); redistribution of blood flow to the leg; change in walking efficiency or increased pain tolerance; or metabolic changes in the muscles.[32,33] It has been suggested that exercise training may also reduce mortality in claudicants, possibly owing to a reduction in blood pressure or an increase in high-density lipoprotein cholesterol levels.[33]

It therefore seems reasonable to encourage regular exercise in patients with claudication, on the basis of epidemiological studies as well as controlled studies of benefit in walking distance.

Drug therapy

Anaemia, heart failure and diabetes can each contribute to leg ischaemia, so appropriate investigation and therapy is required for each of these conditions. Anticoagulant or antiplatelet therapy should be considered in patients with proven thrombophilia, to reduce the risk of thrombotic events. Likewise, immune suppression should be considered in arteritis. As previously discussed, drug treatment of hypertension and hyperlipidaemia may be indicated, based on the total cardiovascular risk profile, in patients who do not respond to diet and exercise.

There are surprisingly few studies of the effects of antihypertensive or lipid-lowering drugs in patients with claudication. The choice of antihypertensive drug in claudicants is problematical: beta-adrenergic blockers may reduce leg blood flow and walking distance, especially in combination with nifedipine.[35] The Medical Research Council trial in mild hypertension[36] found that beta-adrenergic blockers were ineffective in preventing arterial events in smokers, who comprise a high percentage of claudicants. Claudicants also have a high prevalence of renal artery stenosis at angiography,[37] which may lead to renal hypoperfusion following use of angiotensin converting enzyme inhibitors. Thiazide diuretics or vasodilators may therefore be the drugs of choice.

The role of antithrombotic drugs, and of drugs which aim to increase walking distance by either lysis of thrombotic arterial obstructions, or increase in leg blood flow at microcirculatory level, will now be considered.

Antithrombotic drugs

There is now evidence from epidemiological studies that peripheral arterial disease is associated with activation of platelets and blood coagulation,[8,9] each of which may play a role in both progression of peripheral arterial disease, and in increased risk of myocardial infarction and thrombotic stroke in patients with peripheral arterial disease. It is therefore logical to consider the use of either antiplatelet drugs or anticoagulants in patients with peripheral arterial disease.

A recent meta-analysis of randomized controlled trials of antiplatelet drugs in patients with peripheral arterial disease[38] showed substantial reductions in risk of arterial events (myocardial infarction, stroke or death), as well as in risk of arterial occlusion following peripheral arterial bypass grafting or angioplasty. Furthermore a recent report from the Physician's Health Study in the USA (a randomized controlled trial of aspirin) showed a substantial reduction in need for peripheral arterial surgery.[39] This effect was even more striking in subjects who had intermittent claudication at baseline (85% risk reduction).[39] These results are consistent with a previous report that aspirin reduced angiographic progression of peripheral arterial disease,[40] and suggest that antiplatelet agents should be given routinely to all patients with intermittent claudication unless contraindicated (e.g. by bleeding disorders or history of peptic ulcer). Aspirin is the drug of choice: a dose of 150 mg/day (or 300 mg on alternate days) appears as effective as any. In patients in whom aspirin is contraindicated (e.g. allergy) or not tolerated (e.g. gastrointestinal adverse effects), ticlopidine may be substituted as and when it is licensed in the UK.[38,41] Patients on ticlopidine should be monitored for adverse effects such as neutropenia and diarrhoea.

There is less evidence that long-term oral anticoagulants are beneficial in patients with peripheral arterial disease; although they have been shown to reduce the risk of cardiovascular events in patients with femoropopliteal grafts, previous myocardial infarction, or atrial fibrillation, and could be considered in such patients.[42]

Thrombolytic drugs

These agents (streptokinase, urokinase and alteplase) are progressively establishing a place in the management of critical leg ischaemia, especially when given by local infusion into the acute thrombotic occlusion, with or without clot aspiration and/or angioplasty.[7] They have also been used in patients with claudication, not unreasonably as arterial thrombosis often precipitates claudication (Fig. 5.1) and remains lysable for several months.[43] Both systemic and local thrombolysis have been used,[43] but the bleeding complications and the lack of randomized controlled trials caution against use in noncritical leg ischaemia at present.

Drugs increasing leg blood flow at microcirculatory level

This is the most controversial area of conservative management of peripheral occlusive arterial disease. Annual prescription of these vasoactive and/or rheologically active drugs costs millions of pounds in the UK each year and accounts for a large part of drug expenditure by general practitioners; it reflects the high prevalence of claudication in the population and the limited role of vascular surgeons and interventional radiologists. The great majority of patients with claudication are unsuitable for, unfit for, do not benefit from, or do not want arterial procedures. Furthermore, increasing financial limitation of the National Health Service means that such expensive interventions are rationed progressively to those with critical leg ischaemia. Angioplasty or bypass grafting can have adverse effects (including acceleration of occlusive disease in some patients), and of course they do nothing for the progression of atherosclerosis and ischaemia elsewhere in the body. By contrast, drugs acting on ischaemic microcirculatory vessels, or which increase the ability of blood to flow through such vessels, are more generally applicable to arteriopaths in the population; are more generally applicable to all ischaemic organs (heart, brain and limbs) in an arteriopath ('reaching the parts that surgeons and catheter-pushers cannot reach'); and constitute a rational approach to the generalized ischaemic problems of the arteriopathic patient.

As previously noted, epidemiological studies have supported the concept that blood viscosity, as well as arterial resistance, is a determinant of symptomatic leg ischaemia.[2,8,10] Hence drugs with rheological effects have a rational basis for use in claudicants. As regards vasoactive drugs, they have lived for years in the shadow of the concept that arterial disease is all-important in leg ischaemia: 'It is no good opening the tap further if there is an obstruction in the main water pipe'.[44] Such statements are predicated upon visualization of the leg circulation as a simple plumbing system, which is understandable for surgeons and interventional radiologists whose main interest is in opening or bypassing blocked major arteries. However, recent microcirculatory studies show that vasoactive drugs can increase nutritional *skin* blood flow (a much better predictor of skin necrosis than arterial pressures) in the absence of any change in leg arterial pressure. This shows that drugs can have selective effects on the ischaemic microcirculation, and may broaden the 'plumbing' approach to leg ischaemia.[45] Microcirculatory studies are much more difficult to apply to exercising *muscle* than to static skin; however, the increasing application of techniques for assessing ischaemic muscle blood flow (such as magnetic resonance imaging) may clarify the effects of vasoactive drugs in claudicants.

Most clinical trials of vasoactive and/or rheologically active drugs in patients with claudication have used walking distance as the major endpoint. Assessment of this endpoint is difficult, owing to inter- and intra-patient variability; and the design and results of many of these studies have been criticized.[15,46] It is, however, interesting that much of such criticism comes from vascular surgeons who routinely perform procedures which have *never* been evaluated by randomized controlled trials![7] As in many other areas of medicine, trial methodology is improving for studies of claudication, and guidelines have been suggested.[46,47] Contrary to the statement in a recent British National Formulary that 'no controlled studies have shown any improvement in walking distance',[48] large controlled studies have shown positive results for oxpentifylline,[47,49] naftidrofuryl,[50] and ticlopidine[51] (which may have rheological as well as antiplatelet effects, through its ability to reduce fibrinogen levels). Though the mean increase in walking distance compared with patients receiving a placebo is often small, some individual patients do show impressive responses. Furthermore it seems inappropriate to have a double standard for claudication and for angina pectoris, whose placebo response (to drugs *or* to operation) is also well documented. Patients are as frustrated if they cannot walk because of a sore lower half as because of a sore upper half, hence doctors who discriminate at the umbilicus may hit below the belt. While the anticipated benefits of time, stopping smoking, and regular exercise are awaited, it may therefore be worth trying one or more of these agents in patients whose daily activities are severely curtailed.[51]

Conclusions

The major risk in a person with claudication is of heart attack and stroke; the risk of critical leg ischaemia and amputation is small, especially if the person complies with conservative management (regular aspirin use in particular appears to reduce six-fold the need for vascular surgery). As with angina, the mainstay of management is therefore conservative medical therapy. The clinician's advice should be: consider your lifestyle; stop smoking; take regular exercise and aspirin; and avoid invasive procedures unless your limb is threatened, or unless you are impatient enough about your lifestyle limitation to risk their complications.

References

1. Dormandy J, Mahir M, Ascady G, Balsano F, De Leeuw P, Blombery P, *et al.* Fate of the patient with chronic leg ischaemia: a review article. *J Cardiovasc Surg* 1989; **30:** 50–7.
2. Fowkes FGR (ed). *Epidemiology of Peripheral Vascular Disease.* London: Springer Verlag, 1991.
3. Fowkes FGR, Housley E, Cawood EHH, Macintyre CCA, Ruckley CV, Prescott RJ. Edinburgh Artery Study: prevalence of asymptomatic and symptomatic peripheral arterial disease in the general population. *Int J Epidem* 1991; **20:** 384–92.
4. Mitchell JRS, Schwartz CJ. *Arterial Disease.* Oxford: Blackwell, 1965.
5. Dormandy JA, Murray GD. The fate of the claudicant – a prospective study of 1969 claudicants. *Eur J Vasc Surg* 1991; **5:** 131–3.
6. Fowkes FGR, Housley E, Riemersma RA, Macintyre CCA, Cawood EHH, Prescott RJ, Ruckley CV. Smoking, lipids, glucose intolerance, and blood pressure as risk factors for peripheral atherosclerosis compared with ischemic heart disease in the Edinburgh Artery Study. *Am J Epidem* 1992; **135:** 331–40.
7. European Working Group on Critical Limb Ischemia. Second European consensus document on chronic critical leg ischemia. *Circulation* 1991; **84** (Suppl IV): 1–26.
8. Lowe GDO, Fowkes FGR, Dawes J, Donnan PT, Lennie SE, Housley E. Blood viscosity, fibrinogen and activation of coagulation and leucocytes in peripheral arterial disease: Edinburgh Artery Study. *Circulation* 1993; **87:** 1915–20.
9. Smith FB, Lowe GDO, Fowkes FGR, Rumley A, Rumley AG, Donnan PT, Housley E. Smoking, haemostatic factors and lipid peroxides in a population case-control study of peripheral arterial disease. *Atherosclerosis* 1993 (in press).
10. Dormandy JA, Hoare E, Khattab AH, Arrowsmith DE, Dormandy TL. Prognostic significance of rheological and biochemical findings in patients with intermittent claudication. *Br Med J* 1973; **iv:** 581–3.
11. Wiseman S, Kenchington G, Dain R, Marshall CE, McCollum CN, Greenhalgh RM, Powell JT. Influence of smoking and plasma factors on patency of femoropopliteal vein grafts. *Br Med J* 1989; **299:** 643–6.
12. Reilly DT, Wolfe JHN. The young patient with claudication. *Br Med J* 1991; **303:** 845–8.
13. Lowe GDO, Forbes CD. Predisposing and aggravating factors in arterial disease and venous thrombosis. In: *Surgical Management of Vascular Disease,* Bell PRF, Jamieson CW, Ruckley CV (eds). London: WB Saunders, 1991: 47–62.
14. Coffman JD. Intermittent claudication – be conservative. *N Engl J Med* 1991; **325:** 577–8.
15. Housley E. The non-operative treatment of lower limb ischaemia. In: *Surgical Management of Vascular Disease,* Bell PRF, Jamieson CW, Ruckley CV (eds). London: WB Saunders, 1991: 197–204.
16. Marston A. Clinical evaluation of the patient with atheroma. In: *Surgical Management of Vascular Disease,* Bell PRF, Jamieson CW, Ruckley CV (eds). London: WB Saunders, 1991: 119–30.
17. Housley E. Treating claudication in five words. *Br Med J* 1988; **296:** 1483.
18. Tunstall-Pedoe H. The Dundee coronary risk-disk for management of change in risk factors. *Br Med J* 1991; **303:** 744–7.
19. Greenhalgh RM. The effect of smoking on arterial disease and venous thrombosis. In: *Surgical Management of Vascular Disease,* Bell PRF, Jamieson CW, Ruckley CV (eds). London: WB Saunders, 1991: 103–9.
20. Jonason T, Bergström R. Cessation of smoking in patients with intermittent claudication. *Acta Med Scand* 1987; **221:** 253–60.
21. Jonason T, Ringqvist I. Changes in peripheral blood pressures after five years of follow-up in non-operated patients with intermittent claudication. *Acta Med Scand* 1986; **220:** 127–32.
22. Gordon T, Kannel WB, McGee D, Dawber TR. Death and coronary attacks in men after giving up cigarette smoking: a report from the Framingham Study. *Lancet* 1974; **ii:** 1345–7.
23. Shinton R, Beevers G. Meta-analysis of relation between cigarette smoking and stroke. *Br Med J* 1989; **298:** 789–94.
24. Allen DR, Browse NL, Rutt DL, Butler L, Fletcher C. The effect of cigarette smoking, nicotine and carbon monoxide on the permeability of the arterial wall. *J Vasc Surg* 1988; **7:** 139–45.
25. Rose G. Randomised trial of antismoking advice: 10 year results. *J Epidem Commun Hlth* 1978; **32:** 275–81.
26. Abbott RD, Yin Y, Dwayne MA, Reed MD, Katsuhiko Y. Risk of stroke in male cigarette smokers. *N Engl J Med* 1986; **315:** 717–20.
27. Ernst E, Matrai A. Abstention from chronic smoking normalises blood rheology. *Arteriosclerosis* 1987; **64:** 75–7.
28. Rothwell M, Rampling MW, Cholerton S, Sever PS. Haemorheological changes in the very short time

after abstention from tobacco by cigarette smokers. *Br J Haematol* 1991; **79:** 500–3.
29. Meade TW, Imeson J, Stirling Y. Effects of changes in smoking and other characteristics on clotting factors and the risk of ischaemic heart disease. *Lancet* 1987; **ii:** 986–8.
30. Housley E. Exercise. In: *Epidemiology of Peripheral Vascular Disease,* Fowkes FGR (ed). London: Springer-Verlag, 1991: 227–34.
31. Wannamethee G, Shaper AG. Physical activity and stroke in British middle aged men. *Br Med J* 1992; **304:** 597–601.
32. Ernst E, Matrai A. Intermittent claudication, exercise and blood rheology. *Circulation* 1987; **76:** 1110–14.
33. Holm J. The effect of exercise on intermittent claudication. In: *Surgical Management of Vascular Disease,* Bell PRF, Jamieson CW, Ruckley CV (eds). London: WB Saunders, 1991: 111–18.
34. Lundgren F, Dahllöf AG, Lundholm K, Schersten T, Volkmann R. Intermittent claudication – surgical reconstruction or physical training? A prospective randomized trial of treatment efficiency. *Ann Surg* 1989; **209:** 346–55.
35. Solomon SA, Ramsay LE, Yeo WW, Parnell L, Morris-Jones W. Beta-blockade and intermittent claudication: placebo controlled trial of atenolol and nifedipine and their combination. *Br Med J* 1991; **303:** 1100–4.
36. Medical Research Council Working Party. Stroke and coronary disease in mild hypertension: risk factors and the value of treatment. *Br Med J* 1988; **296:** 1565–70.
37. Choudhri AH, Cleland JGF, Rowlands PC, Tran TL, McCarty M, Al-Kutoubi MAO. Unsuspected renal artery stenosis in peripheral vascular disease. *Br Med J* 1990; **301:** 1197–8.
38. Antiplatelet Triallists Collaboration. Secondary prevention of vascular disease by prolonged antiplatelet treatment. *Br Med J* 1993; in press.
39. Goldhaber SZ, Manson JE, Stampfer MJ, LaMotte F, Rosner B, Buring JE, Hennekens CH. Low-dose aspirin and subsequent peripheral arterial surgery in the Physicians' Health Study. *Lancet* 1992; **340:** 143–5.
40. Hess H, Mietaschk A, Deischsel G. Drug-induced inhibition of platelet function delays progression of peripheral occlusive arterial disease: a prospective double-blind arteriographically controlled trial. *Lancet* 1985; **i:** 415–19.
41. Boissel JP, Peyrieux JC, Destors JM. Is it possible to reduce the risk of cardiovascular events in subjects suffering from intermittent claudication of the lower limbs? *Thromb Haemost* 1989; **62:** 681–5.
42. Hirsh J. Oral anticoagulant drugs. *N Engl J Med* 1991; **324:** 1865–75.
43. Martin MM. Peripheral arterial thrombotic disorders. In: *Clinical Thrombosis,* Kwaan HC, Samama MM (eds). Boca Raton: CRC Press, 1989: 181–205.
44. Boyd M. Quoted by Richards RL, *Peripheral Arterial Disease: A Physician's Approach.* Edinburgh: Livingstone, 1970: 63.
45. Bollinger A, Fagrell B. *Clinical Capillaroscopy.* Toronto: Hogrefe and Huber, 1990.
46. Cameron HA, Waller PC, Ramsay LE. Drug treatment of intermittent claudication: a critical analysis. *Br J Clin Pharmacol* 1988; **26:** 569–76.
47. Lindgarde F, Jelnes R, Bjorkman H, Adielsson G, Kjellstrom T, Palmquist I, Stavenow L. Conservative drug treatment in patients with moderately severe chronic occlusive peripheral arterial disease. *Circulation* 1989; **80:** 1549–56.
48. British Medical Association and Royal Pharmaceutical Society of Great Britain. *British National Formulary, No. 22.* 1991: 85.
49. Porter JM, Cutler BS, Lee BY, Reich T, Reichle FA, Scogin JT, Strandness DE. Pentoxyfylline efficiency in the treatment of intermittent claudication: multicenter controlled double-blind trial with objective assessment. *Am Heart J* 1982; **104:** 66–72.
50. Lehert P, Riphagen FE, Gamand S. The effect of naftidrofuryl on intermittent claudication: a meta-analysis. *J Cardiovasc Pharmacol* 1990; **16** (Suppl 3): S81–S86.
51. Arcan JC, Panak E. Ticlopidine in the treatment of peripheral occlusive arterial disease. *Sem Thromb Hemost* 1989; **15:** 167–70.
52. Lowe GDO. Drugs in cerebral and peripheral arterial disease. *Br Med J* 1990; **300:** 524–8.

6

Aortoiliac occlusion

Anthony DB Chant

Peripheral vascular surgeons are concerned, for the most part, with aneurysmal or occlusive disease below the renal arteries. This chapter will confine itself to infrarenal disease, its presentation, assessment and treatment. It will also cover the treatment of some of the complications of aortoiliac vascular operations. Reference to the upper aorta in renal disease will be found in Chapter 24 and to aneurysmal disease in Chapter 11. The references for the most part are confined to recent articles from the international literature; through these, more interested readers will find their way back into a literature which first burgeoned in the early 1960s following the introduction of prosthetic vascular grafts.

Presentation

Patients presenting with aortic disease tend to be below 60 years of age. This contrasts with patients with femoropopliteal disease, who tend to be older. As well as classical calf claudication, buttock claudication and impotence may be a feature if the internal iliac vessels are also involved. It was this combination of problems which Leriche described in his original contribution on the subject. If found in combination with femorodistal disease (and these are the most high-risk cases), patients can present with rest pain or gangrene. On rare occasions aortic disease presents itself as visceral ischaemia, for instance with ischaemic colitis or renal failure.

Diagnosis

Despite exciting new diagnostic developments, history-taking and the physical examination still play important roles. Specific points in the history relate firstly to the pain, and secondly to the patient's lifestyle and general health. Knowledge of the characteristics of the pain, if clearly defined, can save patients from much distress and unnecessary investigations. *Vascular claudication* is usually confined to muscle groups, made worse with increased effort and eased by rest. On rare occasions 'the feet go numb'. *Neurological claudication*, by contrast, is frequently associated with numbing of the feet and, importantly, is often made worse by standing up *prior* to exercise or by climbing stairs. The other important part relating to the pain is its influence on lifestyle: Is the patient confined to the house? Can he hold down his job? Does he *really* need to play golf? The importance of both patient and doctor understanding the symptoms before embarking on investigations which can lead the patient into potentially high-risk surgery cannot be emphasized too much.

The characteristic of bruits is especially important. Since the development of angioplasty, clearly defined bruits are often interpreted as good evidence of short stenoses. Their presence might suggest the possibility of angioplasty, when previously no investigation or treatment would have been deemed necessary for a patient with claudication. Lastly, of course, a careful examination of the neurological and muscular skeletal system is essential, for not only can disease in these systems mimic aortoiliac disease, *they can also coexist.*

Investigations

Since the early 1970s, continuous-wave Doppler examination of blood vessels has proved its worth in noninvasive assessment. More recently, the addition of B-scans in so-called duplex scanners has made aortoiliac assessment even more accurate.[1] To *rule out* aortoiliac disease is as important as diagnosing it, particularly when infrainguinal reconstructions are being considered. However, despite the success of duplex scanning, aortography in one form or another remains at the time of writing, the cornerstone investigation in most instances prior to treatment decisions.

Details of such investigations appear elsewhere in this book, but Fig. 6.2 illustrates the three common problems presenting to vascular surgeons in this area: unilateral iliac disease, complete aortic occlusion with severe peripheral ischaemia, and 'classic' aortoiliac disease.

Indications for treatment

The basic indications for treating any vascular disease (the three L's – Life, Limb and Lifestyle) provide a simple framework for deciding on an aortic reconstruction. My own decision pathway is summarized in Fig. 6.1.

Many of the patients seen by vascular surgeons will not have been through this very simple decision matrix. Not everyone understands either the risks or benefits of aortic surgery; certainly many patients do not. A cavalier attitude may be excusable when life or limb are threatened, but the decision to operate is often best postponed until both patient and his doctors have had an opportunity to discuss matters thoroughly. This is especially apt when lifestyle changes in those reaching retirement years almost certainly can suffice.

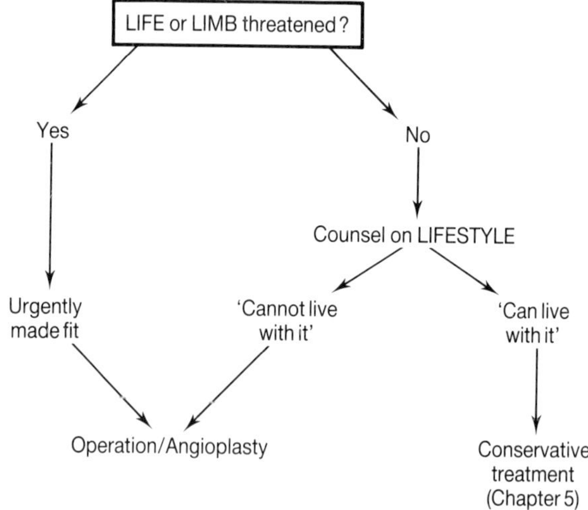

Fig. 6.1 The 3-L decision pathway.

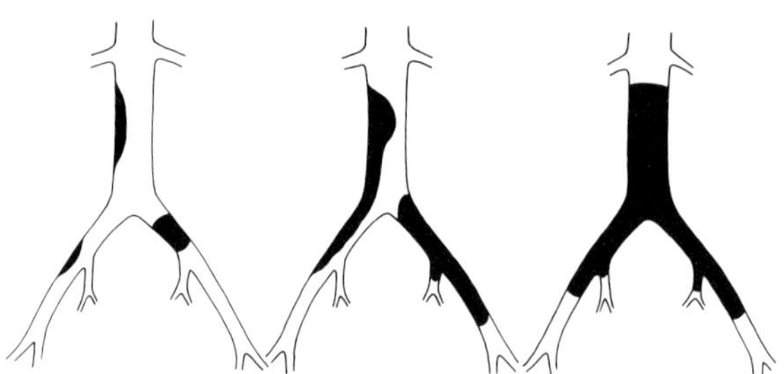

Fig. 6.2 Diagram showing unilateral iliac disease (left), extensive bilateral disease (middle) and a complete aortic occlusion (right).

Treatment options

'Conservatism', of course, has its place (see Chapter 5) and is in many ways more important in this group of patients than others. These patients tend to be younger, and even if they do require an operation an altered lifestyle and maximized cardiovascular condition will augur well for graft patency and increased longevity. This kind of holistic approach can make these major procedures worthwhile.

Percutaneous angioplasty (PTA)

In the first instance, if the patient is lucky, the block or stenosis will be sufficiently short for percutaneous transluminal angioplasty (PTA) to be performed (see Fig. 6.2, left). This is normally carried out with an overnight stay, following percutaneous puncture of the femoral artery in the groin under local anaesthetic. The lengths of stenosis that individual radiologists and vascular surgeons are willing to dilate do vary. In general, dilatation of stenoses produce good results compared with that of even short occlusions (Chapter 27). The addition of stents appears to confirm benefits but, as in many areas of vascular intervention, *hard* evidence is difficult to come by.

Aortic operations

Patients whose X-rays are similar to those in Fig. 6.2 (middle and right) would, on my unit, be offered aortic reconstructions. Conventionally the abdominal aorta is still approached through a midline or paramedian incision. Other surgeons use transverse incisions and still others use the retroperitoneal approach. This latter, of which I have limited experience, does theoretically offer great advantages in both exposure for the surgeon and comfort for the patient. So far, however, limited trials have failed to produce convincing evidence either way.[2]

The easier of the two cases (Fig. 6.2, middle) would almost certainly have an aortobifemoral graft from just below the renals to the bifurcation of the profundas. The technique I use (Fig. 6.3) consists of an end-to-end anastomosis at the top as opposed to an onlay where the graft is sewn end-to-side. The choice of graft is often determined by historical rather than rational factors. There appears to be little point in choosing knitted grafts unless sealed.[3] However, despite the poorer handling characteristics of woven grafts, no-one has proved that they are inferior from the point of view of patency. On this issue, therefore, 'the jury is still out'. I use Prolene sutures and 'parachute' a gelatin sealed graft down into position, following the insertion of the first key stitches. In those difficult cases where doubt exists regarding mesenteric perfusion, I occasionally perform onlay grafts[4] (Fig. 6.4), but in my hands this reconstruction seldom 'sits nicely'. Personally I find side-clamping the abdominal aorta difficult, and my incidence of so-called 'trash foot' on the relatively good side is unacceptably high.

In cases of complete aortic block (Fig. 6.2, right), aortic endarterectomy is indicated at least at the top end. This technique, described by Courbier,[5] then allows the graft to be sewn well below the renals in comparative safety and ease.

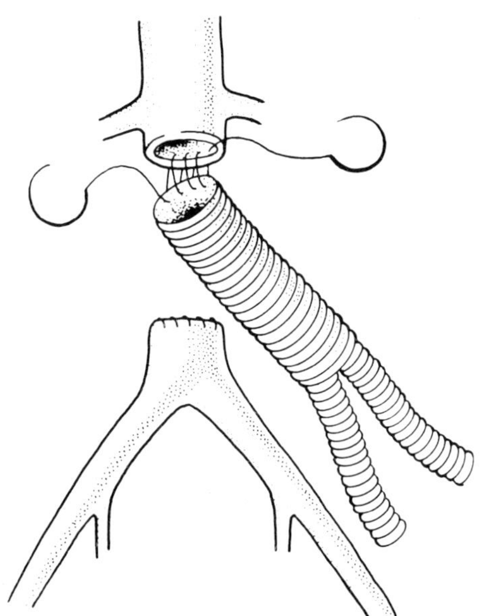

Fig. 6.3 Diagram showing graft being 'parachuted' into place for end-to-end anastomosis. The distal end of the aorta has been oversewn.

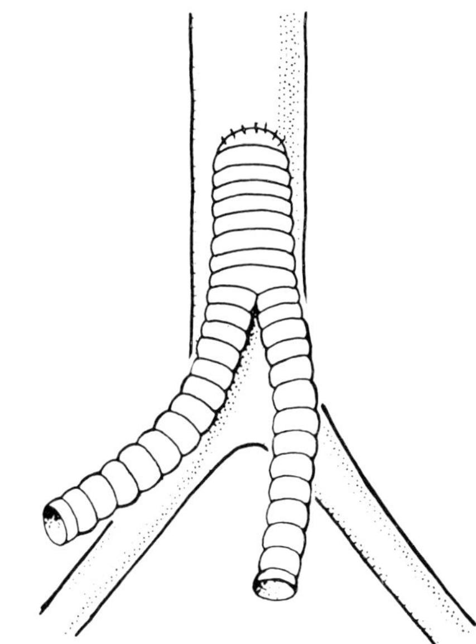

Fig. 6.4 An end-to-side (onlay) anastomosis.

Endarterectomy of the whole of the aorta is still practised in certain centres. Its advantage is cheapness and no danger of graft infection. Its disadvantage is that it can be tedious, with increased blood loss. It has worse patency rates, largely owing to difficulties experienced with the external iliac arteries and the so-called 'break-off' points in the profunda.[6] Many of us still insist on draining the abdominal cavity and groins postoperatively. However, the literature suggests that this is unnecessary and possibly counterproductive.[7]

Unilateral iliac lesions

The management of this type of lesion is still controversial.[8] Five treatment options are available: angioplasty, a unilateral graft, endarterectomy, a crossover graft, or (perhaps surprisingly for the non-vascular reader) an aortobifemoral graft. Dealing with the latter, this somewhat radical view (to which I actually lean) is proposed by Rutherford,[9] the reason being that the aorta, and almost invariably the other iliac system, is involved in the early stages of the disease, so 'why not do a proper operation from day one?' The other options do, in fact, have a relatively lower patency rate, and 're-do operations' also have their problems;[10] thus in the younger patient a case certainly can be made for the radical approach.

Extra-anatomic bypass in unfit patients

In certain unfit patients where, for example, infection precludes abdominal surgery, so-called extra-anatomic bypasses are sometimes indicated. On the whole, these are done for critical ischaemia rather than claudication. As far as I am aware, no comparative trial has been undertaken; but even in so-called high-risk patients, patency rates are surprisingly good[11] (see Chapter 27). The most commonly performed are the femorofemoral crossover and axillo-bifemoral grafts. Rarely, in cases of infection at the groin level, the obturator route is used. Lastly (in my experience with less success), aortoiliac disease can be bypassed with axillopopliteal bypasses.

Complications

Possible complications are similar to those threatened after any major abdominal operation, with the addition of course of 'vascular complications'. A recent review from Edinburgh[10] suggested that, in those operations where re-do surgery was indicated, 56% were for graft thrombosis, 22% for false aneurysms and a further 22% for graft complications such as infection and aortoenteric fistulae.

Graft thrombosis

Early thrombosis is almost certainly due to poor patient selection or poor technique. Failures to do with the former are often due to poor 'runoff' and may need correction by the addition of profundaplasty or femoral distal bypass. Prevention of this complication is theoretically easy in that both segments could, if affected, be treated simultaneously. A recent British series confirms this,[12] but even so, many vascular surgeons would shrink from such radical surgery, especially in the elderly. Delayed thrombosis is more likely to be due to progression of disease. In both early and delayed thromboses (unless occurring immediately postoperatively), rather than re-explore the old graft, extra-anatomic reconstructions should be considered.

False aneurysms

False aneurysms most frequently occur in the femoral region and may be associated with endarterectomy of the femoral vessels, inappropriate suture material and grafts placed too tightly. Small asymptomatic aneurysms can safely be left and observed, but the larger ones require interposition of more Dacron.[13] Prevention is best achieved by the use of sutures such as Prolene; resisting endarterectomy unless absolutely necessary; having the graft tension correct; and possibly splitting the inguinal ligament.

Infection

This is the most menacing of all complications.[14] Its treatment should be left to experts, but even in the best hands morbidity (amputation) and mortality are high.[15] Various techniques have been offered to overcome the problem. The more recent conservative methods include percutaneous drainage under CT guidance, and instillation of antibiotics.[16] The conventional treatment, however, is excision of the graft, closure of the aortic stump and extra-anatomic bypass. The aortic stump closure poses enormous problems and secondary haemorrhage from this is a common cause of death. Prophylactic antibiotics and careful technique offer the patient the best prognosis; prevention is better than cure.

Haemorrhage

Certain technical details should be noted regarding aortic operations. *The danger points are not the arteries but the veins.* The surgeon should aim, therefore, to dissect planes of cleavage as close to the artery as possible and start the dissection away from danger points. Thus, in the iliac region the lower common iliac is a better place to start developing planes rather than at the point where the artery crosses the caval confluence. Similarly, the vena cava starts to leave the aorta as it approaches the level of the renals, and at the bifurcation they are often closely adherent.

Whilst bleeding can be minimized, a certain amount of blood loss is almost inevitable.[3] How this can best be dealt with is described in Chapter 12.

Mesenteric ischaemia

Almost invariably in the aortoiliac segment, disease exists either in the inferior mesenteric or internal iliac vessels, posing a possible problem for gut perfusion. Fig. 6.5 shows very clearly just how closely involved the mesenteric circulation can be in maintaining limb perfusion, and vice versa.

In the large majority of aortoiliac reconstructions, even using end-to-end anastomoses at the top, gut perfusion is rarely a problem. There are sophisticated pH determinants of potential ischaemia,[17] but

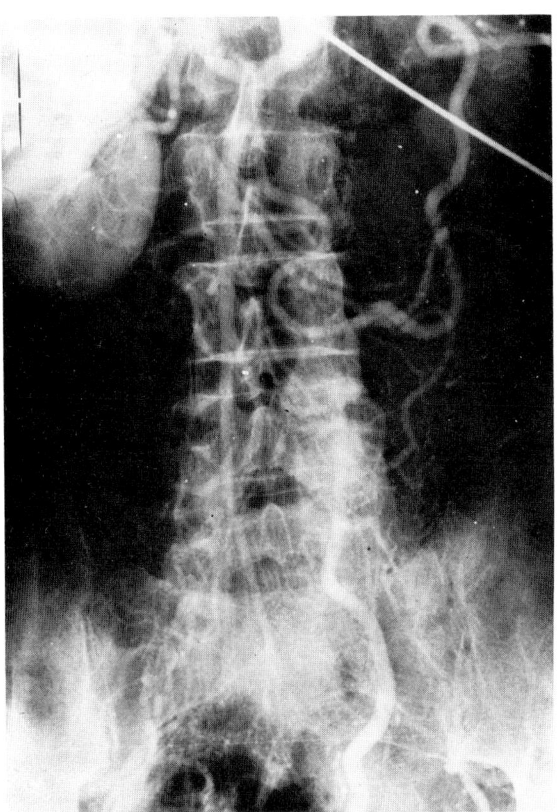

Fig. 6.5 High translumbar aortogram for high aortic occlusion. Note the collateral circulation to legs by mesenteric artery.

my own rule of thumb consists of back-bleeding the detached inferior mesenteric artery. If it bleeds, I do nothing; if it doesn't I review the X-rays and either re-implant it into the graft or ensure that the internal iliacs are separately perfused with jump grafts.

Impotence

We end as we began: it is perfectly possible to replace a Leriche-style vascular impotence with iatrogenic impotence caused by unnecessary division of autonomic nerves in the pelvis. Despite this, with care, potency can be preserved in 94% of cases.[18] Aortic endarterectomy is especially prone to this complication; conversely, an aortobifemoral graft from just below the renals rarely is. If from the aortogram I expect problems, I discuss the possibility with the patient; if not, then to worry patients unnecessarily is unkind, particularly in cases where the indication for surgery is critical ischaemia.

Conclusions

In cases where an absolute indication for surgery exists (threat to life or limb), modern grafts and techniques mean that in most instances the aortoiliac segment can be either bypassed or reconstructed. Percutaneous angioplasty is the treatment of choice in the shorter (especially iliac) lesions, for the claudicant. As with all surgery, however, patient selection is the key to success. Five minutes talking will often save five hours unnecessary operating!

References

1. De Smet AA, Kitslaar PJ. A duplex criterion for aorto-iliac stenosis. *Eur J Vasc Surg* 1990; **4:** 275–8.
2. Cambria RP, Brewster DC, Abbott WM, Freehan M, *et al.* Transperitoneal versus retroperitoneal approach for aortic reconstruction. *J Vasc Surg* 1990; **11:** 314–24.
3. Chant ADB, McEleney P, Machin D, Clifford PC. Risk factors and transported requirements in aortic surgery. *J Cardiovasc Surg* 1988; **29:** 208–10.
4. Melliere D, Labastie J, Becquemain JP, *et al.* Proximal anastamosis in aorto-bifemoral bypass: end-to-end or end-to-side? *J Cardiovasc Surg* 1990; **31:** 77–80.
5. Courbier R, Jausseran JM. Juxta-renal aortic occlusion. In: *Vascular Surgery Techniques*, Greenhalgh RM (ed). London: Butterworth, 1984.
6. Naylor AR, Ah-See AK, Engeset J, *et al.* Aorto-iliac endarterectomy: an 11-year review. *Br J Surg* 1990; **77:** 190–3.
7. Dunlop MG, Fox JN, Stonebridge PA, Clason AE, *et al.* Vacuum drainage of groin wounds after vascular surgery: a controlled trial. *Br J Surg* 1990; **77:** 562–3.
8. Hanafy M, McLoughlin GA. Comparison of iliofemoral and femorofemoral crossover bypass in treatment of unilateral iliac arterial occlusive disease. *Br J Surg* 1991; **78:** 1001–2.
9. Piotrowski JJ, Pearce WH, Jones DN, Whitehill T, Bell R, Patt A, Rutherford RB. Aortobifemoral bypass: the operation of choice for unilateral iliac occlusion. *J Vasc Surg* 1988; **8:** 211–18.
10. Haiart DC, Callam MJ, Murie JA, Ruckley CV, *et al.* Re-operations for late complications following abdominal aortic operations. *Br J Surg* 1991; **78:** 204–6.
11. Edwards JM. Axillo-femoral bypass in poor risk patients. In: *Extra-Anatomic Bypass and Re-do Arterial Surgery*, Greenhalgh RM (ed). London: Pitman, 1982: 117–21.
12. Harris PL, Cave-Bigley, McSweeney L. Aorto-femoral reconstruction and the role of concomitant femoro-distal bypass. *Brit J Surg* 1985; **72:** 317–20.
13. Ochsner JL. Management of femoral pseudo-

aneurysms aneurysms. *Surg Clin N Amer* 1982; **62:** 431–40.

14. Newington DP, Houghton PW, Baird RN, Horrocks M. Groin wound infection after arterial surgery. *Br J Surg* 1991; **78:** 617–19.
15. O'Kelly TJ, Collin J, Murie JA, Morris PJ. Which deaths in vascular surgery are avoidable? A review of 150 consecutive deaths on the Oxford Regional Vascular Service. *Eur J Vasc Surg* 1990; **4:** 395–9.
16. Matley JP, Beningfield SJ, Lourens S, Immelman EJ. Successful treatment of infected thoraco-abdominal graft by percutaneous catheter drainage. *J Vasc Surg* 1991; **13:** 513–15.
17. Nevelsteen A, Beyens G, Duchateau J, Suy R. Aorto-femoral reconstruction and sexual function: a prospective study. *Eur J Vasc Surg* 1990; **4:** 247–51.

7

Femorodistal grafts

W Bruce Campbell

Bypass grafts distal to the inguinal ligament continue to excite discussion, controversy and difficulties because of their chance of failure. If the graft fails, one in four claudicants will be worse than before operation.[1] The patient with a critically ischaemic foot will have suffered a long and unsuccessful operation, he will still require an amputation. Amputation level may not have been compromised[2], but the patient's morale is sapped by a failed bypass.

Success with femorodistal grafts requires careful patient selection, good planning, and meticulous surgical technique. Even after the operation, sophisticated follow-up methods may help to prevent grafts from blocking.

In this chapter, 'femorodistal' will be used to refer to all grafts from the femoral artery, which will then be subdivided into femoropopliteal and femorotibial.

Patient selection

Palpating the femoral and popliteal pulses provides basic information about whether a patient is a candidate for femorodistal bypass grafting. Usually these patients have a good femoral and an absent popliteal (although the popliteal may be present in some patients still suitable for more distal bypass procedures). Severe ischaemia causing rest pain or tissue necrosis is the clearest reason for operation, but disabling intermittent claudication may also be a reasonable indication. However, the decision to perform a femorodistal bypass depends on many factors, which have to be balanced against one another in each individual case.

Intermittent claudication

For patients with intermittent claudication the pain needs to constitute a real disability and must have been present for some months. Furthermore the patient himself must press for an operation. Patients with bilateral symptoms of equal severity are a particular problem, because dealing with one leg will not increase their walking distance. If both legs are grafted, then the long-term failure rates are additive, and there must be some compelling reason to embark upon bilateral bypass surgery.

The general condition of the patient, and associated medical conditions, are important factors. If the patient has angina and shortness of breath, these not only increase the risk of operation, but they may also limit the benefit of bypass grafting. It is vital to find out how severe they are before embarking on an operation.

Continued smoking should be an absolute contraindication to surgical treatment of claudication. The 25–30% of patients who lie about their smoking habits remain an unsolved problem. Other special risk factors, such as polycythaemia or thrombocythaemia, which might well cause a graft to block, should be corrected or be regarded as militating strongly against operation (see also Chapter 5).

The nature of the operation required plays a major part in the decision to operate on a claudicant. An above-knee graft to a good popliteal artery with three-vessel runoff is a reasonable option for any disabled claudicant. Below-knee grafts, or the presence of poor runoff, may be associated with a higher failure rate, and symptoms need to be very disabling to justify operation. Femorotibial bypass is very rarely done for claudication, but there may be the occasional special case. For grafts below the knee, the availability of autogenous vein is always desirable.

Several other factors will influence the decision. Obese patients, and particularly those with deep groin creases, are unattractive candidates. Previous failed bypass operations should sound a note of caution. By contrast, claudicants with low ankle pressures (less than 70 mmHg) have a poorer prognosis if treated conservatively,[3] and this may provide an added reason to consider surgical treatment.

Rest pain, ulcers, and gangrene

When associated with severe ischaemia, these symptoms and signs are usually persuasive reasons to attempt whatever distal bypass surgery is reasonably possible. It is, however, important to appreciate that not all of these patients need immediate 'limb salvage', and a selective approach is vital. As with claudicants, the decision to operate is a balance between the severity of the problem, the nature of operation required, and the circumstances of the patient. If a straightforward graft to the popliteal artery is possible, with fair runoff, then this is usually worthwhile for any patient with rest pain or trophic lesions. However, if a graft is required to a poor tibial artery, if autogenous vein is not easily available, or if other adverse factors mentioned above are present, then an immediate decision to perform bypass grafting may not be the best for the patient.

Ischaemic rest pain is an unlikely diagnosis with an ankle pressure above about 70 mmHg, and with pressures above this level ulcers may heal, albeit slowly. A period of good local care and observation may be the best option in the first instance. The patient with mild pain at rest, controlled by the occasional analgesic, may also improve, and so there is no need for immediate operation, especially if this would mean a procedure with a significant risk of failure. Dry gangrene of digits alone is not neccessarily an indication for operation.

Primary venous ulcers, which are indolent on account of concomitant arterial ischaemia, may be worth treating by femoropopliteal bypass when possible. Superficial venous surgery and/or skin grafting may be done at the same operation with success. Patients with ulceration or skin changes over the area required for access to distal arteries pose a special problem, and this may make them unsuitable for operation.

Finally, it is important to recognize those patients for whom primary amputation is the best treatment, rather than bypass grafting. Examples include those with fixed flexion contracture of the knee, or inability to stand on the limb because of frailty or paralysis. Conversely, patients who have already lost the other leg should be considered for reconstruction if they have even minimal use of the remaining threatened limb (for transferring from wheelchair to bed), because bilateral amputation is such a gross disability.

Aneurysms

Popliteal aneurysms are the commonest requiring a bypass graft in this segment of the arterial tree, but they will not be considered here (see Chapter 3).

Planning the operation

Inflow

Good inflow is a prerequisite for a graft from the femoral artery,[4] and an obviously reduced femoral pulse would make the surgeon review the arteriogram. (Absence or gross reduction of the femoral pulse is, however, a good omen for the patient with an ischaemic limb, because it indicates that proximal bypass grafting or angioplasty is likely to be possible, with their good and durable results.) Sometimes a femorodistal bypass graft may be required as an adjunct or sequel to correction of serious inflow disease.

Occasionally, doubt remains about the quality of the inflow after pulse palpation and arteriography (an aortogram is essential if there is the slightest doubt about the aortoiliac segment). Doppler waveform analysis and other non-invasive methods have been advocated to assess inflow, but in practice doubt about this is not common, and in these cases the best method for resolving the issue with easily available equipment is direct measurement of femoral artery pressure, before and after injection of 20 mg papaverine. This is done with a needle and three-way tap attached to a pressure transducer. A resting femoral pressure 10 mmHg lower than brachial, or a pressure 25 mmHg lower after papaverine, is abnormal. If the pressure is only marginally reduced, then a femorodistal graft may still be a reasonable option, although the chance of graft thrombosis is increased.[4] Whenever possible, iliac stenoses should be corrected by angioplasty before femorodistal bypass.

Runoff

The state of the runoff vessels has long been recognized as an important influence on patency of femorodistal bypass grafts.[5] In general, grafts should be taken to an artery with uninterrupted continuity into the foot. When this is the popliteal artery, then the number of patent tibial arteries influences long-term success. Grafts should be anastomosed to the popliteal artery beyond any obvious areas of disease in that vessel. Grafts to an 'isolated popliteal segment' have generally been abandoned, and a graft to a good tibial artery is probably a better option.

Grafts to tibial arteries tend to do badly when the vessel does not cross the ankle joint. Continuity of a tibial artery into an intact foot arch is a good prognostic sign.[6,7]

Runoff assessment can be done with a simple Doppler probe and good arteriograms. Listening with a Doppler probe over arteries at the ankle and foot will detect patency. Some vessels may only be audible with the foot dependent when the pressure is very low.[8] The best arteriograms are obtained by direct antegrade puncture of the femoral artery (easier and quicker for the radiologist than an aortogram) in the patient with a good femoral pulse. Digital subtraction provides particularly good pictures of the distal arteries. Views should extend to the ankle, and the counsel of perfection is to obtain images of the foot vessels as well when contemplating femorotibial reconstruction, although this is not always practical, and arteriograms may fail to show some patent distal arteries.

Other techniques which may help in assessment include preoperative pulse-generated runoff; and intraoperative arteriograms and peripheral resistance measurements. In most cases, however, decisions can be made on the basis of Doppler and arteriograms.

There are considerable advantages to having made firm plans preoperatively, but in occasional cases it will prove neccessary to explore two, or even three of the tibial arteries, to find the best one for grafting, or occasionally to decide against reconstruction altogether. Intraoperative methods for measuring peripheral resistance are not in widespread use, and pose the problem of what to do if the results predict graft failure on account of high distal resistance. Should the operation proceed in the light of this bad prognosis? Should it be abandoned? Should patients be prepared for amputation at the same procedure? There are no established answers to these questions, but they should be considered carefully before embarking on any of the predictive intraoperative tests which have been described.

Marking the vein

In the patient with an easily visible and palpable saphenous vein, this can simply be marked in durable felt-tip pen at the bedside.

For the patient whose vein is not obvious, and especially before femorotibial grafting, duplex scanning and marking of the vein is a major advantage. Absence of an adequate saphenous vein may sway the decision against operation in doubtful cases. Preoperative marking makes the operation quicker and avoids unnecessary dissection with elevation of flaps searching for the vein. If a good vein is not present in the affected limb, the contralateral long saphenous, the short saphenous, or arm veins can be mapped, so that they can be selected and marked before operation.

The operation

This section will not describe how to do these operations in exhaustive detail, but will highlight certain points that are important, possibly helpful, or controversial.

Reversed or *in situ* vein bypass grafts?

There is no significant difference between the results of these two methods for femoropopliteal grafting.[9] The main advantage of the *in situ* technique is with bypass to tibial arteries, when the large end of the vein can be joined to a large artery and the small end to an artery which is often very small. This means that veins which would be much too narrow at their distal ends for reversed vein bypass can be used quite satisfactorily. There is also less chance of the vein twisting when performing an *in situ* bypass.

In practice, surgeons who perform few bypasses distal to the popliteal artery tend to use traditional reversed vein bypass, while those who do a lot of tibial grafts frequently opt for the *in situ* technique for all grafts. I advocate a selective policy. Femorotibial bypasses are clearly best done *in situ*, but I prefer reversed vein bypass to the popliteal for three reasons. First, the upper end of an *in situ* graft is often difficult to approximate to the common femoral, which seems the best place for the proximal anastomosis. Second, there is less risk of damage to the vein wall or of valve cusp problems using the reversed technique. Third, passing a reversed vein through a subsartorial tunnel removes any risk of kinking (which can happen to an *in situ* graft plunging deeply into the popliteal fossa).

Preparation

A good technique for preparation and towelling is essential. Sudden exposure of the patient's genitals or an unsterile operating table in these often long operations is undesirable. A transparent plastic bag on the foot is helpful (with at least the forefoot spared from colouring by antiseptic so that its true colour can be seen).

Incisions

Practice varies. Some surgeons make a single long incision exposing the whole vein which is probably safest for avoiding any damage to the vein graft when dissecting beneath skin bridges, or when passing a valvulotome during *in situ* grafting. It allows easy identification and ligation of all tributaries. However, both reversed and *in situ* bypass can be done through several short incisions, which may make for less problems in wound healing. This is the technique I usually employ.

Access to the popliteal, posterior tibial, and peroneal arteries is achieved by a medial approach, through the incision made over the saphenous vein. There is no real advantage to the lateral approach for the peroneal artery, which involves excising a segment of fibula. The anterior tibial is simply exposed by an approach between extensor hallucis longus and extensor digitorum. The posterior tibial and peroneal arteries in particular are best approached in the distal part of the calf, beyond the bulk of the calf muscle bellies.

The recipient artery

As a rule, it is best to expose the distal artery first, especially if there is any doubt about its quality. Otherwise a 'two surgeon' approach, one working proximally and one distally, makes for efficient use of time, if only during the initial dissection and vein harvesting. I open the recipient vessel at an early stage, to check that it is adequate, both by local inspection, and by passing a soft (number 6) umbilical catheter down it, followed by flushing of the distal vascular bed with heparin saline. Systemic heparin can be given later, before clamping the common femoral artery.

Preparation of the vein

In preparing the saphenous vein the use of small Ligaclips on tributaries saves time, but ligatures are safest next to the vein if tributaries are to be divided. When preparing a vein for *in situ* bypass it is wise always to leave it well anchored to the tissues in the region of the knee, but freeing it for some distance in the upper thigh can help approximation to the common femoral artery.

It is seldom easy to anastomose an *in situ* vein graft well up onto of the common femoral artery: indeed, the best landmark for the level of the saphenofemoral junction is the profunda origin. It is helpful to conserve as much vein length as possible by applying a narrow (e.g. DeBakey paediatric) arterial clamp flush with the femoral vein, dividing the terminal long saphenous with a scalpel along the edge of this, and then closing the femoral vein with a continuous Prolene suture placed initially over the clamp. If the proximal superficial femoral artery is patent and soft, then this can be used for the anastomosis. Some surgeons are prepared to perform endarterectomy of this vessel to use it for the proximal anastomosis. In general I favour good mobilization of the saphenous vein to reach the common femoral artery.

Preventing twists and kinks

During *in situ* grafting, the proximal anastomosis is carried out first, followed by valve disruption if a Hall or similar valvulotome is used (a quick and satisfactory method which seldom causes damage). When the distal end of the vein has been placed adjacent to the recipient artery (which will involve tunnelling for the anterior tibial), blood flow should always be allowed to ensure that there are no twists or kinks. For reversed vein bypass, some surgeons mark one side of the vein with dye to guard against twisting, but I prefer simply tunnelling it (deep to sartorius), and then flushing it forcefully with heparin saline to abolish any twisting. Alternatively the top anastomosis can be done first, followed by distal flushing with blood.

The anastomoses

Magnification (e.g. 2.5x or more) is an advantage in dissecting out tibial arteries, and anastomosing grafts to them. To remain comfortable in the use of magnifiers it is probably worthwhile using them for all femorodistal anastomoses. Even those with excellent uncorrected vision confess to their advantage after getting used to them (I say this as a convert).

For femoral anastomoses, a 4/0 or 5/0 polypropylene suture is generally adequate. The 4/0 suture is commonly supplied with a heavier needle which is useful if the femoral artery is thickened or calcified. Distally, a 5/0 suture is usual for the popliteal artery. For tibial arteries, 6/0 or 7/0 sutures are satisfactory.

A continuous suture technique, starting with the graft 'heel' by a parachute technique, is common practice and works well for the femoral and popliteal arteries. This may also be appropriate for good-calibre tibial arteries, but interrupted sutures (perhaps five in all) at the apex of the tibial anastomosis, inserted under good vision, left long, and then tied down, provide a safe and meticulous method of ensuring that this vital part of the operation is perfect.

Some surgeons recommend performing the distal anastomosis over a cannula, passed distally down the vessel, and small occlusive stents are becoming available for this purpose. It certainly is a way of ensuring that the lumen is not obliterated during the placement of sutures. I seldom do this, but routinely slide an umbilical catheter through the distal part of the anastomosis before final closure to check that it passes through easily.

It is important to allow an external flush of blood before final closure of the distal anastomosis, both to confirm good blood flow and to expel any clots.

Checking the final result

There is no single foolproof technique. If there is an excellent pulse in the artery beyond the distal anastomosis and the foot rapidly becomes pink, then further intraoperative tests are generally superfluous, although it is always a good rule to measure the Doppler ankle pressure before the patient leaves the operating table.

If the result seems less than perfect for any reason, then an arteriogram should be done (with a proximal clamp in place). This usually shows the nature of the problem. There is no point leaving an unsatisfactory situation, because the graft will almost inevitably fail, even though revising anastomoses to miniscule and calcified tibial arteries at the end of a long procedure is exhausting. Perseverance should not prevent unscrubbing for a cup of tea before tackling this.

A sterile Doppler probe can be useful for assessing flow in the artery distal to the anastomosis. It can also be used in the localization of residual tributaries to an *in situ* vein, and earlier in the operation it may help if there is any doubt about which tibial artery is patent. I have yet to be convinced that any more sophisticated tools for intraoperative flow detection or measurement are genuinely helpful.

Alternatives to saphenous vein

There is no argument that autogenous vein is the most long-lasting conduit, especially for femorotibial grafts,[10,11] but surgeons vary in the lengths to which they will go to obtain this, if the saphenous vein is absent or inadequate. Some will search for contralateral long saphenous vein, short saphenous veins, arm veins (forbid venepunctures in these if you may need them), and even the superficial or deep femoral vein.[12] Segments of various veins may be joined together to produce adequate length. If good vein is in short supply, then a distal graft origin site, such as the popliteal artery, should be used if possible.[13] Finally, what is 'adequate' saphenous vein? Those with diameter less than 3–4 mm tend to do poorly for grafts to the popliteal artery, but narrower distal ends are quite satisfactory for femorotibial grafts.

Polytetrafluoroethylene (PTFE) gives satisfactory results to the popliteal artery,[10] and I seldom hesitate to use this above the knee in the absence of good saphenous vein. Some surgeons advocate a policy of preferential use of PTFE in this situation, so saving the vein for more distal grafting at a later date,[14] but this is controversial. PTFE also gives reasonable results to the below-knee popliteal, but it is less good than vein in the long term. It is probably worthwhile using ring-reinforced PTFE when crossing the knee joint. Use of a Miller vein cuff[15] (or Taylor vein patch[16]) probably improves the results of PTFE grafts, and certainly seems worthwhile on the occasions when PTFE is taken to tibial arteries.

There is evidence to support the use of human umbilical vein (HUV) as an alternative (possibly superior) to PTFE.[17] It is expensive, and less easy to suture to tibial arteries than a vein cuff, followed by a thin-walled PTFE graft. The long-running struggle for supremacy between PTFE and HUV as the best alternative to vein for femorodistal bypass is likely to continue for the foreseeable future. Recently, there has been renewed interest in the use of Dacron for grafts distal to the inguinal ligament.[18]

Complications

Early signs

Haemorrhage in the recovery room is a dramatic early complication, and is almost always due to a ligature slipping from a vein graft. Bleeding later in the postoperative period is rare and occurs secondary to infection.

Early occlusion is usually caused by technical error or some correctable problem unrecognized at operation. In general these grafts should be re-explored, thrombectomy performed, and a search made for the cause, which should then be corrected. Thrombectomy alone occasionally suffices, but if the situation is not somehow improved, re-occlusion is usual. I empirically anticoagulate all patients who require re-operation for blocked grafts (early or late).

If there is any doubt about whether or not a graft has failed in the day or two after surgery, it usually has.

The long wounds involved in femorodistal bypass are prone to delayed healing, and wound problems are the commonest medical reason for delayed discharge from hospital after successful reconstruction. Redness and oozing of thigh wounds (but without frank infection) and areas of superficial dehiscence (particularly in deep groin creases) are not uncommon. Lymphatic leaks occasionally occur in the groin; both these and haematomas can be guarded against by sound groin wound closure with at least two subcutaneous layers.

Some ankle (and leg) swelling is common, and may be partly due to disturbance of lymphatic channels at the time of the operation. Patients should be reassured that this is not serious and that it will gradually diminish over a few weeks.

Late graft occlusion and graft surveillance

From a pragmatic point of view there are two approaches to follow-up of femorodistal grafts:

1. The patient should be told explicitly the signs of graft occlusion and instructed to return directly and immediately to the vascular surgical ward if his graft ever blocks. Outpatient follow-up is largely superfluous. Long-term clinic appointments seem more for the sake of the surgeon than for the patient, but a single postoperative clinic visit a month or two after discharge from hospital is reasonable.
2. The alternative is an aggressive policy of close follow-up (e.g. by duplex scanning) to detect any stenoses which may develop in the graft, especially during the first few months when the occlusion rate is highest.[19] This is done with a view to correcting any stenoses found (by angioplasty or operation), thereby theoretically preventing graft occlusion[20] (see Chapter 8).

There do seem to be definite benefits from the second approach, although it is still not certain whether all stenoses detected really would lead to graft occlusion if left. Few vascular surgeons have yet established a comprehensive system of graft surveillance, but this is likely to become an important function of the clinical vascular laboratory in the future.

References

1. Brewster DC, LaSalle AJ, Robison JG, Strayhorn EC, Darling RC. Femoropopliteal graft failures: clinical consequences and success of secondary reconstructions. *Arch Surg* 1983; **118:** 1043–7.
2. Cook TA, Davies AH, Horrocus M, Baird RN. Amputation level is not adversely affected by previous femoro-distal bypass surgery. *Eur J Vasc Surg* 1992; **6:** 599–601.
3. Jelnes R, Gaardsting O, Jensen KH, Baekgaard N, Tonnensen KH, Schroeder T. Fate in intermittent claudication: outcome and risk factors. *Br Med J* 1986; **293:** 1137–9.
4. Charlesworth D, Harris PL, Cave FD, Tyalor L. Undetected aorto-iliac insufficiency: a reason for early failure of saphenous vein bypass grafts for obstruction of the superficial femoral artery. *Br J Surg* 1975; **62:** 567–70.
5. Cutler BS, Thompson JE, Kleinsasser LJ, Hempel GK. Autologous saphenous vein femoropopliteal bypass: analysis of 298 cases. *Surgery* 1976; **79:** 325–31.
6. Dardik H, Ibrahim IM, Sussman B, Greweldinger J, Alder J, Kahn M, Dardik I. Morphologic structure of the pedal arch and its relationship to patency of crural vascular reconstruction. *Surg Gyne Obst* 1981; **152:** 645–8.
7. Karacagil S, Almgren B, Bowald S, Eriksson I. A new method of angiographic runoff evaluation in femorodistal reconstructions. *Arch Surg* 1990; **125:** 1055–8.
8. Campbell WB, Fletcher EL, Hands LJ. Assessment of the distal lower limb arteries: a comparison of arteriography and Doppler ultrasound. *Ann Roy Coll Surg Eng* 1986; **68:** 37–9.
9. Harris PL, How TV, Jones DR. Prospectively randomised clinical trial to compare *in situ* and reversed saphenous veingrafts for femoropopliteal bypass. *Br J Surg* 1987; **74:** 252–5.
10. Veith FJ, Gupta SK, Ascer E, *et al.* Six-year prospective multicenter randomized comparison of autologous saphenous vein and expanded polytetrafluoroethylene grafts in infrainguinal arterial reconstructions. *J Vasc Surg* 1986; **3:** 104–14.
11. Taylor LM, Edwards JM, Porter JM. Present status of reversed vein bypass grafting: five-year results of a modern series. *J Vasc Surg* 1990; **11:** 193–206.
12. Schulman ML, Badhey MR, Yatco R. Superficial femoral-popliteal veins and reversed saphenous veins as primary femoropopliteal bypass grafts: a randomised comparative study. *J Vasc Surg* 1987; **6:** 1–10.
13. Ascer E, Veith FJ, Gupta SK, *et al.* Short vein grafts: a superior option for arterial reconstructions to poor

or compromised outflow tracts? *J Vasc Surg* 1988; **7**: 370–8.

14. Quinones-Baldrich WJ, Busuttil RW, Baker JD, *et al.* Is the preferential use of polytetrafluoroethylene grafts for femoropopliteal bypass justified? *J Vasc Surg* 1988; **8**: 219–28.
15. Miller JH, Foreman RK, Ferguson L, Faris I. Interposition vein cuff for anastomosis of prosthesis to small artery. *Aust NZ J Surg* 1984; **54**: 283–5.
16. Tyrell MR, Chester JF, Vipond MN, Clarke GH, Taylor RS, Wolfe JHN. Experimental evidence to support the use of interposition vein collars/patches in distal PTFE anastomosis. *Eur J Vasc Surg* 1990; **4**: 95–101.
17. Eickhoff JH, Bromme A, Ericsson BF, *et al.* Four years' results of a prospective, randomized clinical trial comparing polytetrafluoroethylene and modified human umbilical vein for below-knee femoropopliteal bypass. *J Vasc Surg* 1987; **6**: 506–11.
18. Mosley JG, Marston A. A 5-year follow-up of Dacron femoropopliteal bypass grafts. *Br J Surg* 1986; **73**: 24–7.
19. Taylor PR, Wolfe JHN, Tyrell MR, Mansfield AO, Nicolaides AN, Houston RE. Graft stenosis: justification for 1-year surveillance. *Br J Surg* 1990; **77**: 1125–8.
20. Moody P, de Cossart LM, Douglas HM, Harris PL. Asymptomatic strictures in femoro-popliteal vein grafts. *Eur J Vasc Surg* 1989; **3**: 389–92.

8

Graft occlusion

NJW Cheshire and JHN Wolfe

In this chapter we consider the causes and effects of arterial bypass graft occlusion. The surgical correction of lower-limb ischaemia accounts for a large proportion of the vascular surgeon's work-load. Most of the data described will be based on infrainguinal grafts, although many of the principles outlined may be applied to grafts in other locations.

In the UK over the last two decades there has been a shift away from arterial reconstruction for intermittent claudication, with the result that a higher proportion of grafts are now performed for critical leg ischaemia. Recognition and treatment of impending failure in this group of grafts is important. Occlusion may have calamitous consequences for the patient. Any contemporary description of infrainguinal graft failure must also consider the wider issue of the surgical and economic value of arterial reconstruction in the leg. Reports of low graft patency rates combined with anecdotes of numerous reinterventions prior to amputation or death, serve to strengthen the beliefs of pessimists. Those who believe in reconstruction and reintervention must produce data to justify their policies.

Incidence

The incidence of graft failure is described by the the European Concensus Document on Critical Leg Ischaemia,[1] which estimates average 1-year graft patency rates for femoro/above-knee popliteal grafts of 85% when vein is used and 80% for PTFE or other prosthetic grafts. Femorocrural grafts in the lower third of the calf yield success rates of 55% and 25% for vein and prostheses respectively. It must be appreciated that these are concensus results from many centres in different countries, and individual units with a specialist interest in lower-limb reconstruction may achieve better results.

The figures provided in the European Document include grafts that have thrombosed but have undergone secondary intervention which has restored patency. The success of reintervention is of major clinical and economic importance and will be considered further later. The document highlights the basic premise that both increased graft length and the presence of prosthetic material increase the likelihood of graft failure.

The perfect graft

The perfect graft should afford high patency rates to medium- and long-term follow-up, provide the vascular surgeon with virtually unlimited conduit length (to allow bypass to any of the crural vessels in the lower calf), be easy to handle and suture, and be cheap and easily available. At present autologous vein is the graft of choice as this gives optimal patency rates, is ideal for difficult anastomoses and is cheap. Unfortunately, sufficient lengths of suitable graft are not always available, and in a series of over 130 femorocrural grafts at St Mary's Hospital we were only able to use vein grafts in approximately two-thirds of cases.[2] However, a high proportion of patients in this series had undergone prior peripheral or coronary arterial reconstruction (thus using available autologous vein), and other groups have been able to use vein in a higher percentage of reconstructions.[3]

Of prosthetic grafts for infrainguinal bypass, expanded PTFE (Impra/Gortex) seems to give superior patency rates at medium- and long-term follow-up when compared with Dacron. The newer thin-walled grafts are easier to handle and anastomose than their predecessors. The addition of a removable spiral external support allays fears of graft kinking or compression. The success rates of PTFE below the knee, however, compare very poorly with those of vein grafts (cf. 1-year patency for femorodistal–tibial bypass: 25% prosthetic grafts, 55% vein grafts[1]). The use of distal vein collars[4,5] may improve PTFE patency, and the 3-year patency in our series of full length femorodistal–tibial PTFE grafts, all con-

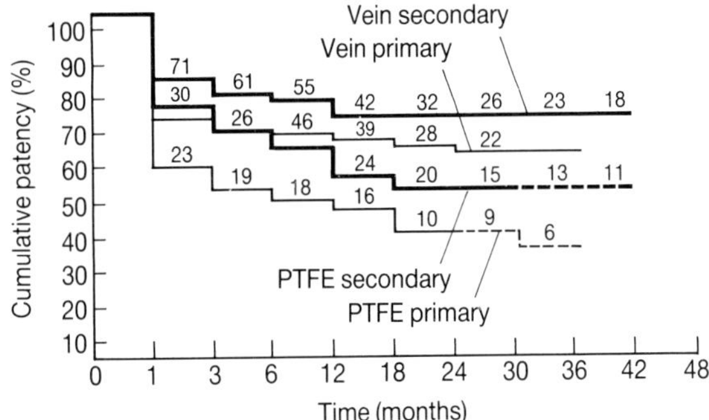

Fig. 8.1 Life-table analysis of femorodistal tibial bypass graft patency. Vein grafts provide superior patency. Three-year PTFE patency was 50% (including salvaged grafts). (Reproduced from reference 2 with permission.)

structed with a collar, was 50%[2] (Fig. 8.1).

The value of the human umbilical vein graft remains debatable. Reported patency rates for tibial or peroneal bypass vary between 50% at 3 years[6] to 18% at 1 year.[7] Many of these studies have used the early version of the graft (Dardik 1 or 2) which is still in use in the USA, and patency rates for the newer vesions (Dardik 5–7, in use in Europe) are awaited.

All prosthetic grafts are relatively expensive, although it is important to realize that some of the costs of the graft are offset by the shorter operating time required for prosthetic bypass, particularly to the crural arteries. In our study of the economics of femorocrural grafting we were surprised to find little difference in the overall costs of an operation using vein or PTFE.[2]

Causes of graft failure

The timing of graft failure gives a clue to the aetiology. Early failure, occurring within one month of operation, is usually due to technical error such as poor patient selection or operative technique. Approximately 10% of grafts will fail in this time period. When grafts thrombose after 2 years, progression of native vessel atherosclerosis, either proximally or distally, is the usual cause. This accounts for 2–3% of all graft failures each year. The most common time for grafts to fail is between 1 month and 2 years (80% of all graft failures), and this is the same period in which graft stenoses are now known to develop.[8].

The development of graft stenoses in the postoperative period was first described in 1973 by Szilagyi. Many groups have subsequently studied the phenomenon, and although the aetiology of stenoses remain obscure (most are now believed to be due to hyperplasia of smooth muscle cells in the vessel wall), most work has shown that stenoses are common, occurring in 20–25% of grafts (Table 8.1) and tend to develop within the first 1 or 2 years of graft implantation.[8,14] In a study of 412 infrainguinal grafts we demonstrated a graft stenosis incidence of 16%. Subgroup analysis showed stenoses in 20% of the 120 femorocrural grafts studied, and 14% of 292 femoropopliteal grafts.[8]

Table 8.1 Incidence of vein graft stenoses

Authors	Number of grafts	Stenosed
Bandyk *et al.*[10]	197	28%
Thompson *et al.*[9]	94	15%
Moody *et al.*[11]	141	28%
Taylor *et al.*[8]	412	16%
Chang *et al.*[12]	350	20%
Mills *et al.*[13]	379	6%

These grafts were monitored with intravenous digital subtraction angiography (IVDSA) and duplex scanning at 6 weeks and 12 weeks postoperatively, then every 3 months for follow-up ranging between 6 and 48 months. Sixty-five per cent of stenoses developed within 6 months of the primary operation, and surprisingly, no new graft-related stenoses were detected after 12 months (Fig 8.2). Other groups have found late stenoses, but these were in retrospective series and it is possible that these lesions had been present for some time.

Although evidence implicating stenoses in medium-term graft failure remains circumstantial, we have shown a positive correlation between the presence of graft stenoses and graft thrombosis; 19 stenosed grafts had a 42% incidence of haemodynamic deterioration or occlusion compared with a 7% incidence in 56 nonstenosed grafts.[15] Moody *et al.*[16] have calculated a three-fold increase in graft occlusion in association with stenoses.

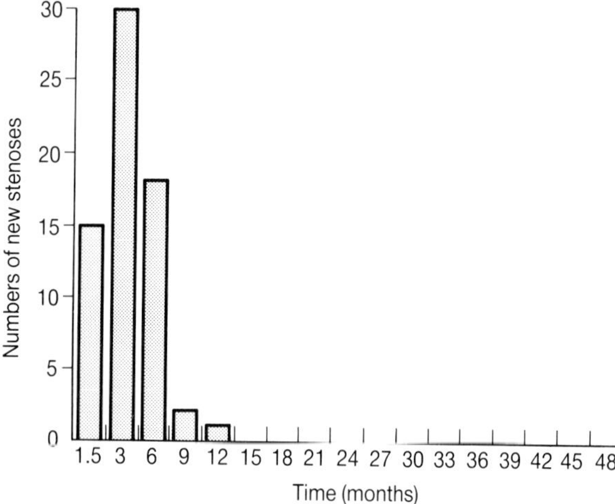

Fig. 8.2 Postoperative time to detection of infrainguinal graft stenoses. Most stenoses were detected within 6 months of reconstruction and no new stenoses developed after one year. (Reproduced from reference 8 with permission.)

Graft stenosis

As stenoses are common and are thought to contribute to a large proportion of graft failures, detection and treatment become important.

Detection

It is likely that improvement in graft survival could be achieved if intraluminal stenoses could be detected and successfully corrected (potentially 80% of all failing grafts). Unfortunately, most stenoses appear to produce minimal changes prior to occlusion of the affected graft. This has led many units to look for methods of early detection of these lesions, before significant haemodynamic compromise occurs.

The ideal stenosis detection programme provides accurate information about the graft and is minimally invasive. It should also be safe, easy to perform and cheap. Numerous techniques have been used with varying degrees of success. Whilst the ideal has not yet been determined, much has been learned of the abnormalities produced in a graft when a stenosis develops. Flow abnormalities are mostly limited to the region of the stenosis until the critical point when flow ceases.

Clinical testing

Early studies used clinical techniques to detect stenoses, chiefly graft pulse palpation supplemented with exercise ankle/brachial pressure ratios.

The presence of a graft pulse means only that a pressure wave is passing along the graft and can occur in the absence of flow; it is therefore insensitive to the minor flow abnormalities associated with early stenoses. The addition of ankle pressure measurements improves sensitivity and can detect stenoses before graft failure. Although the method is cheap and simple, in most studies it detects only about 50% of lesions demonstrable by either duplex scanning or angiography.[17–19]

The duplex Doppler

The availability of duplex scanning in the early 1980s provoked great interest amongst vascular surgeons looking for the ideal graft surveillance tool. A decade later debate continues over the optimal application of this powerful device. Some centres have shown an ability to detect stenoses using a single flow parameter such as peak systolic flow velocity, taken at a single point within a graft.[10] Whilst this technique is simple to execute, in a study of 75 patients we were unable to demonstrate a clear correlation between such a measurement and angiographic findings in normal and stenosed grafts.[15]

As many stenoses are short, the flow abnormalities they produce can be very localized prior to graft failure. We have therefore developed a method of duplex scanning which interrogates the whole of the length of an infrainguinal graft to detect localized flow changes.

Flow at any point in a graft is the product of cross-sectional area and velocity and remains unchanged along the graft, as an arterial conduit is a tube without branches. Any reduction of cross-sectional area must produce a proportional increase in velocity for the flow to remain constant (Fig 8.3). The inaccuracy of direct diameter measurement can therefore be eliminated and one can rely on localized velocity changes to demonstrate alterations in the graft lumen. We sample the velocity at 2 cm intervals along the graft. An increase in velocity greater than 100% (V_2:V_1 ratio >2) is associated with a luminal reduction of 50%. Using this technique in 75 patients, we demonstrated close correlation between V_2:V_1 ratio on duplex scanning, and angiographic stenosis.[15] A stenosis produces a localized

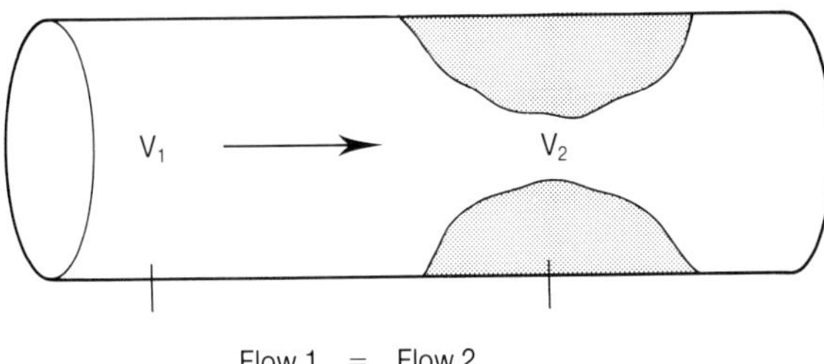

Fig. 8.3 Line drawing of flow in an area of stenosed graft. As the graft is an unbranched tube, flow at all points is equal. Reduction of cross-sectional area by stenosis results in a localized increase in velocity which can be detected by duplex scanning.

increase in velocity which then returns to prestenosis levels downstream. The vein calibre alters at major branch sites so that these are regions of potential error, but this produces a persistant velocity increase, maintained throughout the length of the smaller-calibre vein.

The technique requires time and training. However, we believe that, with experience, a competent operator can examine a whole graft in 30–40 minutes, and that the improved stenosis detection rate obtained using this technique justifies this requirement. New technology, such as colour duplex, enables more efficient $V_2{:}V_1$ scanning for two reasons:

1. The graft is easily detected, which can make difficult areas such as the knee more readily accessible.
2. The whole graft can be rapidly scanned. An increase in velocity shows as a change in shade and these areas can then be interrogated carefully.

One of the weaknesses of the technique is the difficulty in obtaining accurate velocity information from small native vessels distal to the graft (particularly crural vessels), which may be important. We have found an average peak systolic flow velocity under 45 cm/s, as proposed by Bandyk *et al.*,[10] to be of use in the detection of distal native vessel lesions and now use it as an adjunct to $V_2{:}V_1$ measurements. We have not, however, found this measurement alone to be of value in detecting stenoses within the graft.

Angiography

This remains the 'gold standard' against which all new methods of stenosis detection are measured.[17] It must be performed in two planes at 90 degrees to detect all stenoses and is invasive and expensive. Outpatient intravenous digital subtraction angiography, or intra-arterial studies performed through small cannulae, are improving the acceptability of angiography, but cost remains prohibitive for routine screening use. Furthermore the warm flush experienced during contrast infusion can reduce patient compliance to serial monitoring.

Postoperative surveillance

Several centres have already shown that stenoses occur early, within one year of reconstruction.[8,16,17,20] In a study of stenosis progression using duplex and angiography, we demonstrated lesion progression from minor (V_2: V_1 <2) to severe (V_2: V_1 >2) within 3 months.[15] As a result of these studies we have devised a follow-up policy. We begin surveillance at 6 weeks post-reconstruction, repeat it at 12 weeks and then regularly every 3 months for the first year after implantation. If no stenosis is detected by 12 months it is probably not cost-effective to continue to screen all grafts, although this may be desirable to uncover atheroma progression in native vessels. Any graft found to have a stenosis should undergo urgent correction if the stenosis is more than 50% of the lumen area (see below), or continue to be assessed at 3-monthly intervals if less than 50% of the lumen. After secondary intervention the patient starts again at the beginning of the surveillance programme.

Our current practice is to perform both $V_2{:}V_1$ ratios and average peak systolic flow measurement using duplex scanning. Abnormalities detected on noninvasive studies are confirmed on angiography and necessary intervention undertaken.

Reintervention rates and the success of secondary intervention

Any reintervention policy which may improve limb salvage could theoretically have a beneficial effect on large numbers of patients as there is increasing evidence of prolonged survival after reconstruction[2,21] and poor mobility after amputation in this geriatric population.[2,22] In addition, such a policy could be implemented without additional cost. In a recent detailed financial analysis with the support of health economists, we compared reconstruction costs with the cost of primary amputation. Results demonstrated that mean hospital costs generated by reconstruction over medium-term follow-up (including aggressive reintervention) were over 20% less than the cost of amputation.[2] Additionally we studied separately those patients whose primary reconstruction required distal anastomosis to the crural vessels as many doctors (including some vascular surgeons) are suspicious of the value of these operations. We were able to show that even these high-risk procedures cost less to the hospital than amputation.[2] The long-term costs of amputation to the community care budget are difficult to quantify, at least in part because the independance of amputees may vary significantly after discharge from hospital, and the degree of health care required for a given impairment depends on the home and support circumstances of the patient. It is likely that these additional costs contribute substantially to the mean overall cost of amputation.

In another study of 395 primary reconstructions in the leg, we showed that further vascular intervention was required in 44% of reconstructions to all levels, and 67% of femorocrural operations over mean follow-up of 3 years. Importantly, however, a third of these operations were performed in the presence of a functioning primary graft. Therefore, in order to answer the question of whether reintervention was worthwhile following graft failure, we focused on the 30% of all patients and 48% of femorocrural reconstructions in whom secondary operations were performed for recurrent ischaemia. Further vascular reconstruction was undertaken in the majority of these patients. Secondary revascularization was worthwhile in both groups, yielding a 64% success rate for all grafts and a 44% success for crural reconstructions at mean follow-up of 3 years. Reintervention was responsible for almost 20% of all limbs salvaged and a quarter of successful femorocrural grafts.[23]

Our study demonstrates the value of an aggressive approach to reintervention in the salvage of critical legs and supports results from the United States. In a study of the outcome of 202 failed infrainguinal grafts, Bartlett *et al.*[21] described a 59% limb salvage at 5 years after a mean 1.9 further operations per patient. Whittemore *et al.*[24] have suggested a success rate of 50% limb salvage following secondary intervention, although this figure is generated from operations performed on failing and thrombosed grafts, and success in the thrombosed group alone was estimated being as low as 20% at 5 years. More recently, Veith *et al.*[25] have calculated a reduction in overall amputation from 49% to 14% over a 15-year period by adopting a policy of aggressive primary and secondary revascularization. During this time, the primary amputation rate fell from 14% to 5%, whilst secondary amputations remained stable and reintervention rates increased. These figures can only be accounted for by increased success from secondary intervention. Twenty two per cent of patients in this study required reintervention for recurrence of ischaemia, a figure comparable to the 30% recurrence rate found in our study (although not all reconstructions described in this study were performed for critical leg ischaemia).

Management of graft stenosis

Intragraft stenoses are amenable to either open operation or percutaneous transluminal treatment. When stenosis correction was first undertaken, reports of the success of reintervention varied widely between different centres (Table 8.2). Some advocated percutaneous balloon dilatation (PTA) as an almost universal treatment, whilst others treated stenoses by open operation in the form of vein patch angioplasty or jump grafts for perianastomotic lesions. The general uniformity of surgical results became apparent as series showed that success at more than 1 year could be expected in 75% of patients. The results of PTA have been more contentious, with reported patencies varying between 7% and above 90%. A comparison between three centres with widely varying results revealed that the single most important factor predicting outcome after PTA is length of stenosis. Stenoses under 1 cm had a 73% success rate at 2-year follow-up whereas stenoses longer than 3 cm had a significantly reduced success rate of 25% over the same period of follow-up; i.e. PTA yields good results on suitable lesions.[28]

This finding has lead us to alter our reintervention policy and we now only perform balloon angioplasty on stenoses under 1 cm in length. All other stenoses undergo operation. The obvious advantages of percutaneous transluminal angioplasty are its simplicity,

Table 8.2 Results of secondary procedures for graft-related stenoses

Authors	Number of grafts	Balloon dilatation (patency)	Operation (patency)
Berkowitz *et al.*[18]	134	24 (80%)	–
Veith *et al.*[26]	191	30 (90%)	8 (90%)
Cohen *et al.*[27]	322	7 (43%)	22 (82%)
Moody *et al.*[11]	141	17 (93%)	–
Taylor *et al.*[8]	412	14 (50%)	23 (70%)

repeatability and relative inexpense. Whilst open operation is more successful, in most cases it does require general anaesthesia and a longer stay in hospital for the patient.

There is overwhelming evidence that correction of haemodynamically compromised grafts that are still patent is associated with a significant improvement in medium- and long-term patency compared with procedures undertaken after graft thrombosis. Whittemore *et al.*[24] have shown that graft patency after stenosis correction is 82% at 5-year follow-up compared with 28% 5-year patency subsequent to operations following graft thrombosis

In addition, some centres are now able to report the effects of their graft surveillance and stenosis repair programmes. Moody *et al.*[16] have demonstrated a 15% improvement in overall medium-term patency with a policy of aggressive reintervention.

We believe dedication to a programme of graft surveillance combined with the correct intervention following stenosis detection is vital to the survival of infrainguinal bypass grafts. The techniques of surveillance are relatively simple and should be available to all vascular surgeons undertaking regular infrainguinal arterial reconstruction. Although the optimal methods of stenosis repair require clarification, it is hoped that in the future the 80% of graft failures occurring at between 1 month and 2 years can be reduced significantly.

Management of the thrombosed graft

The treatment of patients presenting with a thrombosed infrainguinal graft is dictated by the viability of the leg at presentation. In all cases arteriography should be performed initially to confirm the diagnosis and demonstrate any immediately correctable or unsuspected pathology.

Graft thrombosis with viable limb

The aim of treatment is to restore function to the original graft and correct any lesion within the graft or native vessels which may have caused thrombosis. These circumstances are ideally suited to thrombolysis with streptokinase, urokinase or rtPA (recombinant tissue plasminogen activator). Streptokinase is cheap but may produce anaphylaxis and should not therefore be used twice within 6 months. Urokinase is prohibitively expensive in Britain but slightly cheaper in the USA. rtPA is more expensive and there is no evidence that it is more efficient at clot lysis than streptokinase, although it probably works more quickly.

All agents are administered through an intra-arterial cannula, preferably within a sheath with side holes through which low-dose thrombolytic agent can also be infused. Such an arrangement facilitates easy change of cannula whilst minimizing chances of bleeding around the puncture site and vessel trauma. The secondary infusion along the sheath prevents thrombus forming around the catheter.

The tip of the main cannula delivering thrombolytic agent should be impacted in the thrombus to be lysed under angiographic control, and the progress of thrombolysis monitored with 6- or 8-hourly angiography until the graft is cleared and clinical improvement occurs.

The advantage of this form of treatment is that the cause of the occlusion can be identified by arteriography once the graft is cleared. When a graft stenosis is detected, it can be corrected without need for replacement of the whole graft and loss of valuable autogenous vein. The value of salvaging a thrombosed vein graft has been questioned and most would agree that lysis more than 1 month after occlusion is of little value. Patients are now more aware of graft occlusion, and when they present within 2–3 days of occlusion we have had some long-term success with vein graft lysis.

Another advantage of vein graft thrombolysis is its relatively noninvasive nature (compared with open thrombectomy) and the ability to lyse thrombus in both the graft and smaller distal vessels, which are not be amenable to standard balloon thromboembolectomy.

The most obvious disadvantage of the technique is the danger of bleeding associated with systemic escape or localized build-up of the thrombolytic agent. Groin haemorrhage is the most common complication and is reported in 10–30% of cases when thrombolysis is used for leg ischaemia. Some have suggested that rtPA may be associated with fewer bleeding complications than other agents,[29] but the recent major trial of coronary artery thrombolysis did not provide evidence to support the use of rtPA over other agents.

Even if the leg is viable some patients require fasciotomy, and this may present a considerable problem until the effects of the thrombolytic agent have worn off. If fasciotomy is obviously indicated then this is a relative contraindication to the use of thrombolysis. Perhaps the major contraindication is the use of thrombolysis in a limb that will not survive the 12 hours required for revascularization. Immobility and sensory alterations are therefore contra-indications to the use of thrombolysis.

Graft thrombosis with non-viable limb

In these circumstances emergency operation is required to salvage the limb. The patient should be prepared for operation immediately. After administration of antibiotic prophylaxis and systemic heparin further action depends on the type of graft.

Thrombosed vein grafts

If a thrombosed vein graft can be operated on within 6 hours of onset of acute symptoms, then the aim of treatment should be the restoration of graft flow with detection and correction of any underlying abnormalities. At operation the hood of the distal and proximal anastomosis should be opened and the graft and distal vessels cleared of thrombus using standard techniques. Once flow is established, on-table angiography is performed and any graft or native vessel abnormality corrected with a vein patch or jump graft as described previously. Infusion of 100 000 units of streptokinase into the graft may lyse distal thrombi if these are visualized on the arteriogram.

In the more usual case when operation is undertaken more than 6 hours after thrombosis, a further bypass with vein from another site or a PTFE graft may be needed. In the latter case retention of the distal 1–2 cm of the original graft and its use as a vein cuff may be advantageous.

We have adopted this policy because few of our vein grafts which have been cleared more than 6 hours after failure have remained patent.

Thrombosed PTFE grafts

With PTFE grafts the timing of reoperation in relation to thrombosis is not as critical to further graft survival, and in all cases the surgeon should aim to restore function to the original graft with or without a stenosis-correcting procedure. Since PTFE is more thrombogenic than vein, the critical Reynolds number is reached at higher flow rates and the graft can thrombose without any obvious local pathology.

In all circumstances both proximal and distal graft hoods need to be opened. Thrombus can then be cleared using saline. If good back-flow from distal vessels is obtained, the 'graftotomies' can be closed and an on-table arteriogram performed. Once again any lesion in the graft or native vessels must then be corrected. In a study of 104 failed PTFE grafts, corrective procedures (such as patch angioplasty), were required in 70% of cases.[3]

Prevention of stenosis and failures: the role of drugs

As long ago as 1963, dextran was shown to reduce thrombosis[30] and has since been shown to have a beneficial effect on outcome after arterial reconstruction.[31] The mechanism of action of this colloid involves intravascular volume expansion, antileucocyte and antiplatelet functions and anticoagulant effects. Dextran has few side-effects if cardiac function is normal, and we use it whenever possible for grafts to crural vessels. A multicentre femoropoliteal trial in the UK has shown that low-dose aspirin is associated with improved patency in PTFE grafts.[32] We therefore prescribe aspirin for all prosthetic femorocrural grafts (or persantin, if there are contra-indications to aspirin).

The current interest in subintimal hyperplasia of smooth muscle cells as a cause of graft and anastomotic stenoses has led many groups to look for an agent to block this unwanted response. There is intense research in this area, concentrating on alpha-adrenergic blocking agents and low-molecular-weight heparins. It is to be hoped that this work will have major practical implications in the future.

Other studies are investigating the long-term effect of the combined vasodilator/platelet inhibitor, Iloprost, a synthetic prostacycline analogue. Early results from Birmingham are very encouraging[33] and suggest a prolonged beneficial action.

Conclusions

Based on an incidence of between 25 and 50 thousand critical legs per year in the UK,[1] the figures outlined in this chapter demonstrate that a policy of arterial reconstruction with aggressive secondary intervention could salvage an additional 4000–8000 legs annually compared with a policy of amputation after graft failure. Furthermore, as amputation is more expensive than reconstruction, energetic reintervention would result in savings to the National Health Service of over £20 million a year.[2] It is worth noting that a primary reconstruction policy without femorocrural operations would result in greater losses and expense.

When these data are combined with the obvious advantages of limb salvage to a patients' wellbeing and mobility, we believe that all involved in the management of leg ischaemia should view reoperation after primary reconstruction as an integral part of a successful limb salvage policy. Although we appreciate that unsuccessful secondary reconstruction may be detrimental to patient morale, we believe that the success of reintervention justifies a policy of aggressive approach to the management of recurrent ischaemia after arterial grafting.

References

1. Dormandy J (ed). *European Consensus Document on Critical Limb Ischaemia.* Berlin: Springer-Verlag, 1989.
2. Cheshire N, Wolfe J, Noone M, Davies L, Drummond M. The economics of femorocrural reconstruction for critical leg ischaemia with and without autologous vein. *J Vasc Surg* 1992; **15:** 167–76.
3. Veith F, Ascer E, Gupta S. Secondary arterial reconstructions in the lower extremity. In: *Vascular Surgery,* Rutherford R (ed). Philadelphia: WB Saunders, 1989: 744–53.
4. Miller J. The use of the vein cuff and PTFE. In: *Vascular Surgical Techniques: An Atlas,* Greenhalgh R (ed). London: WB Saunders, 1989: 276–86.
5. Tyrell M, Wolfe J. New prosthetic venous collar anastomotic techniques: combining the best of other procedures. *Br J Surg* 1991; **78:** 1016–17.
6. Largiader J. Experience with 350 crural arterial reconstructions: analysis and conclusions. *Thorac Cardiovasc Surg* 1985; **33:** 146–56.
7. Batt M, Avril G, Gagliardi J, *et al.* Femorodistal bypass using the chemically processed human umbilical vein graft. *Can J Surg* 1990; **33:** 61–5.
8. Taylor P, Wolfe J, Tyrell M, Mansfield A, Nicolaides A, Houston R. Graft stenosis: justification for 1-year surveillance. *Br J Surg* 1990; **77:** 1125–8.
9. Thompson JF, McShane MD, Gazzard V, Clifford PC, Chant ADB. Limitations of percutaneous transluminal angioplasty in the treatment of femorodistal graft stenoses. *Eur J Vasc Surg* 1989; **3:** 209–11.
10. Bandyk D, Seabrook G, Moldenhauer R, *et al.* Haemodynamics of vein graft stenosis. *J Vasc Surg* 1988; **8:** 688–95.
11. Moody P, de Cossart LM, Douglas HM, Harris PL. Asymptomatic strictures in femoropopliteal vein graft. *Eur J Vasc Surg* 1989; **3:** 389–92.
12. Chang B, *et al.* Characteristics of failing infrainguinal grafts. *J Vasc Surg* 1990; **12:** 596–600.
13. Mills J, Harris J, Taylor L, Beckett C, Porter. The importance of routine surveillance of distal bypass grafts with duplex scanning: a study of 379 reversed vein grafts. *J Vasc Surg* 1990; **12:** 379–89.
14. Grigg M, Nicolaides A, Wolfe J. Femorodistal vein bypass graft stenoses. *Br J Surg* 1988; **75:** 737–40.
15. Grigg M, Nicolaides A, Wolfe J. Detection and grading of femorodistal vein graft stenoses: duplex velocity measurements compared with angiography. *J Vasc Surg* 1988; **8:** 661–6.
16. Moody P, Gould A, Harris P. Vein graft surveillance improves patency in femoropopliteal bypass. *Eur J Vasc Surg* 1990; **4:** 117–21.
17. Wolfe J, Thomas M, Jamieson C, Browse N, Burnand K, Rutt D. The early diagnosis of femoropopliteal vein graft stenoses: a prospective 1-year follow-up. *Br J Surg* 1987; **74:** 268–70.
18. Berkowitz H, Hobbs C, Roberts B, Freiman D, Oleaga J, Ring E. Value of routine vascular laboratory studies to identify vein graft stenosis. *Surgery* 1981; **90:** 971–9.
19. Campbell W, Wolfe J. The role of noninvasive tests in arterial disease. *Br J Surg* 1987; **74:** 1075–6.
20. Bell P, Brennan J. Vein graft surveillance by duplex scanning and pressure measurement. In: *The Maintenance of Arterial Reconstruction,* Greenhalgh R, Hollier L (eds). London: WB Saunders, 1991: 135–42.
21. Bartlett S, Olinde A, Flinn W, McCarthy W, Fahey V, Bergan J, Yao J. The reoperative potential of infrainguinal bypass: long term and patient survival. *J Vasc Surg* 1987; **5:** 170–9.
22. Houghton A, Thurlow S, Rootes E, McColl I. Our success in rehabilitating vascular amputees. *Br J Surg* 1991; **78:** 752.
23. Cheshire N, Noone M, Wolfe J. Re-intervention after vascular surgery for critical leg ischaemia. *Eur J Vasc Surg* 1991; **6:** 545–50.
24. Whittemore A, Clowes A, Couch N, Mannick J. Secondary femoro-popliteal reconstruction. *Ann Surg* 1981; **193:** 35–42.
25. Veith F, Gupta S, Wengerter K. Changing atherosclerotic disease patterns and management strategies. *Ann Surg* 1990; **212:** 402–14.
26. Veith FJ, Weiser RK, Gupta SK, *et al.* Diagnosis and management of failing lower extremity arterial reconstructions prior to graft occlusion. *J Cardiovasc Surg* 1986; **25:** 381–4.
27. Cohen JR, Mannick JA, Couch NP, Whittemore AD. Recognition and management of impending vein graft failure. *Arch Surg* 1986; **121:** 78–9.
28. Taylor PR, Gould D, Harris P, Al-Kutoubi A, Wolfe JH. Balloon dilation of graft stenoses. – reasons for failure. *BR J Surg* 1990; **7:** 371.
29. Dawson K, Dex E, Platts A, Hamilton G. Groin haemorrhage complicating intra-arterial thrombolytic therapy: choice of technique and agent. *Br J Surg* 1991; **78:** 363.
30. Moncrieff J, Dain J, Canizaro P, *et al.* Use of dextran to prevent arterial and venous thrombosis. *Ann Surg* 1963; **158:** 553.
31. Rutherford R, Jones D, Bergentz S, *et al.* The efficacy of dextran 40 in preventing early post-op thrombosis following difficult lower extremity bypass. *J Vasc Surg* 1984; **1:** 765.

32. McCollum C, Kenchington G, Alexander C, Franks PJ, Greenhalgh RM. PTFE or HUV for femoro-popliteal bypass: a multi-centre trial. *Eur J Vasc Surg* 1991; **5:** 435–43.

33. Smith FCT, Tsang GMK, Watson HR, Shearman CP. Iloprost reduces peripheral resistance during femoro-distal reconstruction. *Eur J Vasc Surg* 1992; **6:** 194–8.

9

Sepsis

John Chamberlain

Infection following arterial surgery may result in catastrophe, particularly where prosthetic grafts are involved. Diagnosis and treatment of such infection is often difficult and it is therefore imperative that every method possible is used to prevent it. Over the last 35 years, patients with both aneurysmal and occlusive arterial disease have benefited from the implantation of vascular prostheses. However, even with the development of modern materials infection still occurs in a significant percentage of patients which may result in tissue death with subsequent disability, and not infrequently loss of life. This chapter will review current views on the diagnosis, management and prevention of these infections.

The incidence of wound infection reported after arterial operations varies from 1% to over 20%. The actual infection of prosthetic material is lower than this, being in the region of 1% in most series, but has been reported in up to 6% of cases. In a review of 2000 cases in which prosthetic material had been implanted, Szilagyi *et al.*[1] reported an overall incidence of graft infection of 1.1%. This was higher in femoropopliteal bypass with an incidence of 2.5%. The mortality rate of those patients with infected grafts was 35% with an amputation rate of 25%. This important study set a baseline for future comparison but it was carried out before the era of routine antibiotic prophylaxis. Operations requiring groin incisions are particularly associated with infection due not only to direct contamination, but also to division of infected inguinal glands and lymphatics. Johnson *et al.*[2] reported a 33% groin wound infection rate but of these only 2% had prosthetic graft involvement.

Over the last two decades the incidence of graft infection has fallen, probably owing to the routine use of antibiotic prophylaxis and to improved surgical techniques. As with other 'clean' surgical procedures, the expected wound infection rate should be less than 2%. With antibiotic prophylaxis, Goldstone and Moore[3] have shown that graft infection can be reduced from 4.1% to 1.5%, and a number of other reports indicate that prosthetic graft infection can be reduced from around 12% to less than 1%. Many graft infections occur late, which makes the true incidence difficult to determine. The reasons for this are uncertain but may be related to initial suppression of bacterial flora by prophylactic antibiotics. However, porous graft materials may sequestrate organisms, protecting them from host defences.

Microbiology

Infection following arterial operations may be due to almost any organism, but *Staphylococcus aureus* is the most common. Szilagyi *et al.*[1] in their initial series reported that most were due to *Staph. aureus*, the second most common group being Gram-negative bacteria. Gram-positive infections tend to occur soon after operation, but infection due to other organisms may occur later. Beard and Wilmshurst have summarized the bacteria implicated in prosthetic graft infection (Table 9.1). In recent years *Staph. epidermidis* has been recognized as being frequently related to late infection.[4] Strachan[5] emphasizes that there should be greater awareness of the possible presence of this organism in graft infections, particularly those involving the groin. He emphasizes the need for isolation and identification techniques to separate contaminants from pathogenic organisms, and warns that prophylactic antibiotics may encourage the emergence of resistant *Staph. epidermidis* strains.

In the presence of suppuration it may not be too difficult to obtain culture and sensitivity of the organism. However, in more chronic and late infections, particularly if they are deep infections associated with a graft, this may be more difficult. Every effort should be made to obtain appropriate culture material even, if necessary, with aspiration of fluid or tissue from around the graft using CT or ultrasound guided techniques. Bandyk[4] reported results of antibiotic sensitivity in *Staph.* epidermidis: a large

Table 9.1 Principal infecting organisms

Organism	Incidence in graft infections (%)
Staphylococci (coagulase +ve and −ve)	44
Proteus genus	11
Escherichia coli	10
Streptococcus faecalis	8
Pseudomonas genus	7
Serratia marcescens	5
Klebsiella and *Corynebacterium* genera	4
Bacteroides genus	3
Streptococcus viridans	1
Diphtheroides	1
Salmonella genus	1

From Beard JD and Wilmshurst CC. In: *Vascular Surgery – Current Questions*, Barras D'Sa (ed). Oxford: Butterworth–Heineman, 1991.

number are resistant to antibiotics, particularly penicillin, but all were sensitive to gentamicin and 91% to cephalosporins.

Clinical presentation

The clinical presentation varies greatly. It may be early or late and can be associated with both general and local symptoms and signs.

As with any other infection following operation, there may be early signs of wound infection, with erythema, local tenderness and swelling and discharge of serosanguinous fluid or even pus. This may be associated with anastomotic dehiscence causing haemorrhage or a false aneurysm. All of the systemic signs of infection, including fever, tachycardia and hypotension, may also be present. Infection may be associated with occlusion of the graft and disappearance of pulses. Distal septic emboli with mircro-infarcts at the extremity of the limb can also occur. Early infection in deep abdominal prostheses may be associated with local signs and abdominal tenderness. There may be evidence of retroperitoneal bleeding or even external blood loss via an enteric fistula. Local wound infection may or may not progress to sloughing of the wound, with deep infection and subsequent exposure of the graft.

The presence of a bloody discharge from an operation wound associated with prosthetic insertion is pathognomic of graft infection. Gastrointestinal bleeding in a patient who has had a graft inserted should be assumed to be associated with an aortoenteric fistula until proved other wise by appropriate investigations, such as CT scanning and if necessary laparotomy.

Late infections are often extremely difficult to diagnose. There may be little systemic upset with occasionally just a moderately raised temperature. The patient may feel generally unwell. There may be little in the way of local signs, although there is sometimes local tenderness over previous wounds or there may be an anastomotic aneurysm. In any patient who has had a vascular prosthesis inserted and presents with vague symptoms, graft infection should be considered and investigated.

Fortunately a large number of wound infections that are associated with the initial operation remain superficial and respond to local treatment without subsequent prosthetic involvement.

Diagnosis

Diagnosis of graft infection can be difficult. Suspicion may arise from a knowledge of the risk factors present during previous management of the patient, but in order to establish the diagnosis it is usually necessary to rely on complex investigations. Even when in a relatively superficial wound the graft is exposed, further investigation may be required to establish the true extent of the infection, and to define whether this is localized or involves the entire length of the graft. This can have an important bearing on management.

Simple tests such as white cell count and erythrocyte sedimentation rate may be raised in cases with systemic upset, but often they are normal. Blood cultures are useful particularly in patients who have intermittent fever. In patients who have aortic grafts where there is a suspicion of enteric fistula, examination of stools for blood may give a clue as to the nature of the infection. In such patients upper GI endoscopy may be helpful in excluding other causes of gastrointestinal bleeding.

Most helpful are various imaging techniques. A plain X-ray film may show the presence of soft tissue shadows, including fluid collections or even gas alongside the region of a graft; this is indicative of infection. Modern scanning techniques have proved particularly helpful in the assessment of these patients. Ultrasound scanning,[6] computerized tomography and MRI[7] may all demonstrate the graft, and the presence of fluid or gas around it. The first two techniques are now available in most hospitals.

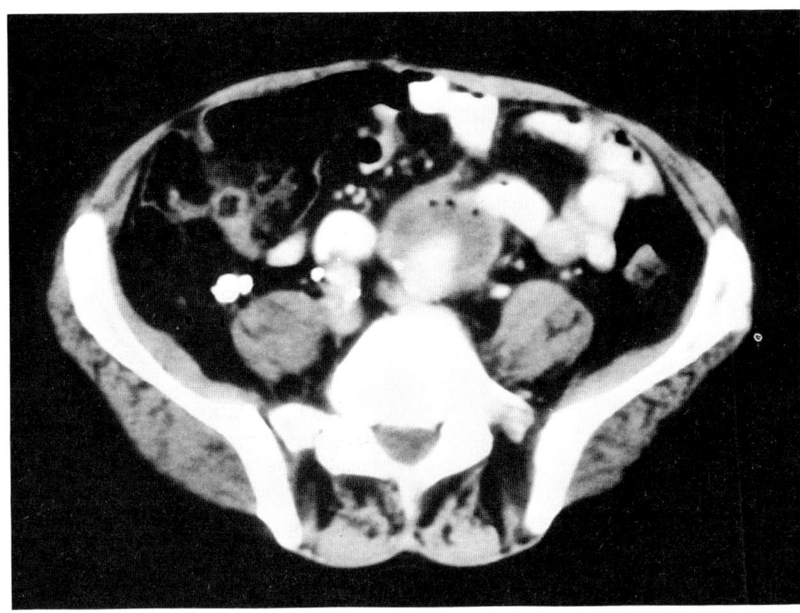

Fig. 9.1 CT scan showing fluid and gas in a periaortic space above upper aortic anastomoses.

Fig. 9.1 shows fluid and gas associated with an infected graft and aorto-enteric fistula.

If there is any doubt as to the nature of a peri-graft fluid collection, then needle aspiration of this may be carried out with ultrasound or CT scanning guidance.[8] This fluid can be examined bacteriologically. Such aspiration should be carried out under careful aseptic control as there is also the possibility of introducing infection by these techniques. Both indium-labelled and technecium-labelled leucocyte imaging have been shown to be of value.[9,10] The latter test has been found useful as a rapid method for assessing the presence of graft infection (Fig. 9.2).

Angiography has been of relatively little value in assessing graft infection. It rarely shows any evidence of aortoenteric fistula but may demonstrate the extent of graft occlusion associated with infection, or may show the presence of pseudoaneurysms

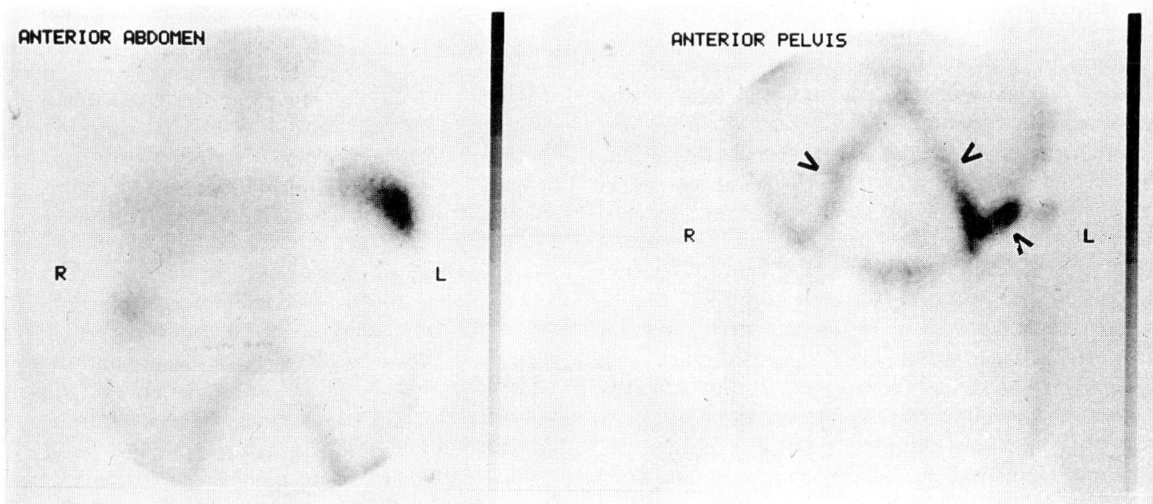

Fig. 9.2 Technetium $^{99}Tc^{m}$ hexametazine scan (HMPAO) showing infection in an aortofemoral graft with maximum activity in the left groin.

which are perhaps more easily diagnosed by other scanning techniques. However, if further reconstruction is contemplated then angiography will be required either pre- or perioperatively, particularly to assess distal vessel patency.

To determine the diagnosis of graft sepsis, a number of the above techniques are often used and in some patients re-exploration of a sinus or even the graft itself may be necessary to exclude infection.

Treatment

Once infection occurs it is unlikely to resolve without interventional measures. The management of these patients falls into two categories, these being general supportive care of the patient and local management of the infected wound or prosthesis.

General management

Early infection may be apparent within a few days of a major vascular operation. Some patients might be in a catabolic state and require full general support, including correction of fluid balance and treatment of any systemic disease, particularly cardiac and respiratory conditions. Adequate nourishment should be provided, if necessary, by intravenous means in very ill patients. Diabetes should be well controlled. Complications associated particularly with vascular operations (such as ischaemic ulcers on pressure points) should be prevented.

Every effort should be made to isolate the infecting organism. Repeated swabbing of wounds for bacteriological culture, blood cultures and needle aspiration of any potentially infected sites must be carried out under aseptic conditions. If there is any local cellulitis or deep infection, and particularly if it is suspected that the graft is involved, then systemic antibiotics will be required, usually given intravenously in the first instance to be sure of adequate serum levels. While awaiting cultures, antibiotics may have to be chosen based on likely causative organisms. In the early days after operation, *Staph. aureus* or coliforms are the most likely infecting organisms. These may be treated by flucloxacillin or a cephalosporin together with gentamicin, although care must be taken with the latter antibiotic, particularly if the patient has renal impairment. When culture and sensitivity of the organisms is obtained, antibiotic therapy should be changed if necessary.

These general measures are particularly important to reduce morbidity and mortality from any further operation which may need to be quite extensive.

Local management of superficial wound infection

If the wound infection, particularly involving groin incisions, is superficial without any associated cellulitis, then local antiseptic dressings (particularly the use of povidone-iodine) may be all that is required. However, once the infection extends down to the graft then it will not usually resolve without more radical treatment. This may involve removal of all infective prosthetic material with revascularization of the extremity by alternative bypass. If the graft is occluded, removal will still be necessary to remove the focus of infection although in some cases revascularization may not be necessary.

Should reconstruction be necessary after an infected graft is removed, then it is desirable that any new graft is placed well away from the infected site, usually by an extra-anatomic approach and where possible using autogenous vein. Short segments of larger arteries can be replaced using strips of vein to construct a large-diameter tube or a spiral vein graft can be constructed.[11] It may be possible in some patients to carry out thromboendarterectomy of the original native vessel, thus revascularizing the extremity when an infected graft has to be removed, the previous arteriotomies being repaired using a saphenous vein patch. This may be particularly appropriate when an aortofemoral graft is removed followed by disobliteration of the native iliac vessels.

Aortoiliac/femoral graft infections

These major infections are life-threatening and are often associated with haemorrhage from anastomotic sites. Complete removal of the graft is nearly always necessary. The patients should be well prepared for operation which, if possible, should be carried out electively. The previous incision should be reopened, the graft excised and the aorta closed, oversewn and sealed off by omentum. Femoral arteriotomies should be closed with vein patches. It may be possible to carry out a disobliteration procedure to revascularize the lower limb but this is not often easily done. Occasionally if the infection is localized to one segment of the graft then local excision and *in situ* replacement may be feasible, particularly if associated with an aortoenteric fistula with little sign of gross infection.[12] However, once the graft is removed, revascularization of the lower limbs is necessary by an extra-anatomic (usually axillobifemoral) bypass. The distal anastomoses should be taken on to the profunda or superficial femoral artery below the previous groin incisions. Some authors advise that an axillofemoral graft should be inserted and then the infected aortoiliac graft removed 3–5 days later. However, this does risk infection of the new prosthesis and most surgeons would probably carry out both procedures at the same time. It is usual to remove the infected graft and then proceed directly to an axillobifemoral bypass. It is important that the original graft and all of the infected tissues undergo microbiological analysis.

Aortic graft infection is often associated with an enteric fistula. This sometimes needs an emergency operation because of massive haemorrhage. The first step is control of the aorta, placing the clamp in the supracoeliac position initially with removal of the prosthesis and oversewing of the aortic stump. The aortic stump should be closed with two layers of monofilament Prolene and covered with omentum as there is always a risk of stump infection and dehisience after this procedure. Complete excision of all infected tissue and appropriate intensive antibiotic treatment is required together with local irrigation with antiseptics such as povidone-iodine or antibiotic solutions. The intestinal fistulous opening should be carefully closed and separated from the aortic stump by omentum. The morbidity and mortality from these revisional procedures is high and some patients may be considered too unfit for them. However, it is unlikely that the patient will survive without operation.

Other methods of treating infected abdominal aortic grafts have been tried and there are reports of successful treatment by percutaneous catheter irrigation. The catheter is inserted under CT or ultrasound control into the perigraft cavity. Antibiotic solutions are irrigated through this and may, in the patient who has less gross infection, enable the graft to heal.[13] However, such treatment rarely provides permanent resolution of the infection.

Groin infections

Infections in the groin, related to aortofemoral or femoropopliteal bypass grafts, are the most common. Superficial wound infections are also common here, and as has already been mentioned, these may respond to local treatment. If, however, the graft are exposed, then usually its removal and revascularization of the limb is necessary. If the infection in a femoropopliteal graft involves the whole length of that graft, then the latter should be removed and replaced with a vein graft if that is feasible. Some patients may survive on collateral circulation and so avoid immediate reconstruction.

If graft infections seem to be localized to the groin and do not extend down the entire length of the graft, then local treatment may be of value. Locally infected grafts may be successfully treated by insertion of gentamicin beads after thorough debridement.[14] Other authors have achieved success using local irrigation with antibiotic or povidone-iodine solutions. Simple repeat packing with iodine-soaked gauze in an open wound may eventually lead to granulation and coverage of the graft. In one series[15] of 56 patients with localized groin wound infection after arterial operations, 30 had superficial and 19 deep wound infections. The remaining patients had infected lymph fistulae. In the patients with superficial infections, the majority settled completely after treatment with specific antibiotics initialy given intravenously and then orally for up to 6 weeks. Overall, 16 patients required debridement and excision of the necrotic wound edges. Graft excision was necessary in 7 patients, 5 of whom required an extra-anatomic bypass. Graft excision was more frequent with Dacron or PTFE than for vein. These results suggest that many groin infections if *localized* can be managed conservatively and radical graft excision is only necessary for a few cases.

Other alternative procedures include the use of an obturator bypass. In a study comparing this method with local biologic cover using local muscle flaps, better healing and fewer complications resulted from bypass.[16] Calligaro *et al.*[17] reported 28 patients with 33 groin infections and managed to preserve complete grafts in 11 of these cases treated locally. In 16 cases they were able to carry out subtotal graft removal at the groin combined with an extra-anatomic aortodistal bypass. They emphasized the need to carry out full operative wound excision and debridement of all infected necrotic tissue which often resulted in a lengthy hospital stay. For many of these patients, after removing all dead tissue, and irrigating the wound with iodine or antibiotics at frequent intervals, the entire graft was covered and the wound healed by delayed secondary healing or by split skin grafts placed on to healthy granulation tissue. It is quite clear that some patients can be treated by these local measures. Anastomotic bleeding, however, is an absolute indication for removal of the graft and appropriate revascularization where necessary.

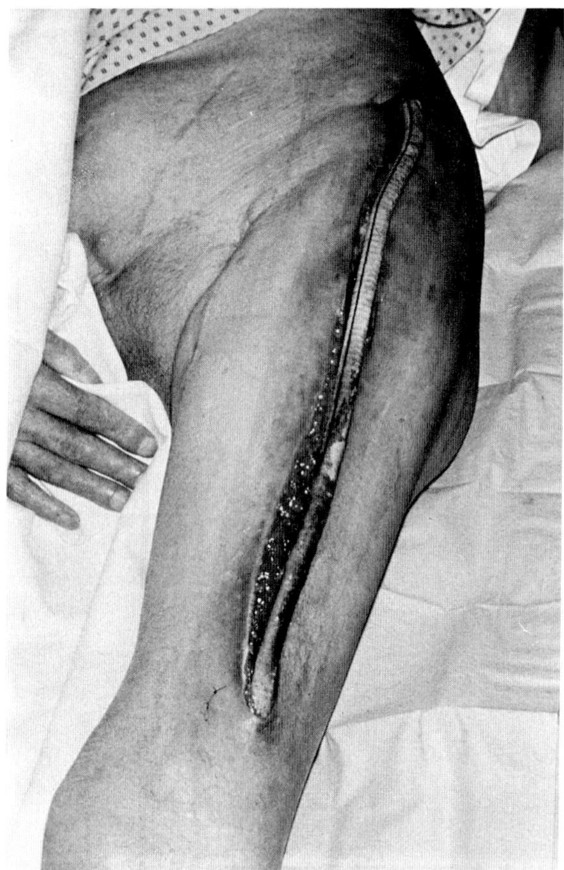

Fig. 9.3 Secondary iliopopliteal bypass with extruded Dacron graft. (Courtesy NAG Jones, Freeman Hospital, Newcastle upon Tyne.)

The more distal infected wounds in the lower limbs are usually superficial, often associated with skin necrosis and may be treated by local therapy and antiseptics. Appropriate antibiotics are given with debridement of the wound, and if the underlying prosthesis is vein then eventually healing will occur with granulation tissue. Occasionally, surgical excision of the necrotic skin and resuture and skin grafting may be necessary. Deep infection of distal wounds usually presents with wound breakdown and the presence of pus within 7–10 days of the bypass being inserted. There may be little systemic upset, but often the infection is associated with haemorrhage. In this situation the wound should be explored and all necrotic tissue removed. If the prosthesis is patent, local antiseptics or irrigation with antibiotics may resolve the infection. Often the graft needs to be removed and a further bypass carried more distally, preferably using vein. Massive haemorrhage, of course, requires urgent operation and ligation of any bleeding vessel to save life followed by revascularization where possible. Even using all of these techniques the morbidity and mortality associated with graft infection remains high. Mortality still ranges from 10–25% and many of these patients come to amputation. Aggressive treatment is therefore vital if these catastrophic complications are to be avoided.

Other alternatives for the management of localized infections of vascular bypass grafts particularly in the groin region include the use of rotational muscle flaps[18] and subsequent skin grafts (see Figs 9.3 and 9.4). If the wound is adequately debrided and there are repeated negative cultures from the wound, then rotational muscle flaps either from the rectus abdominis or from rectus femoris can be turned to cover the wound. If clean granulation tissue has covered the graft, then split skin may be applied. The vascular surgeon should seek the help and guidance of an experienced plastic surgeon in the management of these cases. With care, even extensive graft exposure may be covered.

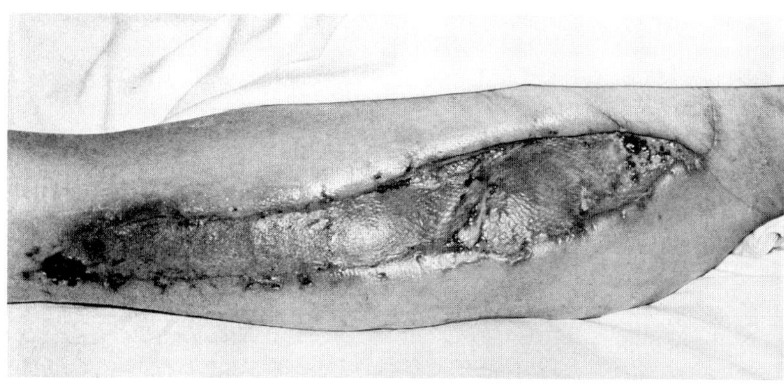

Fig. 9.4 Extruded iliopopliteal graft covered with rectus femoris and split skin grafts. (Courtesy NAG Jones and N McLean, Freeman Hospital, Newcastle upon Tyne.)

Prevention

In view of the serious consequences of infection in arterial surgery, prevention is most important. This is particularly so following insertion of prosthetic vascular grafts such as Dacron, PTFE or biological grafts which usually have a Dacron mesh support. Vein grafts are usually more tolerant to infection but nevertheless the same principles apply.

The usual preoperative methods should be taken to prevent contamination of the graft. Direct contamination usually occurs at the time of the operation and may result from handling with contaminated instruments or the graft being allowed to come into contact with infected tissues such as skin or bowel. It is most important that grafts should be handled carefully and free from contact with all potentially infected tissue. The prosthesis should be handled with instruments as far as possible.

In order to avoid both wound and deeper infections, many attempts have been made to minimize infection from the patient's skin. Total body 'disinfection' with preoperative chlorhexidine baths has been tried, but seem to have little effect on the eventual infection rate.[19] However, good general skin hygiene prior to operation is obviously desirable. Good surgical technique with avoidance of haematomas and of transecting lymph glands and vessels in the groin is particularly important.[20]

Another source of graft infection may be bacteraemia occuring during the procedure. Buckels *et al.* were able to culture organisms from the aortic wall in patients undergoing abdominal aortic aneurysm operations.[21] On this basis a number of surgeons have advocated soaking the prosthesis in antibiotic solutions. However, this is not effective as the antibiotic tends to be washed off the graft very rapidly. Recently, Dacron grafts with a gelatine seal have become available. Rifampicin can be bonded to these grafts and retains significant anti-staphylococcal activity for some weeks.[22]

A number of studies have now shown that high-dose prophylactic antibiotics given intravenously immediately prior to the operation are effective in reducing graft infection.[23] Herbst and his colleagues demonstrated that in patients undergoing elective vascular operation prophylaxis with cefuroxime was effective in keeping graft infection to a minimum. The use of a regimen effective against the most likely infecting organisms is now established practice. The American College of Surgeons' committee on the control of surgical infections recommends that for clean surgical wounds in an ideal operating theatre environment the infection rate should be less than 5%. The committee feels that prophylactic antibiotics cannot be recommended except when the consequent infection will be grave or where permanent implants are inserted.[24] Obviously insertion of vascular prostheses falls into this category in the same way as insertion of an artificial hip joint or a prosthetic heart valve. A number of studies have clearly demonstrated the efficacy of prophylactic antibiotics in keeping wound infections down to low levels. As the most common organisms are staphylococci, such studies have concentrated on prophylaxis for this organism; however, certain coliforms are also prevalent. My regimen is 1 g of flucloxaxillin with 120 mg of gentamicin IV at the beginning of the operation, and then flucloxacillin for 24–48 hours or until any drains are removed. A cephalosporin may be equally effective.

Other factors which should be taken into account in the prevention of infection include the avoidance of operating on patients electively if there are other infections present. Urine and respiratory infections should be dealt with aggressively and operation deferred until these have been resolved. There is some evidence that groin infections are increased if the operation is carried out shortly after angiography which has been carried out by a transfemoral approach. If reconstruction is urgent, angiography should be carried out through the opposite groin.

Simultaneous nonvascular operations should also probably be avoided as there is always a risk, particularly in abdominal surgery, of infection of the graft. If other pathology is found at the time of laparotomy then this should usually take precedence over the arterial operation.

There is some argument about the use of suction drainage. If drains are used they should not be laid directly against the graft. A recent trial[25] showed no difference in lymph leakage, haematoma or wound infection rates whether or not suction drains were used.

Conclusions

Infection following arterial surgery is an infrequent but serious problem. Prevention is the ideal and all care should be taken both preoperatively and during the operation to prevent sepsis. The use of prophylactic antibiotics is now mandatory and has been shown to be effective in reducing infection rates. If infection does occur urgent intensive investigation and aggressive treatment are required. Delay may allow local infection to become more widespread. Once a prosthetic graft is infected, removal of part or all of the it is usually necessary and few patients will escape with local therapy alone.

Recommended further reading

1. Bernhard VM, Towne JB (eds). *Complications in Vascular Surgery.* New York: Grune & Statton, 1985.
2. Baird RN. Infective complications following reconstructive arterial surgery. In: *Surgical Management of Vascular Disease*, Bell PRF, Jamieson CW, Ruckley CV (eds). Philadelphia: WB Saunders, 1992.

References

1. Szilagyi DE, Smith RF, Elliott JP, Vrandecic MP. Infection in arterial reconstruction with synthetic grafts. *Ann Surg* 1972; **176:** 321–3.
2. Johnson JA, Cogbill TH, Strutt PJ, Gundersen AL. Wound complications after infrainguinal bypass. *Arch Surg* 1988; **123:** 859–62.
3. Goldstone J, Moore NS. Infection in vascular prostheses. *Am J Surg* 1974; **128:** 225–33.
4. Bandyk DF, Berni GA, Thick BL, Towne JB. Aortofemoral graft infection due to Staphylococcus epidermidis. *Arch Surg* 1984; **119:** 102–8.
5. Strachan CJI. Current thoughts on Staphylococcus epidermidis in vascular surgery. *J Hosp Infect* 1988; **11** (Suppl B): 33–41.
6. Gooding GAW, Effeney DJ, Goldstone J. The aortofemoral graft, detection and identification of healing complications by ultrasonography. *Surgery* 1981; **89:** 94–101.
7. Olofsson PA, Auffermann W, Higgins CB, Rabahie GN, Tavars N, Stoney RJ. Diagnosis of prosthetic aortic graft infection by magnetic resonance imaging. *J Vasc Surg* 1988; **8:** 99–105.
8. Rabmovici R, Fields S, Bertatzky Y, Shinkin EE, Romanoff HCT. Guided peri-aortic fluid aspiration diagnosing aortic graft infection. *J Cardiovasc Surg* 1988; **29:** 318–19.
9. Reilly DT, Grigg MJ, Cunningham DA, Thomas EJ, Mansfield AO. Vascular graft infection: the role of indium scanning. *Eur J Vasc Surg* 1989; **3:** 393–7.
10. Insall RL, Jones NAG, Chamberlain J, Lambert D, Keavey PM. A new isotopic technique for detecting prosthetic arterial graft infection: $^{99}Tc^{m}$-hexametazime-labelled leucocyte imaging. *Br J Surg* 1990; **77:** 1295–8.
11. Fowl RJ, Merhn KD, Sax HC, Kempezinski RF. Use of autologous spiral vein grafts for vascular reconstructions in contaminated fields. *J Vasc Surg* 1988; **8:** 442–6.
12. Jacobs MJHM, Reul GJ, Gregorie I, Cooley DA. In-situ replacement and extra-anatomic bypass for the treatment of infected abdominal aortic grafts. *Eur J Vasc Surg* 1991; **5:** 83–6.
13. Matley PJ, Beningfield SJ, Lourens S, Immelman EJ. Successful treatment of infected thoraco-abdominal aortic graft by percutaneous catheter drainage. *J Vasc Surg* 1991; **13:** 513–15.
14. Bailey IS, Bindred NJ, Pearson HJ, Bell PRF. Successful treatment of an infected vascular graft with gentamicin beads. *Eur J Vasc Surg* 1987; **1:** 143–4.
15. Navington DP, Houghton PWJ, Baird RN, Horrocks M. Groin wound infection after arterial surgery. *Br J Surg* 1991; **78:** 617–19.
16. Kretschmer G, Niederle B, Hule I, Karner J, Piza-katzer H, Polterauer P, Walzer LR. Groin infections following vascular surgery: obturator bypass (BYP) versus 'Bidogic Coverage' (TRP) – a comparative analysis. *Eur J Vasc Surg* 1989; **3:** 25–9.
17. Calligaro KD, Veith FJ, Gupta SK, Ascer T, Dietzek AM, Franco CD, Wengerter KR. A modified method of management of prosthetic graft infections involving an anastomosis to the common femoral artery. *J Vasc Surg* 1990; **11:** 485–92.
18. Mixter RC, Turnipseed WD, Smith DJ, Acher CW, Rao VK, Dibbell DG. Rotational muscle flaps: a new technique for covering infected vascular grafts. *J Vasc Surg* 1989; **9:** 472–8.
19. Earnshaw JJ, Berridge DC, Slack RCB, Makin GS, Hopkinson BR. Do pre-operative chlorhexidine baths reduce the risk of infection after vascular reconstruction? *Eur J Vasc Surg* 1983; **3:** 323–6.
20. Rubin JR, Malone JM, Goldstone J. Role of the lymphatic system in acute arterial prosthetic graft infections. *J Vasc Surg* 1985; **2:** 92–5.
21. Buckels JAC, Fielding JWL, Black J, Ashton F, Slaney G. Significance of positive bacterial cultures from aortic aneurysm contents. *Br J Surg* 1985; **72:** 440–2.
22. Strachan CJL, Newson SWB, Ashton TR. The clinical use of an antibiotic-bonded graft. *Eur J Vasc Surg* 1991; **5:** 627–32.
23. Herbst A, Kamme C, Norzren L, Quarfordt P, Ribbe E, Thörne J. Infections and antibiotic prophylaxis in reconstructive vascular surgery. *Eur J Vasc Surg* 1989; **3:** 303–7.
24. Altemeier WA, Burke JF, Pruitt BA, for the American College of Surgeons. *Control of Infection in Surgical Patients.* Philadelphia: JB Lippincott, 1976.
25. Dunlop MG, Fox JN, Stonebridge PA, Clason AE, Ruckley CV. Vacuum drainage of groin wounds after vascular surgery – a controlled trial. *Br J Surg* 1990; **77:** 542–63.

10

Amputations

Ken Callum

Should amputations be done by vascular surgeons?

Eighty to ninety per cent of amputations are done for peripheral vascular disease, including those patients with diabetes.[1,2] The remainder are done for trauma, tumours, deformities, chronic infections, etc. In the last century Sir William Ferguson said: 'amputation – one of the meanest and yet one of the greatest operations in surgery: mean, when resorted to where better may be done, great as the only step to give comfort and prolong life'. He must have had vascular surgeons in mind since it would be mean indeed to amputate a patient's leg when a straightforward bypass might save it. No patient should have a major amputation for ischaemia without having been assessed by an experienced vascular surgeon to be certain that nothing can be done to save the leg. Some clinicians may refer the patient to an orthopaedic surgeon for amputation, but it must make for better continuity for the same clinician to look after the patient. This is particularly true when, for example, a patient has had a failed bypass where a synthetic graft has been used. Under these circumstances it may be advisable to remove at least the distal part of the graft so that it is not close to the stump in case wound breakdown occurs. Thus it is right for the initial assessment and subsequent operations to be done by a vascular surgeon.

Limb salvage versus amputation

A successful limb salvage procedure is obviously preferable to a major amputation, and a recently reported study from a district general hospital[3] showed a similar operative and 6-month mortality, but a considerable advantage in favour of vascular reconstruction over amputation in other respects. The bed occupancy was much shorter and only 12% of patients having had a vascular reconstruction required long-term care compared with 58% of amputees. Ninety per cent of patients having had a vascular reconstruction were independently mobile at 6 months compared with 42% of amputees. Other studies[4,5] have shown similar results and it has been estimated that the cost of a successful vascular reconstruction is less than that for amputation,[6] particularly when you consider the high cost of supply and maintenance of artificial limbs, and the need for prolonged physiotherapy.

Does failed bypass result in a higher level of amputation?

There is conflicting evidence on this. Some of the earlier studies suggested that it does,[7,8] more recent studies have shown no difference[9,10] although the mortality is probably slightly higher.[11] Also, healing may take longer where an amputation is preceeded by a long incision down a limb for a femoro-popliteal bypass.

In practice you cannot expect every graft to succeed, but it is reasonable when operating for critical ischaemia to expect an early graft patency at 30 days of about 90%, with a 2-year patency in the region of 75%. When grafts fail, an amputation usually results if the limb was really threatened at the time of the reconstruction. If results are better than this then almost certainly some patients who are suitable for reconstruction are being refused, and if they are significantly worse then too many patients are being submitted to procedures that are doomed to fail. Obviously, it is a matter of clinical judgement as to which limbs to try to salvage. This will only come with time and experience.

Mortality

A number of studies have shown similar mortality for arterial reconstruction and amputation, both for 30-day operative mortality and survival after a few years.[3,12,13] It is often said that if a study of arterial reconstruction is reported where the percentage of patients still alive after 5 years is better than 40% then many of the patients probably had their operation done for claudication rather than for critical ischaemia. In fact, the 5-year patient survival in a number of studies has been more like 25%,[14,15] showing that ischaemic gangrene carries a prognosis as bad as many cancers. The majority of deaths are due to ischaemic heart or cerebrovascular disease.

Operative mortality varies with the level of amputation. At the above-knee level it is probably between 15 and 20%, although published results vary between 3 and 42%.[16,17] For below-knee, Grit–Stokes and through-knee amputations the rate is probably nearer 10% with a slightly narrower variation in reported series. The reason is partly due to higher levels of amputation being required for patients with more severe ischaemia. These patients are generally poorer operative risks. However, the Gritti–Stokes amputation can almost always be done as an alternative to an above-knee amputation and does seem to carry a lower mortality. This may be due to less trauma from muscle cutting and blood loss.[18,19]

Walking and the level of amputation

It is difficult to be absolutely certain of walking rates after amputation in an elderly group of patients. The figures vary widely in different reported series. Mobility grading may be classified as in Table 10.1 Probably only 40% of those patients with an above-knee amputation would have reasonable mobility (i.e. groups 3–5), whereas at the below-knee level the figure is about 80% and for the through-knee or Gritti–Stokes amputation about 60%. However, a recent report of amputations performed in the South East Thames Region suggested that only 5% became totally free of a wheelchair.[20]

When considering bilateral above-knee amputees only a very small proportion will be ambulant. Patients with bilateral below-knee amputation, however, will probably have something in the region of 50–60% chance of a reasonable ambulation, particularly where there is a gap of a year or more between amputations so that they have had a chance to learn to walk well with one artificial limb.

Table 10.1 Mobility grading

0	Bedridden (cannot transfer from wheelchair)
1	Wheelchair mobility
2	Limited household ambulation
3	Unlimited household ambulation
4	Limited community ambulation
5	Unlimited community ambulation

Deciding on the level of amputation

It is obviously desirable to amputate at the lowest level that will heal. In practice the most important decision is whether or not a below-knee amputation will succeed, although occasionally one may have a similar decision about a forefoot amputation. With all the modern technology it ought to be possible to obtain an accurate prediction as to whether or not a particular amputation will heal.

Methods include study of the arteriogram, ankle systolic pressure,[14] transcutaneous oxygen pressure ($TcPO_2$),[21] skin perfusion pressure,[22,23] skin thermography,[23] and the laser Doppler flowmeter.[23,24] De Frang *et al.*[11] have provided an excellent review of these techniques and conclude: 'The reported sensitivities and specificities are inadequate to recommend the clinical use of any of them in selecting amputation level.' However, they go on to point out that current healing rates based on clinical judgement alone exceed 70% for forefoot amputations and 90% for major lower-limb amputations. They conclude that one should 'select the most distal possible level based on clinical judgement alone'.

It is important to remember that not all patients with ischaemic gangrene will need a major amputation. Some cases where the patient's pain can be controlled with analgesics and there is no infection may have spontaneous healing, presumably due to the development of collaterals. In diabetics with small vessel disease and infection, amputation of a toe – perhaps with the adjacent 'ray' to include part of the metatarsal and infected tendon and fibrous tissue – may be all that is required. Obviously, if a patient has uncontrollable rest pain or extensive gangrene, which investigations have shown are not amenable to reconstruction, then a major amputation will be required. Sometimes this may need to be done urgently because of infection or general toxicity caused by the gangrene.

Preoperative preparation

Patients requiring amputation have a high incidence of other medical problems, in particular ischaemic heart disease, cerebrovascular disease, chronic obstructive airways disease and diabetes. Adequate analgesia should be given as this will encourage joint movements and help prevent soft tissue contractures. Bed rest, with elevation of the limb if possible, will help to reduce oedema.

It will not usually be possible to clear an ulcer or infected gangrene prior to operation, which may indeed sometimes be needed urgently to stop the infection spreading. A swab should be taken of any infected areas on the foot so that the organism and antibiotic sensitivities are known prior to operation if possible. When an amputation stump becomes infected it is nearly always with the same organism as that found in the infected lesion in the foot.

Even when there is no obvious infection present, prophylactic antibiotics should be given perioperatively. There is a strong argument for giving penicillin or metronidazole in the absence of other infection to prevent gas gangrene of the amputation stump, which may develop as a result of contamination with bowel organisms.

The rehabilitation team

This consists of the surgical and nursing staff, rehabilitation medicine consultant, physiotherapist, occupational therapist and prosthetist (they do not like being called 'limb fitters' nowadays). In many cases a social worker may be needed, and in some a counsellor/psychologist may be helpful. Obviously the support of the family is very important. Any patient well rehabilitated after an amputation may also be able to reassure and encourage. Preoperative involvement of the team is ideal if there is time and may be helpful in selecting the amputation level in difficult cases.

Physiotherapy

The physiotherapist should always see the patient *before* the operation, both to try to prevent or treat flexion contractures and build up the strength in other muscles. Following the operation, early and intensive physiotherapy is required; this is particularly true in the case of a below-knee amputation, where all the members of the ward staff should encourage the patient to straighten the knee. Adequate analgesia continues to be very important. There is no one regimen of analgesia for every patient as the choice and dosage of drugs varies with the size, age and general condition of the patient. An epidural anaesthetic for a day or two before and after amputation is helpful and recent studies suggest that this reduces the incidence of phantom pain.

Counselling

Psychological problems are more likely when an amputation has been needed as a result of trauma, when there may be resentment about the cause of the accident or the early medical treatment. In the case of children there may be parental guilt. These problems are fortunately much less common when amputation is done for ischaemia, since the majority of patients have suffered severe pain, often for quite a long time. There is a saying that patients should 'earn their amputation' by having the pain for some time before operation, and although this is a very hard attitude there may be an element truth in it.

Certainly, in all cases a careful and sympathetic explanation about the reason for the operation and what the future is likely to hold is essential, particularly where the amputation does have to be done urgently after a short history.

Amputations considered at each level

Toes and forefoot

If the extent of the gangrene involves the distal half of the toe or less, then it is probably wise to leave it alone to separate over some weeks, especially in diabetics. Where no reconstruction has been done it is certainly safer to leave alone, and conversely where one has been done the improvement is often greater than might be thought initially.

Where more than half of the toe is gangrenous then it will save time to do an amputation as it can take months for a whole toe to separate. These can be done under digital nerve block, cutting through healthy skin closest to the line of demarcation. The bone will then need to be nibbled back so that the skin flaps can close easily. If a patient is diabetic or the toe infected it is safer to leave the wound open. In other circumstances the skin can be gently closed, possibly with a Steristrip.

'Ray amputation'

This is a drainage amputation for infected diabetic toes and is particularly useful where the infection extends proximally. The latter occurs more commonly on the sole of the foot although it may occur on the dorsum. The relevant toes are excised, a line of excision is carried back through the infected tissue until healthy, uninfected tissue is reached. The underlying metatarsal (plus any infected tendons and

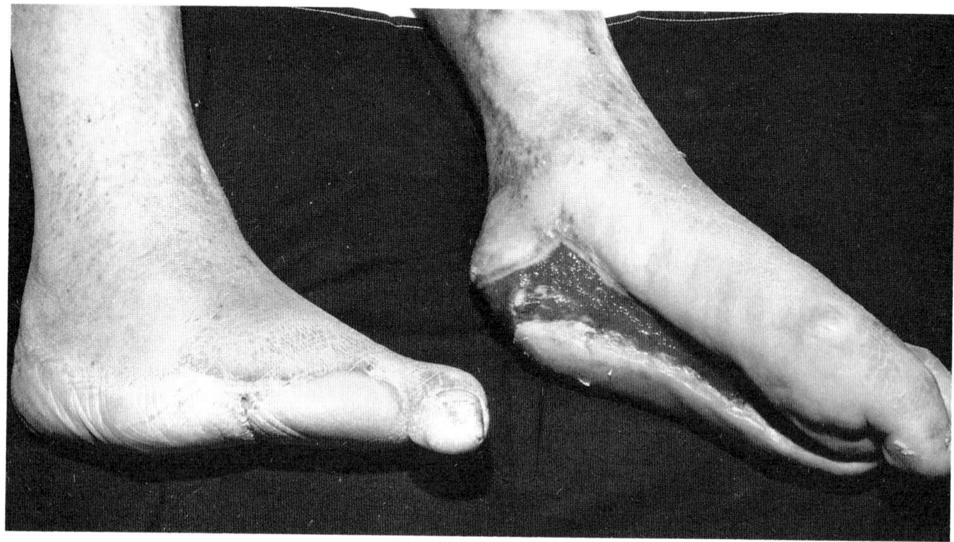

Fig. 10.1 Extended 'ray amputation' in a diabetic. Despite being so radical and on the sole, this went on to heal and the patient was able to walk satisfactorily.

fibrous tissue) is excised. It is very important to avoid damage to the next digital artery which may result in the adjacent toe becoming gangrenous. If the infection tracks back a long way then the skin should be excised to the full extent of the infection, all infected material removed and the wound left open for drainage. Sometimes the procedure may have to be very radical and yet, provided one can eradicate the infection, good healing can be obtained even with long incisions on the sole of the foot (Fig. 10.1).

Transmetatarsal amputation

Where all of the toes and perhaps the distal forefoot are gangrenous, then an incision is made through the most distal healthy skin on the sole of the foot and more proximally on the dorsum. The metatarsals are divided at the level of the dorsal skin incision and the solar skin is then flapped over.

Use of local anaesthetic

Many patients having amputations of the toes and forefoot are elderly and unfit. They may have already had a bypass operation and a proportion of them will have a non-healing amputation stump which needs a more proximal amputation. For all of these reasons it is advantageous to avoid a general anaesthetic.

For amputations of the toes a simple digital nerve block can be done in much the same way as a ring block except that one may need to come a little more proximally on to the distal forefoot. Anything more proximal will require an ankle block.[26] This is actually quite simple to do and involves injecting local anaesthetic (approximately 8 ml of 0.5% lignocaine) into each of the six nerves at the ankle, which are all subcutaneous. (These are the tibial, saphenous, anterior tibial, superficial and deep peroneal and sural nerves.) In order to avoid a complete ring of local anaesthetic it is safer to block the saphenous nerve just below the knee where it should be lying next to the vein just behind the posterior border of the tibia. The secret is to give the anaesthetic plenty of time to work, ideally about half an hour. In order to avoid becoming impatient it is better to give the local anaesthetic on the ward and then take the patient to theatre soon after so that the anaesthetic is working satisfactorily by the time of operation.

A recent study[27] showed no difference in the healing rate of those patients having distal amputations done under local or general anaesthetic.

Tarsal amputations

These are the tarso-metatarsal amputation and the mid-tarsal amputation. These amputations result in both inversion and a slight equinus deformity which makes subsequent walking difficult. It is generally, therefore, better to avoid them.

Syme's amputation

In the presence of gangrene affecting the sole of

the foot a Syme's amputation may be considered. In principle, it is a disarticulation of the talo-tibial joint. The heel pad becomes the weight-bearing surface. The operation is only feasible if the heel pad is healthy and is rarely performed for vascular disease.

Descriptions of the procedure can be found in textbooks of operative surgery.[28] The most important technical point is to keep very close to the bone when dissecting the calcaneum out from the heel skin. The main problem is that there is danger of the medial flap necrosing, particularly when the procedure is done for ischaemia. The theoretical advantage of weight-bearing on the stump without a prosthesis is seldom realized. Any prosthesis used does not have enough room for ankle or sole springs and, therefore, most prosthetists feel the patient is better served with a good below-knee amputation.

Below-knee amputation

In 1968 Burgess[29] wrote: 'It is not possible to over-emphasise the importance of the knee for mobility in amputations of the lower limb.' This is every bit as true today. If there is any chance of healing then it is worth trying a below-knee amputation rather than one at a higher level. Below-knee amputees have double the chance of a succesful rehabilitation compared with those having an above-knee amputation. This is equally true in a patient who already has an amputation on the other side, provided that they have previously been walking satisfactorily with an artifical limb.

The main contraindications are fixed flexion contractures of the knee or if the patient has had a stroke with a spastic limb and is, therefore, liable to develop this. It is difficult to fit a prosthesis if there is more than 15 degrees of fixed flexion; although, of course, it may be possible with intensive physiotherapy, and occasionally with manipulation under anaesthetic to reduce a fixed flexion contracture.

Physiotherapy before and immediatlely after the operation is important in avoiding flexion deformity of the knee. Obviously the physiotherapist has the main role in this, but the nursing and medical staff should also encourage the patient to keep straightening the knee. It is usual to do knee straightening exercises whilst lying prone. A fracture board in the wheelchair to keep the knee straight is also helpful.

A week after the operation it is useful to start using the pneumatic post-amputation mobility (PPAM) aid. If there is any evidence of damage to the suture line them mobilization should be temporarily stopped.

The standard Burgess long posterior flap amputation

There are many good descriptions of this[29,30] and for years it has been the standard operation. Its main disadvantage is that it is relatively easy for inexperienced surgeons to leave a rather bulbous stump. The important technical points are to bevel the anterior edge of the tibia and to file this so that it is well rounded where it becomes subcutaneous. The soleus should be excised back to the level of bone division and the gastrocnemius can then be flapped over the bone end and sutured to the deep fascia and periosteum which is continuous with it. By carefully filleting the muscle one can generally achieve a nicely rounded stump.

Skew flap operation

This was described by Kingsley Robinson in 1982 and there have been further descriptions of it which are helpful to read.[31–33] The theoretical advantage is that the main blood supply to the skin is from the arteries that run with the saphenous vein and sural nerve.[32] Many surgeons have fought shy of this operation because they feel it sounds complicated. In reality it is very simple (Fig. 10.2). A mark is made 10–12 cm below the knee joint at the level of the proposed bone division. A vertical line is then drawn 2–2.5 cm (according to the size of the leg) lateral to the anterior margin of the tibia. A line is then found diagonally opposite to this; the easiest way is to measure the circumference with a piece of thread or silk, halve it and then draw a similar vertical line diagonally opposite the first. These lines form the axes of the flaps which are then drawn equally. The length of the flap can be made a quarter of that of the circumference, but in practice it is normally satisfactory to do this by eye. Having incised the skin flaps the gastrocnemius is cut slightly longer so that it can still flap over the tibia. The soleus is filleted out. In every other way the operation is the same as for the long posterior flap operation. Kingsley Robinson recommends separating the skin slightly from the gastrocnemius so that everything lies well. It is not actually necessary to do this and there is a theoretical argument for not separating them as some of the blood supply to the skin may come through perforating vessels from gastrocnemius.

Skew flap or long posterior flap?

Vaughan Ruckley organized a multicentre trial[34] which showed no difference in the healing rate between the two operations. A further study in Derby[35]

Table 10.2 Healing of below-knee amputations

	Skew flap	Long posterior flap	
Total	36	26	
Primary healing	29 (81%)	19 (73%)	NS
Trimming	1	2	
Higher amputation	6 (17%)	5 (19%)	NS

Table 10.3 Limb-fitter's assessment

	Skew flap	Long posterior flap	
Time to heal (days)	18 (10–215)	25.5 (10–168)	
Time to limb-fitting (days)	31.5 (20 146)	52 (28–152)	$p<0.05$
Time to mobility (weeks)	6.5 (4–32)	13.5 (5–49)	$p<0.01$

also showed no difference in the likelihood of failure to heal (Table 10.2). However we did show a significant difference in the time taken to being fitted with an artificial limb and in the time to mobility in favour of the Skew flap operation (Table 10.3). We also concluded that it was easier to obtain a nicely rounded stump with the equal flaps created by the skew flap operation. Figs 10.3 and 10.4 show a typical example of a bulbous stump with the long posterior flap operation and the more rounded stump with the skew flap.

The through-knee and Gritti–Stokes (supracondylar) amputations

For the through-knee disarticulation, medial and lateral U-shaped incisions are made with the medial flap slightly larger than the lateral. Anteriorly the

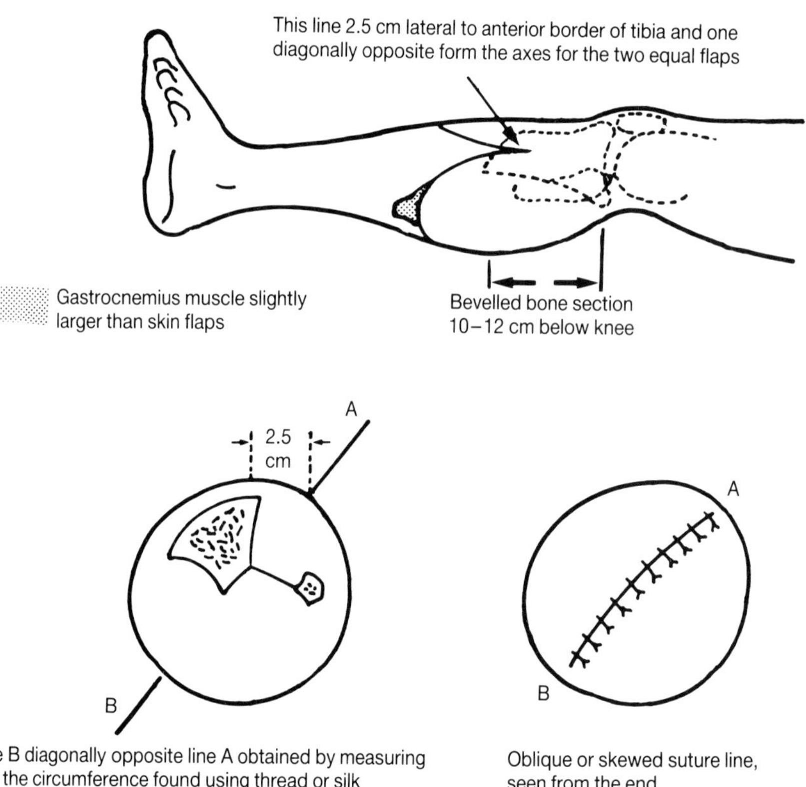

Fig. 10.2 Diagram of skin flaps for the skew flap operation. (Modified from Kingsley Robinson[30] with his kind permission and that of the *British Journal of Surgery* and the publisher, Butterworth & Co.)

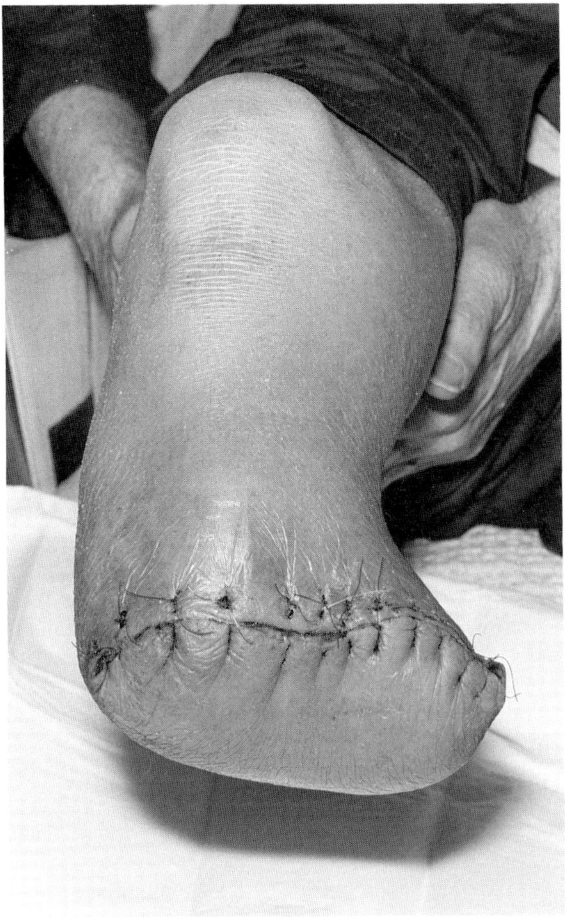

Fig. 10.3 A typical example of a bulbous stump that may occur with the long posterior flap operation.

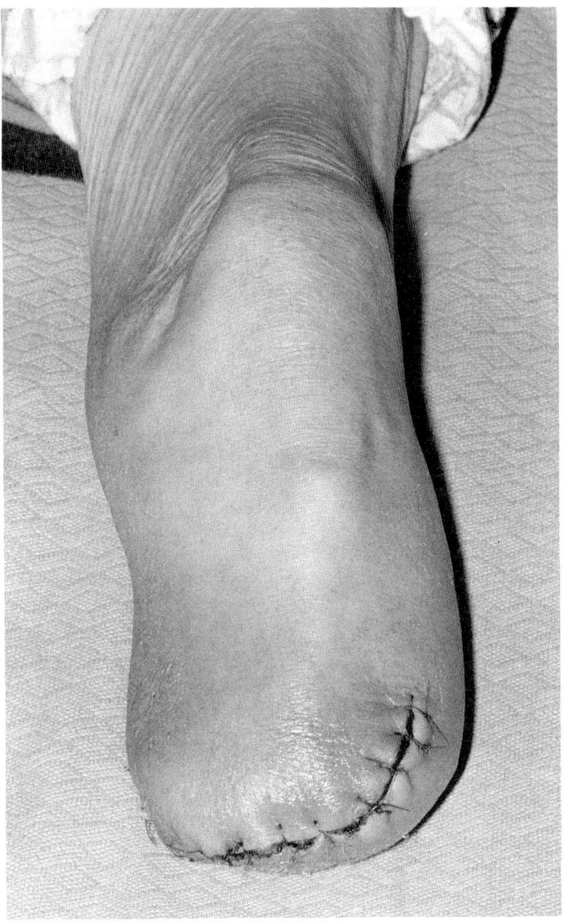

Fig. 10.4 The more rounded stump that is easier to obtain with the skew flap operation.

two flaps meet at the junction of the patellar tendon with the tibia, and posteriorly they meet in the popliteal fossa.[36] The suture line then runs between the condyles and is not involved in weight-bearing.

In the Gritti–Stokes amputation there is a long anterior and short posterior flap. The femur is divided just above the condyles so that the end is not too bulbous yet most of the adductor attachment is still intact. The articular surface is cut off the patella which is then attached to the cut end of the femur. If the femur is bevelled slightly this produces a stable attachment of the patella to the femur[19] (Fig. 10.5).

Although some recent reports[37,38] have shown good healing with the through-knee operation, the general impression (and certainly my personal experience) would suggest that healing is better with the Gritti–Stokes amputation. The only randomized trial, though small, did show a convincing difference in the healing rate in favour of the Gritti–Stokes.[18] The advantage of amputation at this level is that the patient has a longer stump with better muscle attachment and, therefore, better proprioception and control. This is particularly applicable when a patient already has contralateral above-knee amputation or in any patient in whom it is felt that there is really no chance of them learning to walk again. Bilateral above-knee amputations should be avoided because the patient becomes like Humpty Dumpty with not enough length of stump to stop them falling backwards.

The main disadvantage of amputations at this level

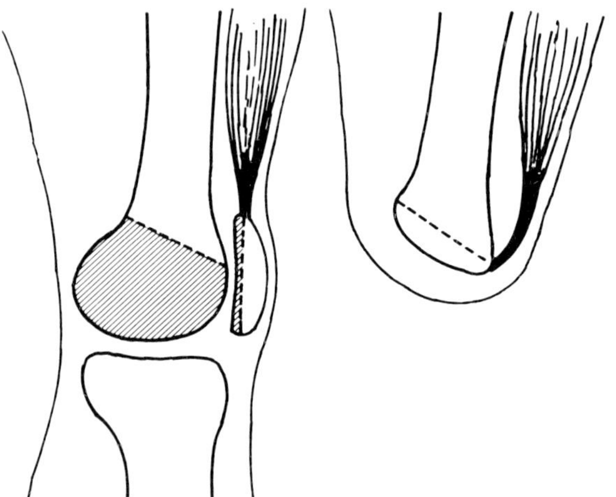

Fig. 10.5 Slight bevelling of the lower cut end of the femur allows a more stable attachment of the patella in the Gritti–Stokes amputation. (With kind permission of Mr BR Hopkinson[19] and of the *British Journal of Surgery* and the publisher, Butterworth & Co.)

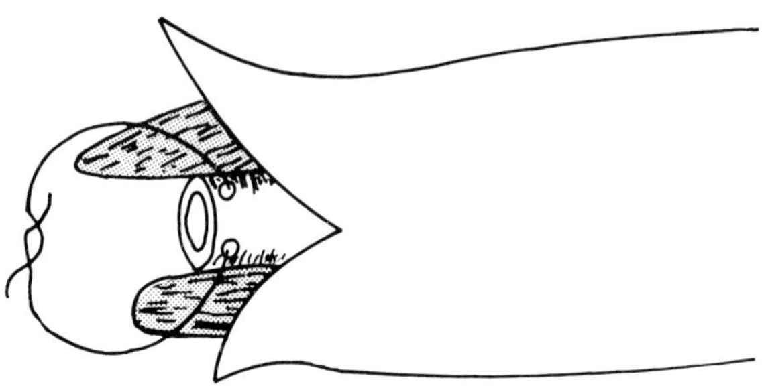

Fig. 10.6 Tunnel drilled in the femur to take the stitches from the muscle to avoid it slipping off the bone end in the above-knee amputation. (With kind permission of Mr JD Lewis[38] and the *Annals of the Royal College of Surgeons of England* and the publisher, Hadley Brothers Ltd.)

is that the knee joint of the artificial limb will be lower than that on the normal side. Thus, when sitting the patients appear to have a longer thigh and shorter shin on the affected side. They tend to walk more awkwardly because of the different level of knee joint. For these reasons prosthetists are not keen on amputations at this level and prefer either below- or above-knee procedures. However, there have been a number of reports[37,38] showing good walking rates with them – I am not aware of any trial comparing Gritti–Stokes and above-knee amputations.

Above-knee amputation

The line of bone division needs to be at least 10 cm above the knee in order to have room to fit a modern knee joint into the prosthesis.[39] If there is going to be satisfactory walking with an artificial limb then the femur length should not be shorter than 20 cm. Between these two limits the length is not critical. Equal anterior and posterior incisions are made and a myoplastic flap performed. One of the disadvantages is that the muscle sometimes slips off the end of the bone but this can be avoided by drilling a tunnel through the femur and taking a stitch from the muscles through it[39] (Fig. 10.6).

The main disadvantage of an above-knee amputation is that walking rates are considerably worse than for lower amputations and there is likely to be a particular problem with bilateral above-knee amputations, as already mentioned. The main advantage is that the healing rate is good. For example, a badly infected Gritti–Stokes or through-knee amputation stump will never heal, but with an above-knee amputation the bone can simply be trimmed back and the wound left open to heal by granulation, or be resutured when the infection is controlled.

Through-hip disarticulation

It is unusual to need to do this procedure for vascular disease and in my limited experience it carries a very high mortality (4 out of 6 to date), mainly because the patients are desperately ill. It is required when all the thigh muscles have infarcted after, for example, an embolism occluding the iliac artery which does not present until the limb is irretrievably dead. Fortunately this is a rare event. (In the minds of many medical students and perhaps some trainee surgeons, the hip disarticulation should not be confused with a hind quarter amputation which is done for tumours of the pelvis where one side of the bony pelvis has to be removed.)

Conclusions

It is vital that all patients with ischaemic gangrene are assessed by a vascular surgeon to see if it is possible to salvage the limb. It makes for better continuity if the amputation is then performed by the same surgeon.

The lower the amputation the better the subsequent walking. If you cannot do a forefoot amputation then the next level is a below-knee amputation.

Every effort should be made to amputate below rather than above the knee if there is any chance of the patient being able to walk again. Methods of predicting the level of amputation have so far been disappointing and clinical judgement remains the mainstay.

The skew flap below-knee amputation may allow earlier limb-fitting and mobilization than the long posterior flap, probably because it is easier to get a nicely rounded stump. The Gritti–Stokes amputation is particularly useful for patients who are bed or wheelchair bound and the lower end of femur should be bevelled to get stable patellar attachment. Although satisfactory walking can be achieved there are problems due to the resulting lower knee joint, and if at all possible it is preferable to amputate at the below-knee level.

If an above-knee amputation is done it is helpful to suture the myoplastic stitches through holes drilled in the end of the femur.

References

1. Coddington T. Why are legs amputated in Britain? In: *Limb Salvage and Amputation for Vascular Disease*, Greenhalgh RM, Jamieson CW, Nicolaides AN (eds). London: WB Saunders, 1988: 331–7.
2. Durham JR. Lower extremity amputation level indications, methods of determining appropriate level, technique and progress. In: *Vascular Surgery*, Rutherford EB (ed). Philadelphia: WB Saunders, 1989: 1687–712.
3. Hosie KB, Kockelberg R, Newbury-Ecob RA, Callum KG, Nash JR. A retrospective view of outcome of patients over 70 years of age considered for vascular reconstruction in a district general hospital. *Eur J Vasc Surg* 1990; **4:** 313–15.
4. Plecha FR, Bertin VJ, Plecha VJ. The early results of vascular surgery in patients 75 years of age and older: an analysis of 3259 cases. *J Vasc Surg* 1985; **2:** 769–74.
5. Coghill TH, Landercasper J, Strutt PJ, Gunderson AL. Late results of peripheral vascular surgery in patients 80 years of age and older. *Arch Surg* 1987; **122:** 581–5.
6. Cheshire NJ, Noone MA, Davies L, Drummond M, Wolfe JHN. Economic options and decision making in the ischaemic lower limb. 'VSS abstracts' in *Br J Surg* 1991; **78:** 371.
7. Szilagyi DE, Hageman JH, Smith RF. Autogenous vein grafting in femoropopliteal atherosclerosis: the limits of this effectiveness. *Surgery* 1979; **86:** 836–41.
8. Kazmers M, Satiani B, Evans WE. Amputation level following unsuccessful distal limb salvage operations. *Surgery* 1980; **87:** 683–7.
9. Light JT, Rice JC, Kerstein MD. Sequelae of limited amputation. *Surgery* 1988; **103:** 294–9.
10. Dardik H, Kahn M, Dardik I. Influence of failed vascular bypass procedures on conversion of below knee to above knee amputation levels. *Surgery* 1982; **91:** 63–9.
11. De Frang RD, Taylor LM, Porter JM. Amputation. In: *Current Problems in Surgery*, Wells SA (ed). St Louis: Mosby Yearbook Inc., 1991: 140–79.
12. Griffith CDM, Callum KG. Limb salvage surgery in a district general hospital: factors affecting outcome. *Ann Roy Coll Surg Engl* 1988; **70:** 95–8.
13. Rush DS, Huston CC, Bivins BA, Hyde GC. Operative and late mortality rates of above knee and below knee amputations. *Am Surg* 1981; **47:** 32–42.
14. Finch DRA, MacDougal M, Tibbs DJ, Morris PJ. Amputation for vascular disease: An experience of a peripheral vascular unit. *Br J Surg* 1980; **67:** 233–7.
15. Dormandy JA, Thomas PRS. What is the natural history of a critically ischaemic patient and without his leg. In: *Limb Salvage and Amputation for Vascular Disease*, Greenhalgh RM, Jamieson CW, Nicolaides AN (eds). London: WB Saunders, 1988: 11–26.
16. Bunt TJ, Manship LL, Byhoe PH, Haynes JL. Lower extremity amputation for peripheral vascular disease; a low risk operation. *Am Surg* 1984; **50:** 581–4.
17. Otteman MD, Stahlgren LH. Evaluation of factors which influence mortality and morbidity following major lower extremity amputations for arteriosclerosis. *Surg Gynae Obst* 1965; **120:** 217–20.
18. Campbell WB, Morris PJ. A prospective randomised comparison of healing in Gritti–Stokes and through-knee amputations. *Ann Roy Coll Surg Eng* 1986; **69:** 1.
19. Doran J, Hopkinson BR, Makin GS. The Gritti–Stokes amputation in ischaemia: a review of 134 cases. *Br J Surg* 1978; **65:** 135.
20. Houghton AD, Taylor PR, Thurlow S, Rootes E, McColl I. Success rates for rehabilitation of vascular amputees: implications for preoperative assessment and amputation level. *Br J Surg* 1992; **79:** 753–5.
21. Kram HB, Appel PL, Shoemaker WC. Multisensor transcutaneous oximetric mapping to predict below knee amputation wound healing: use of a critical PO_2. *J Vasc Surg* 1989; **9:** 796–800.
22. Stockel M, Oversen J, Brochner-Mortenson J, Emneus H. Standardized photo-electric technique as a routine method of selection of amputation level. *Acta Ortho Scand* 1982; **53:** 875–8.
23. Ley JA, Vega ME, Fernandez JI, Ochoa LM, Romero A, Cardova M. The amputation level: noninvasive methods and clinical criteria. *CCR Vasa* 1990; **32:** 320–6.
24. Holloway GA, Burgess EM. Preliminary experience

with laser Doppler velocimetry for the determination of amputation levels. *Prosth Orthot Int* 1983; **7:** 63–6.
25. Kram HB, Appel PL, Shoemaker WC. Prediction of below knee amputation wound healing using non-invasive laser Doppler velocimetry. *Am Surg* 1989; **159:** 29–31.
26. Löfström B. Nerve block at the ankle. In: *Illustrated Handbook in Local Anaesthesia*, Eriksson E (ed). Copenhagen: Sorenson & Co., 1979: 112–15.
27. Byrne RL, Nicholson ML, Woolford TJ, Callum KG. Factors influencing the healing of distal amputations performed for lower limb ischaemia. *Br J Surg* 1992; **79:** 73–5.
28. Fiddian NJ. Amputations. In: *General Surgical Operations*, Kirk RM, Williamson RCN (eds). London: Churchill Livingstone, 1987: 416–28.
29. Burgess EM. The below knee amputation. *Bull Prosth Res* 1968; 19–25.
30. McCollum CN. Posterior-flap below-knee amputation. In: *Vascular Surgical Techniques: An Atlas*, Greenhalgh RM (ed). London: WB Saunders, 1989: 340–6.
31. Robinson KP, Hoile R, Coddington T. Skew-flap myoplastic below-knee amputation: a preliminary report. *Br J Surg* 1982; **69:** 554–7.
32. Robinson KP. Skew-flap below-knee amputation. In: *Limb Salvage and Amputation for Vascular Disease*, Greenhalgh RM, Jamieson CW, Nicholaides AN (eds). London: WB Saunders, 1988: 373–82.
33. Robinson KP. Skew-flap below-knee amputation. In: *Vascular Surgical Techniques: An Atlas*, Greenhalgh RM (ed). London: WB Saunders, 1989: 347–53.
34. Ruckley CV, Prescott RJ. Is there any advantage of skew-flap rather than Burgess below-knee amputation? In: *Limb Salvage and Amputation for Vascular Disease*, Greenhalgh RM, Jamieson CW, Nicolaides AN (eds). London: WB Saunders, 1988: 383–7.
35. Reynolds J, Hind R, Lindsey G, Nash JR, Callum KG. Skew-flap versus the Burgess long posterior flap – a prospective randomised trial. 'VSS abstracts' in *Br J Surg* 1991; **78:** 370.
36. Fulford GE. Amputation in peripheral vascular disease. In: *Tutorials in Postgraduate Medicine: Peripheral Vascular Surgery*, Birnstingl IM (ed). London: Heinemann, 1973: 407–18.
37. Houghton A, Allen A, Luff R, McColl I. Rehabilitation after lower limb amputation: a comparative study of above-knee and Gritti–Stokes amputations. *Br J Surg* 1989; **76:** 622–4.
38. Moran BJ, Buttenshaw P, Mulcahy M, Robinson KP. Through-knee amputation in high-risk patients with vascular disease: indications, complications and rehabilitation. *Br J Surg* 1990; **77:** 1118–20.
39. Chadwick SJD, Lewis JD. Above knee amputation. *Ann Roy Coll Surg Eng* 1991; **73:** 152–4.

11

Aneurysms

Jack Collin

An aneurysm by definition is an abnormal dilatation of a blood vessel. The dilatation may be localized or generalized, in which case it is usually called arterial ectasia or arteriomegaly. In practice the term aneurysm is reserved for dilatations of arteries; dilated veins are simply varicosities. The common sites for aneurysms to develop in descending order of frequency, but excluding intracranial aneurysms, are:

1. infrarenal abdominal aorta
2. abdominal aorta and common iliac
3. common iliac
4. internal iliac
5. femoral
6. thoracic aorta and thoracoabdominal aorta
7. popliteal
8. splenic
9. other visceral arteries.

Strangely, true aneurysms of the external iliac artery appear to be unknown.

Types of aneurysm

True aneurysm

There is stretching of the entire arterial wall so that the aneurysm wall contains all the elements of the normal arterial wall although there may be partial fragmentation of elastic tissue and collagen occasioned by or responsible for initiating the dilatation.

False aneurysm

This aneurysm is lined only by connective tissue formed from the outer layers of the arterial wall. In the UK most false aneurysms occur at the site of graft arterial anastomoses, particularly in the femoral artery; but in the USA, and particularly in South Africa, stab injuries are the common cause.

Fusiform aneurysm

As the name implies, the aneurysm is spindle shaped. These comprise the great majority of aneurysms at all sites.

Saccular aneurysm

This appears as a pouch or sack-like outgrowth from one side of the artery. They are commonly seen in association with severe atherosclerotic occlusive disease beside a large atheromatous plaque, or occasionally in mycotic aneurysms.

Mycotic aneurysm

This term is an historical misnomer. The aneurysms are infective in origin and occur in patients with bacterial endocarditis or septicaemia. The organism is usually a pathogenic bacterium. The disease seemed set to disappear with the decline of rheumatic heart disease, but is now enjoying a renaissance as a consequence of the increasing popularity of intravascular drug addiction and eating white meat. The causative organism in the latter case is usually *Salmonella enteritidis* contaminating the carcass and eggs of hens and infecting its human host by a combination of unwise food storage, inadequate cooking and the cook–chill–warm television dinner of late twentieth century man.

Dissecting aneurysm

The underlying defect is degeneration of the media of the arterial wall which allows blood to track along the length of the aorta. The entry point is almost always in the arch of the aorta and there may be a re-entry point at a lower level, creating a double blood flow channel, or the false channel may rupture externally with fatal consequences. Dissecting aneurysms are a variety of false aneurysm. Most are fatal within hours as a consequence of rupture, cardiac tamponade or visceral infarction. Treatment of survivors involves vigorous hypotensive medication and selective judicious operation, particularly when the aortic valve or heart are compromised.

Inflammatory aneurysm

Inflammatory aneurysms occur in the thoracic and

abdominal aorta and the common and internal iliac arteries. They comprise around 10% of all abdominal aortic aneurysms encountered in clinical practice, but since they are commonly symptomatic this probably over-represents the prevalence of the inflammatory variant of aortic aneurysms in the entire population. The pathogenesis of this disorder is still the subject of debate, but the original suggestion that the inflammation was a response to leakage of blood from contained aortic rupture is not tenable.

The macroscopic appearance at operation may be either an angry hyperaemic periaortic inflammation or a chronic fibrotic 'icing sugar' aortic wall; both types may be seen at different points on the same aneurysm. Histologically the wall of all aortic aneurysms show evidence of an inflammatory response and the difference between the macroscopically inflamed and non-inflamed aneurysm is quantitative rather than qualitative.

The condition is best regarded as a chronic periaortitis and has much in common with idiopathic retroperitoneal fibrosis. Recent work by Mitchinson in Cambridge has advanced the theory that the periaortitis is an immune reponse to antigens, principally ceroid, leaking from atheromatous plaques into the aortic adventitia. There is a widely held belief that inflammatory aortic aneurysms are less likely to rupture than non-inflammatory aneurysms, but all abdominal aortic aneurysms are thin-walled posteriorly where contained ruptures commonly occur. Inflammatory abdominal aortic aneurysm should be suspected in patients presenting with a history of abdominal and back pain and who have a tender aneurysm. An elevated erythrocyte sedimentation rate will be present in half of those with an inflammatory aneurysm, and the diagnosis can be confirmed by demonstrating a thickened aortic wall on computerized tomography.

In some patients the ureters may be obstructed by periaortitis or more commonly where they cross an inflammatory iliac aneurysm. Such patients may present with renal failure or hydronephrosis.

Arteriovenous aneurysm

A direct communication occurs between the arterial and venous systems causing either aneurysmal dilatation of the vein or a false aneurysm. The communication may be congenital, in which case it is usually an arteriovenous malformation; or it may be secondary, when it is generally called an arteriovenous fistula. Arteriovenous fistulae may rarely be spontaneous but usually follow direct arteriovenous trauma which is often iatrogenic.

Abdominal aortic aneurysm (AAA)

Epidemiology

The incidence of aortic aneurysm has changed markedly over the last 100 years. In the early part of the century the majority of aneurysms were caused by tertiary syphilis and predominantly involved the thoracic aorta.[1] Today almost all aortic aneurysms are degenerative in origin, with the infrarenal abdominal aorta being the principal site affected.

In the last 30 years there has been a linear increase in the number of recorded deaths from aortic aneurysm in England and Wales. In part this can be explained by the progressive growth in the number of elderly in the population, but age-specific death rates for aortic aneurysm have also increased.[2] Much of the apparent change may be due to enhanced awareness of the disease, improved diagnosis and altered referral patterns. In the USA a similar increase in mortality for aortic aneurysms occurred between 1951 and 1968, but recorded deaths then plateaued and in white males have declined by 2% per annum since 1976,[3] possibly as a consequence of surgical treatment.

In contrast to occlusive arterial disease, AAA is almost exclusively confined to the elderly. There are few deaths from ruptured AAA before 60 and the disease becomes commoner with advancing years. The annual risk of death from AAA for a man aged 87 is 0.23% and for a woman 0.07%. In men, total deaths from AAA reach a peak in the 70–74 age-group, while in women the peak occurs a decade later.[4] A man aged 67 is ten times more likely to die from this disease than a woman of the same age.

Aetiology

The common AAA of elderly men has traditionally been labelled as 'atherosclerotic' in origin. This classification has for too long stifled thinking and needs to be re-examined. Inevitably in the elderly the abdominal aorta, in common with every other artery, will show obvious features of atheroclerosis; but this is insufficient evidence on which to base a pathological diagnosis which fails to explain so many known facts about the disease.

Tilson and Stansel published a detailed comparison between patients with AAA and those with occlusive aortoiliac disease.[5] They found that the aneurysm patients were nine times more likely to be male, were on average 11 years older and much less likely to have had previous arterial surgery. Patients with occlusive disease were 16 times more likely to require reoperation after aortic surgery.

Attention was first drawn to a familial grouping of AAA in 1977,[6] and the disease has recently been shown to have a prevalence of 29% in first-degree male relatives.[7] There seems little doubt that AAA has a strong genetic base and that with the rapid pace of advance in molecular biology the gene or genes responsible may soon be identified.

The mechanism by which the genetic predisposition interacts with environmental factors, such as cigarette smoking and hypertension, to initiate the pathogenesis of aneurysm formation is not clear. The fact that an atherogenic regimen does not usually induce aneurysmal disease is an issue that is only recently being faced in the experimental literature.[8] Current theories suggest that degradation of collagen[9] or elastolysis[10] may be the proximate cause of aneurysm formation and rupture.

Clinical presentation

Most abdominal aortic aneurysms are asymptomatic and are discovered incidentally during abdominal examination or by ultrasonography. For many patients the first intimation of their disease, when the aneurysm ruptures into the peritoneal cavity, is also their last. Others are more fortunate and experience posterior or lateral ruptures of the aneurysm which are tamponaded to a variable extent by the surrounding connective tissue and intact posterior peritoneum.

In a patient presenting with the classic symptoms of sudden-onset central abdominal and lumbar back pain associated with pallor, vasoconstriction, hypotension and tachycardia, the diagnosis of rupture is seldom in doubt. Incorrect diagnoses of myocardial infarction, aortic dissection, pancreatitis and, commonly, renal colic are all still recorded with monotonous regularity, with consequent delayed treatment. Variations in presentation may legitimately delay diagnosis. In some patients the rupture is so well tamponaded that no haemodynamic disturbance may occur. This interlude should not be wasted since free rupture and death from exsanguination may happen at any moment until the aneurysm is replaced. Ruptured internal iliac artery aneurysms may cause sciatica and rarely present as a haematoma in the buttock.

Most AAAs contain mural thrombus which may occasionally embolise and cause the patient to present with acute ischaemia of one or both legs. Similar symptoms result if the aortic aneurysm thromboses, but in this case the outlook is much worse since restoration of the circulation requires emergency aortobifemoral grafting in a patient already desperately ill from extensive tissue ischaemia.

Equally dramatic but rare presentations result from fistulation of an AAA into the duodenum or inferior vena cava. Aortoenteric fistula presents as sudden upper gastrointestinal haemorrhage usually episodic over days rather than immediately fatal. Diagnosis depends on endoscopic visualization of the duodenojejunal flexure which is almost always the site of communication. Aortoenteric fistula is a very uncommon cause of upper gastrointestinal haemorrhage in a patient who has never had an arterial operation, and the diagnosis is usually suspected in a patient who has had a previous aortic operation, particularly an aortobifemoral bypass graft.

Aortocaval fistula is usually an incidental problem in a patient with coexistent retroperitoneal rupture of an AAA, and consequently in practice this is seldom diagnosed until massive venous haemorrhage is encountered on opening the aorta during emergency surgery. Very rarely the AAA may rupture only into the inferior vena cava, when the patient may present with high-output cardiac failure and venous hypertension.

The commonest clinical presentation is with a pulsatile epigastric mass which the patient may first recognize while lying in bed or his bath. Abdominal and lumbar back pain is suggestive of sudden expansion of the aneurysm or an inflammatory AAA and may be accompanied by aneurysm tenderness. Unless an inflammatory AAA can confidently be diagnosed, the presence of pain and tenderness are indications for urgent repair of the aneurysm.

Management

In the absence of rupture, pain or a tender aneurysm, the decision whether to recommend elective surgery must always be taken advisedly after carefully balancing the risk of premature death from rupture of the aneurysm against the operative mortality and morbidity. There are three factors to consider: the size of the aneurysm, the general health of the patient, and the individual surgeon's audited operative mortality for elective aortic aneurysm repair.

Very small aneurysms (4.0 cm diameter or less)

Very small aortic aneurysms generally enlarge much more slowly than the larger aneurysms which present in routine clinical practice, and median growth rates of 0.2 cm per annum are usual.[11,12] Clinical and autopsy evidence indicates that even these very small aneurysms do sometimes rupture, but there are insufficent data for the risk to be accurately quantified. Several follow-up studies have shown no case of rupture occurring in such patients while the aneurysms remained very small,[12–14] but ruptures did occur as the aneurysms grew.

Elective operation cannot be justified in this group of patients and they should be reviewed with 6-monthly ultrasonography to document any increase in diameter of the AAA.

Small aneurysms (4.0–5.9 cm diameter)

Autopsy studies in patients with an abdominal aortic aneurysm showed that more than a third of those less than 6.0 cm in diameter had ruptured and caused death.[15] Follow-up studies of patients with aneurysms less than 6.0 cm in diameter rejected for operation have demonstrated an annual rupture rate of 6% over three years. Rupture rates will tend to increase progressively with the length of follow-up as the aneurysms continue to expand. It is known that for aneurysms of 4.0–4.9 cm diameter the mean expansion rate is 0.5 cm a year, increasing to 0.7 cm a year for aneurysms of 5.0–5.9 cm diameter.[16]

This wide range of aneurysm sizes covers the extremes of surgical uncertainty. For most surgeons the area of doubt is narrower and covers the middle of the range from 4.5 to 5.4 cm. AAAs under 4.5 cm should be replaced only in the youngest and fittest of patients in institutions with an overall operative mortality of under 3%. It will usually be appropriate to replace an AAA that is over 5.5 cm in all but the oldest and most unhealthy of patients. For aneurysms of 4.5–5.4 cm the decision requires surgical judgement after careful consideration of all the relevant factors in each individual patient.

Large aneurysms (over 6.0 cm diameter)

Patients with aneurysms of more than 6.0 cm are nowadays invariably advised to have an elective operation. What we know of the natural history of large aneurysms comes from studies before 1951 or contemporary studies in patients too ill to undergo a major elective procedure.

The only substantial study before 1951 was that of Estes,[17] who reviewed 97 patients with non-syphilic aneurysms diagnosed at the Mayo Clinic up to 1947. Fewer than half survived for three years and 63% of all deaths were from aneurysm rupture. A follow-up study at Vanderbilt University of patients not offered surgery found that 55% of deaths were due to rupture.[18] Even at an institution where operation was denied only if the patient was very old or had severe coexistent disease, 43% of deaths in patients with unoperated large aneurysms were from rupture.[19]

Fitness for surgery

Replacement of an asymptomatic AAA is an elective operation; it is therefore essential that any coexistent health problems are identified and if possible corrected before operation. Patients with advanced malignancy or degenerative neurological disease are clearly not candidates for aortic surgery. The main risk factors in the majority of patients will be impaired respiratory or cardiac function. Routine respiratory function tests to measure FEV and FEV_1 should always be performed, but more sophisticated tests are seldom necessary.

There has been considerable debate about the most cost-effective method of assessing cardiac performance at rest and on exercise, but this issue is still unresolved. Routine ECG monitoring is essential, but in some patients transient arrythmias or myocardial ischaemia will only be apparent on 24-hour recordings. Our current practice is to perform routine MUGA scanning at rest and after exercise on all patients in sinus rhythm to determine the left ventricular ejection fraction. Ejection fractions of less than 50% give rise to concern, particularly when the fraction falls with exercise. In patients who are in atrial fibrillation, an echocardiogram will allow an assessment to be made of the uniformity of ventricular wall contraction. Evidence of poor myocardial function or ischaemia is an indication for coronary angiography to see if there is a correctable coronary artery stenosis. Current practice is to perform a coronary artery operation first but asymptomatic carotid artery stenosis is ignored since there is no evidence of benefit from prophylactic carotid endarterectomy in this condition.

Operative mortality

In the first few years after AAA replacement became possible, elective operative mortality was around 15%, but in major centres mortality began to fall as operative and anaesthetic techniques and postoperative care improved. As the number of vascular surgeons increased, reports of high operative mortality became less common, a change which in part can be accounted for by reporting and publication bias which ensure that the worst results are never presented and bad results seldom published. In many specialist vascular surgical units the operative mortality is now under 5%; but in district general hospitals without specialist vascular surgeons, operative mortality rates above 15% are still known to occur.[20]

The main justification for elective AAA replacement is to prevent premature death from aortic rupture. It is a poor bargain to exchange possible death at an uncertain date in the future for a high probability of death within hours of prophylactic surgery. Even with an uncomplicated recovery it will be at least 3 months before the asymptomatic AAA patient will feel as well again as he did on the day before operation. It is hard in these circumstances to sell an operative mortality which exceeds the annual risk of death from the untreated disease.

Operative techniques

In the 40 years since the first successful replacement of an abdominal aortic aneurysm, the operation has become easier and quicker, with less blood loss and lower operative mortality and morbidity. The surgical refinements which have contributed to these improvements are a minimal dissection technique, inlay grafting instead of aortic transection, and the use of tube rather than bifurcated grafts in the majority of patients. The techniques of aortic surgery should be taught and well learned in elective operations before the trainee embarks on his first closely supervised ruptured aortic aneurysm replacement. It is often said that with ruptured aneurysms 'there is nothing to lose', since without operation the mortality is 100%. Such *ex cathedra* statements ignore the fact that irretrievable fatal technical errors are much easier to make in an emergency than during an elective aortic operation, and lives will continue to be lost unnecessarily until all emergency aortic operations are performed by trained vascular surgeons.

Elective AAA replacement

A midline full-length abdominal incision permits easy access to the infrarenal aorta and the iliac arteries. Transverse abdominal incisions are popular with some surgeons but exposure of the iliac arteries is restricted. Exteriorization of the small intestines and retraction to the right exposes the abdominal aorta. The peritoneum is incised along the length of the aorta in the midline and over the first 3 cm of the comon iliac arteries. The inferior mesenteric vein lies to the left of the midline and the fourth part of the duodenum to the right; it is unnecessary to divide the former or mobilize the latter. Dissection in a plane between the aortic adventitia and surrounding connective tissue is restricted to a 3 cm length of aorta below the left renal vein and confined to the front and sides of the vessel vertically backwards to the vertebral body. Intravenous heparin is administered and the aorta clamped anteroposteriorly. The common iliac arteries are dissected similarly and clamped anteroposteriorly. Dissection behind the iliac arteries is avoided because of the risk of causing bleeding from the iliac veins. The origin of the inferior mesenteric artery to the left of the midline of the aorta is identified through the peritoneum and ligated with a transfixion suture.

The aneurysm is then incised in the midline from its neck to the aortic bifurcation and its contents of mural thrombus and blood removed. Back bleeding from lumbar vessels is controlled by packing and the incision extended laterally at both ends for half of the aortic circumference. The orifice of each patent lumbar artery is then oversewn in turn to produce a bloodless operative field. An aortic graft of appropriate size is sutured to the neck of the aneurysm using a 00 Prolene continuous suture. Three posterior sutures on each side of the midline are placed carefully and the graft then parachuted into place before completing the anastomosis by direct suture. The distal anastomosis to the aortic bifurcation is fashioned in the same way.

When the common iliac arteries are aneurysmal, a bifurcated 'trouser' graft is necessary. The distal anastomoses may be end-to-end to the common iliac bifurcation or end-to-side to the external iliac arteries with ligation of the common iliac arteries. It is desirable to preserve blood flow through at least one internal iliac artery because in some patients this may be a critical part of the blood supply to the colon and cauda equina. Interestingly the external iliac arteries are never aneurysmal but may be occluded by atherosclerosis, and in this circumstance distal anastomosis to the femoral arteries is unavoidable.

Operation for ruptured AAA

Patients with ruptured AAA survive to operation because aortic bleeding is minimized by hypotension and tissue turgor while blood supply to vital organs is maintained by peripheral vasoconstriction. Induction of anaesthesia will eliminate the protective vasoconstriction and remove the contribution of muscle contraction to aortic tamponade. It is essential, therefore, that all preparations for the operation are made before the patient is anaesthetized.

On exposing the posterior peritoneum distended with haematoma, normal aorta is identified by palpation above the aneurysm and firmly occluded by direct pressure against the vertebral body. Only when blood flow into the aneurysm has been arrested is the posterior peritoneum over the upper part of the aneurysm incised and haematoma with connective tissue cleared until the white wall of the aneurysm is identified. Blunt dissection upwards from this point to the neck will avoid the commonest fatal surgical error of dissecting the aorta too high and too wide, consequently tearing either the left renal, suprarenal or gonadal veins together with the inferior vena cava. After cross-clamping the aortic neck, digital occlusion of the aorta is released and two-handed dissection allows the remainder of the operation to be completed as for an elective operation.

Screening for AAA

In primary referral hospitals in the UK, currently around half of all AAA patients present with aortic rupture. It is known that almost twice as many patients with ruptured AAA die before reaching hospital. This large toll of preventable deaths has provided the stimulus for numerous screening programmes to detect asymptomatic AAA in a variety of population subgroups. The epidemiological data from these studies allows a number of conclusions to be drawn. The following refer to patients in the age range 65–74 years:

1. In otherwise healthy men the prevalence of AAA is 5.0%.[21]
2. In men with occlusive arterial disease the prevalence is 15%.[21]
3. 40% of AAAs detected by screening are clinically significant with a diameter of at least 4.0 cm.
4. AAA is seven to ten times more common in men than women.[2]
5. It is likely that around 50% of first-degree male relatives of patients with AAA will be affected since the prevalence in those relatives over the age of 50 years is known to be 25%.[7]

In the real world of escalating health-care costs and limited resources, for any new screening programme to be viable it should be cheap, cost-effective and restricted to the smallest population group possible. These criteria indicate that routine ultrasonography of the abdominal aorta can be recommended for general application in two population groups:

- all male first-degree relatives of patients with AAA, who should have 5-yearly aortic measurement from the age of 50 onwards;
- all men over 60 years presenting with symptomatic occlusive arterial disease (i.e. intermittent claudication, myocardial infarction, angina or transient ischaemic attacks).

Population screening for all men over 65 years would be expensive and require resources of a similar magnitude to those currently devoted to the national breast screening programme. No government is likely to approve a budget of the size required without clear and unequivocal evidence of benefit, particularly when the target population is largely economically inactive and financially dependent.

Other aneurysms

Thoracoabdominal aneurysms

Crawford has classified these aneurysms into four groups by their anatomical extent:[22]

Type I: Most of the descending thoracic aorta and the abdominal aorta above the renal arteries

Type II: Most of the descending thoracic and abdominal aorta

Type III: Less than half the descending thoracic and the whole or part of the abdominal aorta

Type IV: Confined to the abdominal aorta but including the segment from which the visceral and renal arteries arise.

The operative mortality and morbidity increase with the length of aorta which is replaced; and even in Houston where 75% of all thoracoabdominal aortic aneurysm operations in the USA are performed, the incidence of paraplegia for type II aneurysms is 29% with mortality and haemodialysis rates of 10% each. In centres with less experience, operative mortality rates of 75% have been reported and higher rates are known to occur.

Patients with type III or IV aneurysms believed to be at a high risk of early rupture may be prepared to accept the 5% incidence of paraplegia and an operative mortality that is less than 25%. Operation is appropriate only in major vascular surgical units where the necessary expertise can be accumulated.

Femoral aneurysms

Around two-thirds of all femoral aneurysms are now false aneurysms arising at the site of a vascular anastomosis, commonly to a synthetic graft. Many will be associated with graft infection and present a considerable therapeutic challenge.

The complications of true and false aneurysms are similar, namely rupture, thrombosis or distal embolisation. Surgical repair is indicated when complications occur or prophylactically for large or expanding aneurysms.

Popliteal aneurysms

Aneurysms of the popliteal artery are less common, usually asymptomatic and less likely to be noticed by patients than femoral aneurysms. Rupture can occur, but the usual presentation is with occlusion of the popliteal artery or distal embolisation producing ischaemia of the foot or leg. Treatment of these complications has been transformed by direct intra-arterial thrombolytic infusions which in many cases can restore patency of vessels and allow elective replacement of the aneurysm to be performed.

Visceral aneurysms

Aneurysms of the visceral arteries are rare, most reports in the literature being of single cases. Splenic artery aneurysms account for around two-thirds of the total, with most of the remainder being renal, hepatic, gastric or superior mesenteric artery aneurysms. Iatrogenic aneurysms or arteriovenous fistula can follow hepatic or renal biopsy but when contained within the organ seldom cause problems. Most visceral aneurysms present only if they rupture, but bile duct compression and jaundice, pancreatitis, gut ischaemia, renal failure and hypertension have all been reported.

Most patients are middle-aged; but in contradistinction to other aneurysms, a high proportion of cases occur in young people in their 30s the majority in women. In developed countries with high standards of obstetric care, ruptured visceral artery aneurysm is now one of the major remaining causes of maternal mortality.

References

1. Brindley P, Stembridge VA. Aneurysms of the aorta: a clinicopathological study of 369 necropsy cases. *Am J Path* 1956; **32:** 67–82.
2. Collin J. The epidemiology of abdominal aortic aneurysm. *Br J Hosp Med* 1988; **40:** 64–7.
3. Lilienfeld DE, Gunderson PD, Sprafka JM, Vargas C. Epidemiology and aortic aneurysms. I: Mortality trends in the United States 1951–81. *Arteriosclerosis* 1987; **7:** 637–43.
4. Office of Population Censuses and Surveys, England and Wales. *Mortality Statistics: Cause*. London: HMSO, 1984; series DH2 11.
5. Tilson MD, Stansel HC. Differences in results for aneurysms versus occlusive disease after aortic bifurcation grafts: results of 100 elective grafts. *Arch Surg* 1980; **115:** 1173–5.
6. Clifton MA. Familial abdominal aortic aneurysm. *Br J Surg* 1977; **64:** 765–6.
7. Collin J, Walton J. Is abdominal aortic aneurysm familial? *Br Med J* 1989; **299:** 493.
8. Tilson MD. A perspective on research in abdominal aortic aneurysm disease, with a unifying hypothesis. In: *Aortic Surgery*, Bergan JJ, Yao JST (eds). London: WB Saunders, 1989: 27–35.
9. Busuttil RW, Abou-Zamzam AM, Machleder HI. Collagenase activity of the human aorta: a comparison of patients with and without abdominal aortic aneurysms. *Arch Surg* 1980; **115:** 1373–8.
10. Brown SL, Backstrom B, Busuttil RW. A new serum proteolytic enzyme in aneurysm pathogenesis. *J Vasc Surg* 1985; **2:** 393–9.
11. Collin J, Heather B, Walton J. Growth rates of subclinical abdominal aortic aneurysms: implications for review and rescreening programmes. *Eur J Vasc Surg* 1991; **5:** 141–4.
12. Nevitt MP, Ballard DJ, Hallett JW. Prognosis of abdominal aortic aneurysms: a population-based study. *N Engl J Med* 1989; **321:** 1009–14.
13. Cronenwett JL, Murphy TF, Zelenock GB, *et al.* Actuarial analysis of variables associated with rupture of small abdominal aortic aneurysms. *Surgery* 1985; **98:** 472–83.
14. Scott RAP, Ashton HA, Kay DN. Routine ultrasound screening in management of abdominal aortic aneurysm. *Br Med J* 1988; **296:** 1709–10.
15. Szilagyi DE, Smith RF, De Russo FJ, Elliott JP, Sherrin FW. Contribution of abdominal aortic aneurysmectomy to prolongation of life. *Ann Surg* 1966; **164:** 678–99.
16. Sterpetti AV, Schulz RD, Feldhaus RJ, Peetz DJ, Fasciano AJ, McGill JE. Abdominal aortic aneurysm in elderly patients: selective management based on clinical status and aneurysmal expansion rate. *Am J Surg* 1985; **150:** 772–6.
17. Estes JE. Abdominal aortic aneurysm: a study of one hundred and two cases: *Circulation* 1950; **2:** 258–64.
18. Foster JH, Gobbel WG, Scott HW. Comparative study of elective resection and expectant treatment of abdominal aortic aneurysm. *Surg Gynecol Obstet* 1969; **129:** 1–9.
19. Szilagyi DE, Elliott JP, Smith RF. Clinical fate of the patient with asymptomatic abdominal aortic aneurysm and unfit for surgical treatment. *Arch Surg* 1972; **104:** 600–6.
20. Guj AJ, Lambert D, Jones NAG, Chamberlain J. After CEPOD – aortic aneurysm surgery in the Northern Region. *Br J Surg* 1990; **77:** 344–5.

21. Collin J, Araujo L, Walton J, Lindsell D. Oxford screening programme for abdominal aortic aneurysm in men aged 65–74 years. *Lancet* 1988; **2:** 613–15.
22. Crawford ES. Thoracoabdominal and proximal aortic replacement for extensive aortic aneurysmal disease. In: *The Cause and Management of Aneurysms*, Greenhalgh RM, Mannick JA, Powell JT (eds). London: WB Saunders, 1990: 351–85.

12

Use of blood and blood products in vascular surgery

JF Thompson

Blood transfusion medicine was once a medical backwater. The specialty now has a high profile owing to public concerns about the safety of this important resource. An important offshoot of this increased interest has been re-examination of the pathophysiology, indications and economics of blood transfusion. This is an important area for the vascular surgeon, who is a major consumer of blood and blood products. This chapter advocates a careful approach to blood transfusion, reviews the pathophysiology of hypovolaemic shock, and describes the techniques available to reduce blood transfusion.

History of blood transfusion

The first reference to blood transfusion is attributed to the Roman poet Ovidius (43 BC–18 AD). He related how Princess Medea rejuvenated the aged Prince Aeson by slitting his throat, 'letting the blood run out of him, and filling his ancient veins with rich elixir'. Italian physicians recommended the sucking of blood from arm veins for rejuvenation, and one notable recipient was Pope Innocent VIII, who in 1492 was given a draught of blood from three youths.

Early accounts are confused by a failure to distinguish those who actually did something from those who merely talked about it. In 1656 there are records of Sir Christopher Wren giving intravenous infusions of an impressive array of substances, from opiates to beer, in a series of experiments on dogs. The scientific approach was developed in May 1665 by Bishop Wilkins and his friend Richard Lower, a Cornish physician. They had been stimulated by Harvey's description of the circulation, reported at meetings of the 'Invisible College', later to become the Royal Society.

Wilkins performed a successful transfusion between two dogs, using a syringe. Soon afterwards, in 1669, Lower performed the first direct transfusion, between two Bull Mastiffs, meticulously recorded in his *Tractatus de Corde*. Meanwhile, Louis XIV had founded the Académie des Sciences in response to the formation of the Royal Society. In 1667 the Royal Physician, Jean-Baptiste Denys, performed the first transfusions in humans. He recognized that repeated 'therapeutic' phlebotomy led to anaemia. However, following the death of one of his patients (a philandering husband who was given calf's blood to dampen his high spirits) stringent guidelines were imposed by the Faculty of Medicine of Paris. As the Faculty were bitterly opposed to transfusion, permission was never granted.[1]

Similar sentiments in Britain curbed interest in transfusion, until James Blundell (1790–1878) of Guys' Hospital described the effects of post-partum haemorrhage in humans. He used homologous and autologous transfusion in dogs to prevent the lethal consequences of haemorrhage and studied clotting, infection, rate of bleeding, delay in transfusion, air embolism and incompatibility in a series of experiments that were remarkable for the era (1818). Blundell is thought to have performed the first human-to-human blood transfusion and some credit him with the first use of autotransfusion for post-partum haemorrhage. Even so, sixty years later, Dr William Highmore of Sherborne in Dorset was still faced with the tragedy of watching a young mother bleed to death with post-partum haemorrhage and suggested reinfusion of the defibrinated blood.

The twentieth century was marked by the discovery of blood groups and iso-agglutination by Karl Landsteiner (1868–1943), for which he won the Nobel Prize. The discovery of citrate as an effective, safe anticoagulant led to the blood 'bank' and allowed Robertson in 1918 to store blood for 21 days and use it to treat haemorrhage on the battlefield. He discovered the advantages of adding glucose and that an acid reaction prevented caramelization of the glucose during autoclaving. With the pioneering work of JV Dacie and the establishment of a National Blood Transfusion Service, advanced operations such as those on the heart and blood vessels were possible. Technical advances and national publicity, with a population motivated by wartime austerity, ensured a plentiful supply of donors and this happy situation persisted until comparatively recently.

Haemorrhage and shock

Patients undergoing vascular operations may lose considerable volumes of blood at a rate which is not always controlled. The patient with a ruptured aortic aneurysm is an ideal model for haemorrhagic shock, but situations such as revascularization for acute lower-limb ischaemia result in similar pathophysiological responses.

The neurohormonal responses to hypovolaemia are well known and involve a sympathetic response to increase vasomotor tone and the renin–angiotensin system. One of the most important symptoms of shock, present in most patients with ruptured aneurysms, is thirst, mediated by angiotensin II acting on the sub-forniceal organ of the hypothalamus.

The most significant consequences of haemorrhagic shock involve microcirculatory disturbances, coagulopathy and activation of the cellular and humoral mediators of acute inflammation. Platelets and neutrophil leucocytes are sequestrated in ischaemic peripheral tissues, releasing thromboxane A_2, leukotrienes and platelet activating factor. Thromboxane is a powerful vasoconstrictor, causing redistribution of bloodflow with reduced skin, muscle, intestine and bone perfusion. Platelet and white cell activation causes local microvascular plugging, thrombosis and venoconstriction. Local coagulopathy is worsened by stasis, hypoxia and acidosis. One vulnerable vascular bed which suffers is that of the reticuloendothelial system, where sludging predisposes to sepsis.

Vascular permeability is increased by the release of mediators from tissues, cells and plasma (Fig. 12.1). Local mediators of inflammation can also act as hormones, leading to injury to distant organs. In the lungs, sequestration of platelets and white cells contributes to the development of the respiratory distress syndrome (Table 12.1).

The kidney is vulnerable to the same microvascular insult, which may lead to renal failure. Prolonged hypotension leads to regional infarction and acute tubular necrosis. There is no doubt that other organs experience significant injury even during elective operations. One example is the brain;

Table 12.1 Features of the respiratory distress syndrome

Features
Characteristic mottling throughout lung fields on chest X-ray
Arterial hypoxaemia despite adequate inspired oxygen concentration
Absence of infection
Absence of heart failure

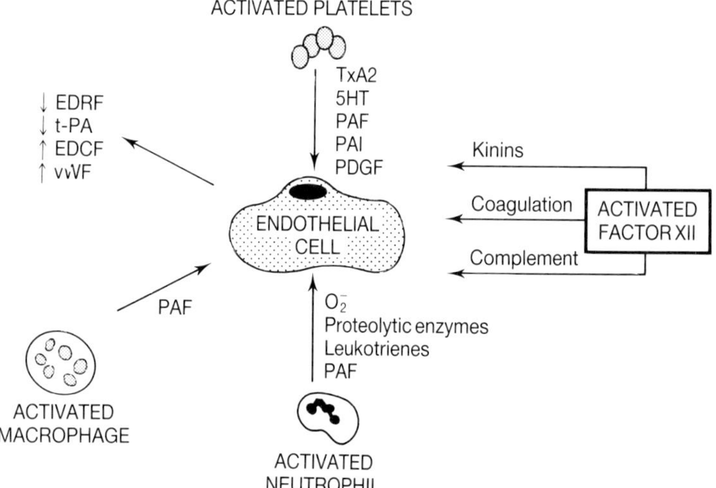

Fig. 12.1 Summary of factors leading to microvascular disturbances in patients with shock. Factor XIIa mediates coagulation, kinin and complement activation. Activation of the cellular components leads to the release of powerful local mediators which can also act as hormones leading to remote organ damage. TxA_2 = thromboxane A_2; PAF = platelet activation factor; PDGF = platelet derived growth factor; EDRF = endothelial cell relaxing factor (nitrous oxide); EDCF = endothelial cell contracting factor; vWF = von Willebrand factor.

elderly patients experience postoperative psychological disturbances ranging from frank psychosis to a subtle inability to concentrate which may persist for several months after aortic surgery.

Red cell transfusion

Indications for red cell transfusion

Humans have evolved with defensive reflexes and a much higher haemoglobin concentration than is needed in normal circumstances, to protect against death due to traumatic blood loss. Most healthy patients can tolerate postoperative haemoglobin levels of 70 g/l without symptoms, but the decision to transfuse should be made with the overall clinical picture in mind. Factors such as age, cardiorespiratory disease and whether or not continued loss is anticipated are important. The indications for red cell transfusion are:

1. maintenance or restoration of oxygen transport by the correction of anaemia
2. restoration of acute loss of more than 20% of the circulating blood volume.

Oxygen transport and tissue oxygen delivery depend on the oxygen affinity of the blood, its packed cell volume (PCV) and cardiac output. The oxygen affinity of bank blood is high, due mainly to a decreased concentration of 2,3 diphosphoglycerate (2,3,DPG) (Table 12.2). Normally, high levels of 2,3,DPG produced by the metabolic demands of glycolysis stimulate the release of oxygen. A compensatory increase in 2,3,DPG occurs in chronic anaemia and explains why these patients can tolerate haemoglobin levels which would result in severe symptoms if the blood loss were acute.

Table 12.2 Factors affecting the oxygen affinity of haemoglobin

Decreased affinity	Increased affinity
↑ pCO_2	↓ PCO_2
↓ pH	↑ pH
↑ 2,3,DPG, ↑ ATP, ↑ Pi	↓ 2,3,DPG, ↓ ATP, ↓ Pi
↑ Temp	↓ Temp
↑ MCHC	↓ MCHC
	↑ HbCO
	↑ Met Hb

MCHC = mean cell haemoglobin concentration; HbCO = carboxyhaemoglobin; Met Hb = methaemoglobin; Pi = inorganic phosphate; ATP = adenosine triphosphate.

The optimum PCV is 30%. At this level the oxygen content of the blood per unit volume has fallen, but blood viscosity decreases due to dilution. Consequently increased microcirculatory flow velocity maintains tissue oxygenation. An increase in ventricular stroke volume occurs which results in an elevated cardiac output but without an increase in heart rate.[2] Tissue oxygen delivery does not fall significantly until the PCV is less than 20%, which is when cardiac output rises sharply. If the heart is healthy, recovery and wound healing is normal at a PCV of 15%.

It is safer to correct preoperative anaemia with haematinics. When an operation is urgent the case should be discussed with the anaesthetist; if the haemoglobin is 80 g/l or less transfusion is usually indicated, but between 80 and 100 g/l it may be possible to withhold blood. Bank blood does not release oxygen efficiently until 2,3,DPG levels are restored, and as this takes at least 24 hours transfusion should not be delayed.

Postoperatively, the recommendation for fit individuals who are not continuing to bleed is that a PCV of 21% is acceptable (Hb 70 g/l).[3] However, vascular surgical patients have a high incidence of ischaemic heart disease and should be managed such that their haemoglobin level on discharge from hospital is approximately 10 g/l. This may involve repeated estimations to determine a trend, and so a microhaematocrit centrifuge is invaluable, especially in theatre. Generally, postoperative blood transfusion should not be ordered on the basis of a single unexpectedly low haemoglobin result (Table 12.3). The decision depends on the likelihood of continued blood loss and factors such as respiratory function, and should be made in collaboration with anaesthetist colleagues.

Table 12.3 Possible errors in haemoglobin determination

Sample dilution due to inadequate line flush or ipsilateral intravenous infusion
Clerical or laboratory error
Haemodilution due to perioperative crystalloid or colloid infusion
Haemodilution due to epidural anaesthesia causing vasodilation
Acute perioperative renal failure (e.g. acute tubular necrosis in ruptured aneurysm)

The volume of blood to transfuse

Blood loss must be estimated accurately, and this can be difficult owing to unmeasured losses on drapes or in haematomata, especially in ruptured aneurysms. The blood volume of the patient must be considered. Blood volume (in ml) is approximately 70 times body weight (in kg). Transfusion of a unit of blood usually increases the haemoglobin by 10 g/l Hb in an average individual, but this may lead to overtransfusion in small (usually female) patients with a low blood volume.

Loss of up to a litre (20% of the blood volume) can be tolerated without blood transfusion if volume replacement is given in the form of crystalloid or colloid solutions. Loss of over 20% of the blood volume is managed by a combination of red cell and volume replacement. Compared with colloid, at least two to three times the volume of crystalloid are required owing to its rapid redistribution. In shocked patients the redistribution of colloid or albumin is enhanced by increased capillary permeability. This decreases intravascular half-life and there is an increased risk of persistent oedema especially in the lungs. Over-enthusiastic preoperative resuscitation is an important cause of postoperative morbidity in shocked patients.

In clinical practice, the degree of filling of the intravascular compartment is difficult to measure accurately. Blood pressure, heart rate, central venous pressure, pulmonary artery wedge pressure and cardiac output all reflect the high-pressure part of the circulation. Central venous pressure is maintained by adrenergic mediated splanchnic venoconstriction which can compensate for a considerable deficit in blood volume. Postoperative patients with a normal pulse, blood pressure, urine output and CVP often feel clammy and shut down due to unrecognized (and unmeasurable) hypovolaemia. When blood volume is restored by recruitment of interstitial fluid, lymph and albumin (synthesized by the liver), peripheral vascular beds open up. This process is synonymous with convalescence; it is frustrating that there is no accurate way of measuring it. Restoration of blood volume can be estimated using ^{51}Cr-labelled red cells, tissue pO_2 or pH measurements; but measuring the difference between peripheral and core temperatures is more practical and deserves emphasis. Feeling the forearm skin temperature with the back of the hand is extremely helpful.

Peripheral venous haemoglobin and haematocrit measurements reflect the concentration of red cells in the peripheral circulation, not the circulation as a whole. For the reasons described above it is difficult to distinguish between anaemia with normovolaemia and hypovolaemic anaemia. Red cell transfusion in the hypovolaemic patient does not increase haemoglobin and haematocrit as much as would be expected. Transfused red cells may increase *plasma* volume by releasing vasodilators such as adenosine and by mechanical stimulation of endothelial cells which release prostaglandins and endothelial derived relaxing factors.

Red cell preparations

Donated whole blood is fractionated by centrifugation and precipitation techniques. This component therapy enables valuable plasma constituents to be preserved, reduces the volume of infusions, increases storage times and enables therapy to be directed by specific needs, such as burns. The common types of red cell preparation are shown in Table 12.4.

Table 12.4 Red cell preparations commonly available in surgical practice

Preparation	PCV	Vol (ml)	Notes
Packed cells	0.6–0.7	200	Plasma reduced; high-viscosity Additional volume replacement needed
Optimal additive	0.5–0.7	300	Plasma replaced with SAG-M (sodium, adenine, glucose, mannitol) Five-week life Lower viscosity
Cell Saver reinfusion product	0.5–0.7	225	Washed autologous red cells resuspended in saline Low-viscosity
Solcotrans unit	0.2–0.4 (same as patient)	500	Non-washed autologous red cells. Contains heparin. Low PCV 40 μm filter mandatory
Whole blood	0.3–0.4	510	Little justification for use

Leucocyte-depleted and thawed, washed frozen cells are available for patients with antibodies or rare blood groups.

Table 12.5 Immediate complications of blood transfusion relevant to surgical practice

Complication	Action required
Circulatory overload due to rapid infusion or heart failure	Frusemide 20 mg/unit of blood Oxygen Diamorphine 2.5–5.0 mg
Hyperkalaemia due to haemolysis (usually due to delay in transfusion)	Transfuse within 6h at ambient temperature. Glucose/insulin infusion if K^+ rises
Haemolytic reactions: fever, tachcardia, loin pain, rigors, vomiting, dyspnoea, hypotension, renal failure and disseminated intravascular coagulation	Usually clerical error Stop transfusion and flush cannula Check identification labels, return blood bag to laboratory and consult haematologist
Non haemolytic reactions: pyrexia, urticaria	Antihistamine, paracetamol If severe may require discontinuation of transfusion
Citrate toxicity, hypothermia, dilutional coagulopathy, acidosis	Warm blood, monitor clotting parameters and platelets Give calcium gluconate (see text)

Acid citrate dextrose (ACD) and citrate phosphate dextrose (CPD) are used to anticoagulate donated blood. The low pH (5.0–5.5) prevents caramelization of the dextrose during sterilisation, but decreases 2,3,DPG levels in bank blood to less than 10% after 14 days storage. Only 40 ml of the 67.5 ml of citrate added to each unit of ACD blood is needed to chelate calcium and prevent clotting. This excess citrate is in the plasma and not the cellular fraction, so packed cells contain less free citrate than whole blood. Rapid transfusion may lower plasma calcium, leading to myocardial depression and ventricular arrhythmias, especially in hypothermia. If in doubt, calcium gluconate (10 ml of 10% solution initially) may be given with ECG monitoring.

Warming of blood and blood products helps to maintain the electrical stability of the heart, improves the function of platelets and clotting proteins, and decreases the toxic potential of excess citrate. Hypothermia is one of the most under-appreciated causes of postoperative bleeding. Platelets in particular are susceptible to temperature; a decreased temperature increases the bleeding time.

Blood administration sets contain a 150 μm screen filter. Additional filtration is not normally necessary, but if a large transfusion is given it may be prudent to add a 40-micron filter to decrease the concentration of microaggregates which may increase pulmonary vascular resistance and predispose to ARDS.

Infection and immune suppression

Concern regarding blood transfusion has centred on the medium- and long-term implications of immune suppression and disease transmission. Blood transfusion leads to depressed cell-mediated immunity in recipients. This effect may be beneficial, such as is seen in the improved survival of renal transplants in transfused recipients; but it may also be detrimental. Perioperative blood transfusion leads to increased septic complications following operation, and recently it has been found that ultrafiltration to remove white cells decreases the incidence of wound infections.[4] HIV-positive individuals progress more rapidly to AIDS if they are transfused whole blood than if they are transfused packed cells. Increased rates of cancer recurrence have been reported in transfused patients but there is as yet no properly conducted trial to confirm the observation. The need for perioperative transfusion depends on so many factors that the effect may be an epiphenomenon.[5]

Blood is now tested serologically for hepatitis A, hepatitis B and non-A non-B hepatitis (now known as hepatitis C), which causes 90% of transfusion-associated hepatitis. The risk of hepatitis C infection following transfusion is small (probably in the region of 1 in 200–400), but the chances that the disease will progress to cirrhosis are high (10–20%). Transmission of HIV by an infected unit of blood is possible despite antibody testing, owing to the window before an infected individual mounts an antibody response. The risk is approximately 1 in 10^6. Many are more concerned about oncogenic viruses which may have a long incubation period, such as HTLV-1 (human T cell lymphoma virus). This virus is more prevalent than HIV but is not tested for. Although the figures are small the diseases themselves are fatal and provoke concern and adverse publicity which may undermine confidence in the blood supply. For all of these reasons it is prudent to minimize blood transfusion.

Reducing blood transfusion

For operations such as carotid endarterectomy, where transfusion is usually not required, a blood sample should be sent for 'group and save'. The blood is typed and screened for clinically important antibodies. If none is found the serum is stored for 7 days after the operation date. If antibodies are found, antigen-negative blood is reserved, even when the chance of transfusion is low. Most physicians cross-match more blood than is necessary. The ratio of blood transfused to blood cross-matched should be audited and the order adjusted according to local and individual requirements; the ratio should be greater than 2:1. Blood released by the transfusion service is out of circulation for several days and often exceeds its expiry date, so a proportion (typically 70%) of the cost of cross-matched blood has to be paid whether it is used or not.

Postoperative transfusion should only be used if clinically indicated. The decision should not be delegated to junior staff; house surgeons do not decide whether or not to perform organ transplants!

Operative techniques such as cutting diathermy and minimal dissection can reduce bleeding. The graft inlay technique minimizes damage to veins, and both the exclusion method of grafting and the retroperitoneal approach to the aorta reduce blood loss. Sealed grafts do not need to be preclotted and may help reduce blood loss, although the benefit is likely to be small compared with woven grafts. Intraoperative heparin makes little difference to overall blood loss, provided it is carefully monitored and reversed if necessary. The activated clotting time (ACT) can be used in theatre to judge the anticoagulant effect of heparin and is useful in adjusting the dose of protamine used to reverse it. Excess protamine is an anticoagulant and inhibits platelet function. Drugs such as nonsteroidal anti-inflammatories and aspirin irreversibly inhibit platelet enzyme systems and increase perioperative blood loss. They should be withdrawn two weeks preoperatively if possible as a new population of platelets is required to re-establish haemostasis.

Platelet and plasma transfusion

Platelets are the most important link in surgical haemostasis. Diminished number or function can lead to excessive bleeding. Circulating platelets are activated by exposure to a variety of stimuli such as collagen, basal membrane structures and microfibrils exposed when vascular endothelial cells are damaged; von Willebrand factor supports this reaction. During the adherence and aggregation of platelets, membrane phospholipid receptors are exposed which stimulate coagulation. These include surface-bound platelet factor III, which binds to factor V. Activated factor X completes the enzyme complex, which catalyses the release of thrombin, leading to further aggregation, adenosine diphosphate release, and the production of thromboxane A_2 and platelet aggregation factor. Fibrinogen is also required for aggregation. One of the mechanisms by which aprotinin (see below) acts is by preserving platelet receptors, which may explain why it reduces bleeding in patients taking aspirin.

Platelets for transfusion are collected by centrifugation of donated whole blood or by apheresis of platelet rich plasma. If operation is planned in patients with thrombocytopenia or a functional platelet disorder, platelet cover should be discussed with a haematologist. During or after operation, platelet transfusion is indicated in dilutional thrombocytopenia, where platelet concentration falls below 50×10^9/l but only if the patient is bleeding.[6] Platelet counts below this level may be acceptable and clinical judgement is imperative, as platelet concentrate may be pooled, thus exposing the patient to a greater number of potentially infected donors. There is no place for 'cook book' prescriptions of a set ratio of platelets or plasma to accompany high-volume red cell transfusion. Finally, it is vital that the patient is warmed postoperatively as platelet enzymes are highly sensitive to temperature.

Plasma transfusion is of very limited value in surgery. The only true indications are the correction of coagulation in an emergency when the patient is receiving oral anticoagulants, or to correct bleeding in a patient with liver disease. Dilutional coagulopathy is a relative indication; surgical bleeding only occurs when clotting protein levels fall to very low levels, corresponding to at least 80% of an exchange transfusion. Plasma must not be administered unless the patient has abnormal clotting studies which reverse *in-vitro* with normal plasma *and* clinically important bleeding.[7]

Autologous blood

The use of the patient's own blood whenever possible is mandatory in the USA and some European countries. Several techniques are relevant to vascular surgery.

Predonation

This involves repeated venesection in the weeks leading up to the time of the operation and can be highly effective. Consent is obtained by the surgeon. The patient undergoes a medical examination and ECG under the auspices of the transfusion medicine department, with measurement of the haematocrit and PCV. If these are acceptable, 450 ml of whole blood is venesected into a standard CPD-A blood-pack, with a shelf-life of 35 days, and the patient is started on oral ferrous sulphate 200 mg twice-daily. The donation is repeated as required, with the final unit being taken at least 4 days preoperatively. An intense marrow response can be stimulated with iron supplementation, so that up to 2 units per week can be donated, with only a slight degree of anaemia.[8] In a review of 11 studies, the mean donation was 2.6 units and 66% of predonors were treated with autologous blood alone. Additional homologous blood was required by only 28%.[9]

There are several techniques available to increase the efficiency of predonation. In the 'leapfrog' approach a patient donates a unit, then at the next hospital visit receives that blood back and donates two units, and so on. Genetically engineered recombinant human erythropoeitin (rHuEPo) stimulates erythropoeisis. In a prospective randomized controlled trial from Ohio,[10] 96% of a rHuEPo-treated group but only 71% of the matched placebo group donated more than 4 units. As rHuEPo is expensive it will probably be reserved for female patients with low blood volumes, or patients requiring large transfusions.

The most important drawbacks to predonation in the United Kingdom are the logistic barrier involved and cancellation of operations due to emergencies and other factors. If the blood is not to be wasted, the admission and operation should be 'ring fenced'.

Isovolaemic haemodilution

Isovolaemic haemodilution involves venesection in the anaesthetic room immediately before the operation, after the insertion of central venous and arterial pressure lines. A colloidal plasma expander is infused simultaneously to avoid hypovolaemia. Bleeding during operation consequently consists of dilute blood, which is replaced with the autologous blood. The volume of blood removed is calculated on the basis of the patient's haematocrit, with a final value of 0.30 usually yielding over 2 units of autologous blood. The blood is kept at room temperature, and is reinfused at the end of the procedure, to maximize the benefit of functional platelets and clotting proteins (Figs 12.2 and 12.3). The technique has been shown to be effective and may actually benefit patients with ischaemic heart disease.[11]

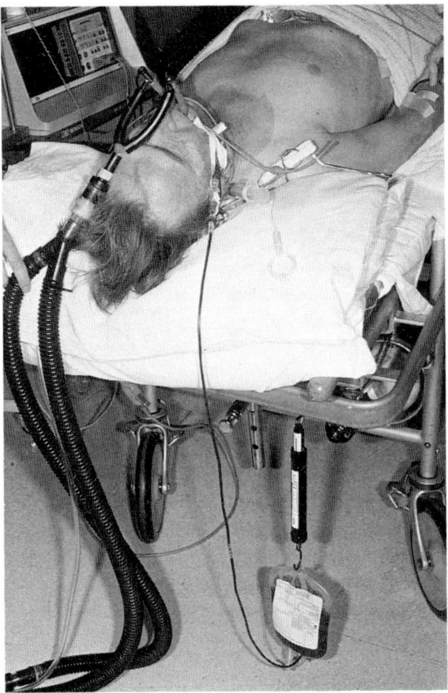

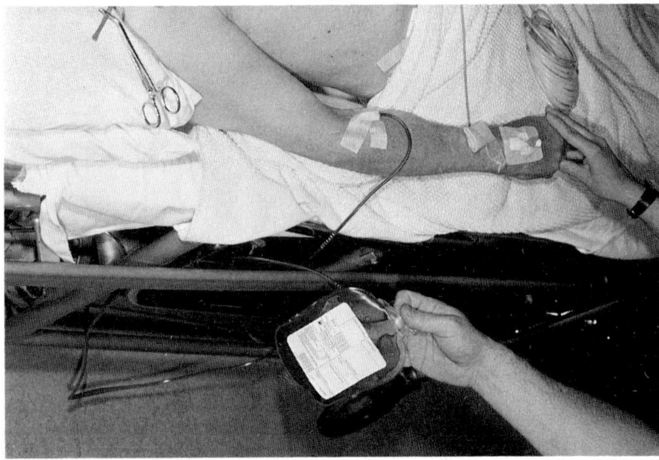

Fig. 12.2 Isovolaemic haemodilution. Two units of blood are withdrawn from the central line (left), or from a peripheral line (right).

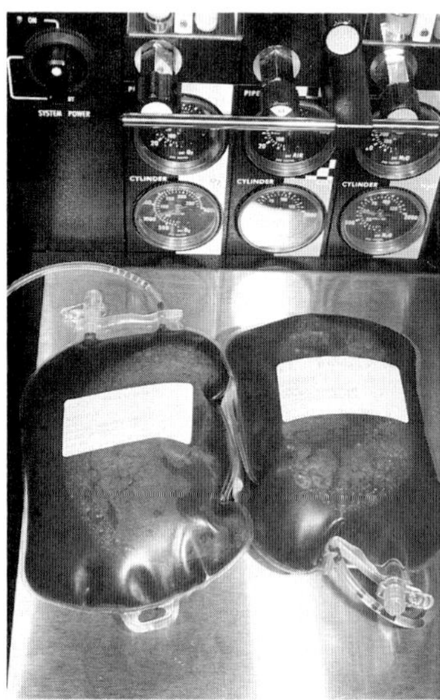

Fig. 12.3 Isovolaemic haemodilution. The blood bags contain CPD anticoagulant and are continuously weighed to ensure isovolaemic replacement with colloid. Blood is clearly labelled and stored at room temperature before reinfusion, in reverse order, after surgical bleeding has ceased.

Salvage autotransfusion

This important technique is useful for abdominal or thoracic surgery as shed blood pools in a natural cavity from where it may be salvaged. Mesothelial lined cavities secrete tissue plasminogen activator which lyses clotted blood, thereby facilitating salvage. The defibrinogenated blood can be reinfused after filtration alone and this simple method has been used for bleeding ectopic pregnancy for many years in Third World countries. Salvage is not suitable for operations where blood does not pool, such as femorodistal reconstruction or carotid endarterectomy. It may be combined with either predeposit or isovolaemic haemodilution. In vascular trauma salvage, systems should not be used if the operative field is contaminated, but if bank blood is not available the technique may save lives. Jehovah's Witnesses may accept cell salvage provided a continuous system is used so that their blood does not lose continuity with the circulation.

In modern devices a suction line is used to retrieve shed blood which is filtered and reinfused, with or without washing. There are several intraoperative systems on the market; either a passive disposable reservoir (Solcotrans, Fig. 12.4) or cell-washing devices such as the Cell Saver (Fig. 12.5). The operating principle of the Cell Saver is shown in Fig. 12.6. It heparinizes shed blood at the sucker tip, enabling salvage to continue throughout the operation and 75–80% of the total loss to be salvaged. Solcotrans autotransfusion requires systemic high-dose heparinization and the ACT should be maintained at twice the baseline figure to inhibit clotting. Solcotrans is an attractive proposition for the smaller hospital as an operator is not required.

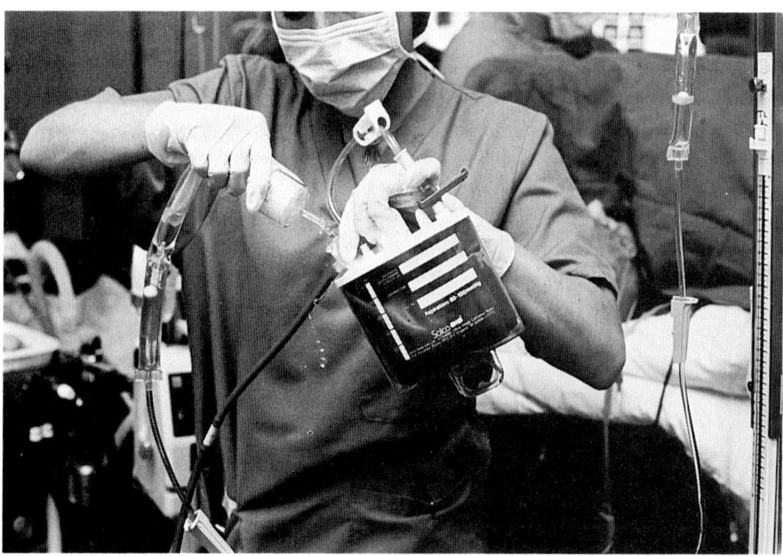

Fig. 12.4 The Solcotrans intraoperative device.

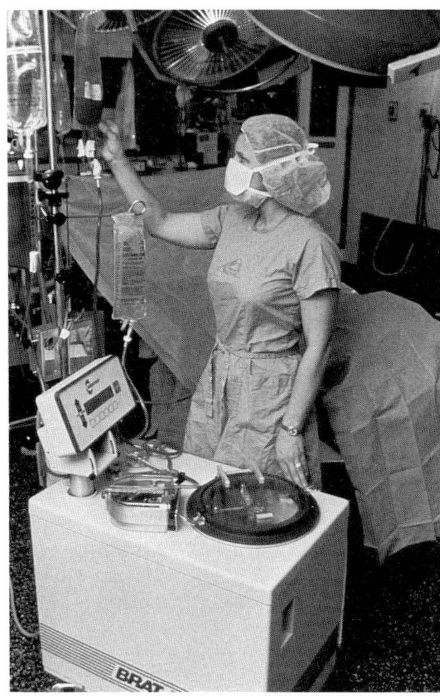

Fig. 12.5 A centrifugal cell-washing device: the Cobe BRAT (Baylor Rapid Autotransfusion) system. Devices such as these can supply a unit of washed red cells resuspended in saline in approximately four minutes.

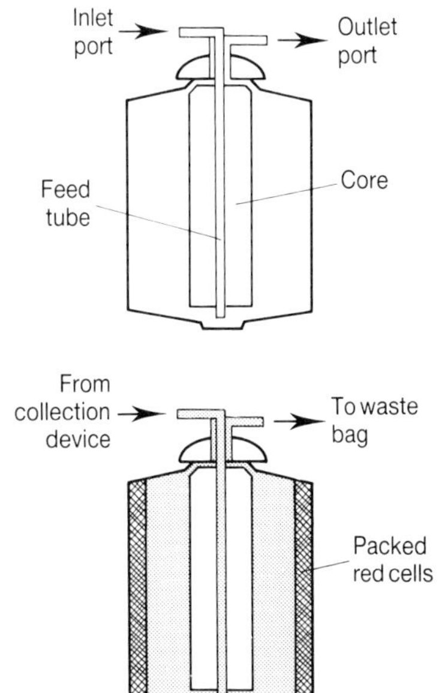

Fluid from the collection device fills the spinning bowl. The denser, heavier red cells are separated from the lighter saline, plasma, and debris

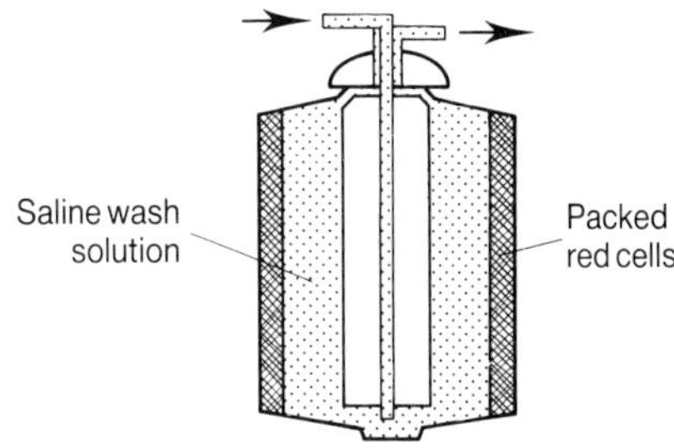

In the wash mode, saline is introduced, displacing the lighter layer containing plasma and debris. The final product consists of red cells resuspended in saline

Fig. 12.6 The operating principle of the Cell Saver.

Pharmacological manipulation of blood loss

Vasopressin and its analogue DDAVP, prostacyclin, dipyridamole and epsilon aminocaproic acid have been used to reduce perioperative bleeding with little proven benefit, but current interest centres on the serine protease inhibitor, aprotinin (Trasylol, Bayer Ltd). After initial studies demonstrating a dramatic reduction in bleeding after re-do cardiac surgery,[12] the effect has been confirmed by a total European experience exceeding 1000 cases. Aprotinin has now been shown to be effective in primary cardiac surgery, orthotopic liver transplantation and hip replacement; and in a pilot study it reduced blood loss in aortic reconstruction.[13] The mechanism of action is unclear, but probably involves preservation of platelet membrane glycoproteins and inhibition of secondary fibrinolysis. A recent report demonstrated inhibition of neutrophil activation during vascular surgery which may be useful in the prophylaxis of ARDS and reperfusion injury.[14]

Final note

Safe and plentiful homologous blood transfusion has enabled the practice of vascular surgery to flourish. The HIV epidemic has, however, stimulated interest into other physiological and pathological consequences of transfusion. All clinicians must use this precious resource wisely and sparingly by conservation and recycling, which is after all the theme of the decade.

Recommended further reading

1. Contreras MC (ed). *ABC of Transfusion.* London: BMA, 1990.
2. Dzik WH, Sherburne B. Intraoperative blood salvage: medical controversies. *Transf Med Rev* 1990; **4:** 208–35.
3. American Association of Blood Banks. *Guidelines for Blood Salvage and Reinfusion in Surgery and Trauma.* Arlington: AABB, 1990.

References

1. Hall RA, Hall MB. The first human blood transfusion. Priority disputes. *Med Hist* 1980; **24:** 461.
2. Messmer K. Acute normovolaemic haemodilution: changes of central haemodynamics and microcirculating flow in skeletal muscle. *Eur Surg Res* 1972; **4:** 55.
3. Office of Medical Applications of Research, National Institutes of Health. Perioperative red cell transfusion. *JAMA* 1988; **260:** 2700–3.
4. Jensen LS, Andersen AJ, Christiansen PJ, Hokland P, Jukl CO, Madsen G, Mortensen J, Moller-Neilsen C, Hanberg-Sorensen F, Hockland M. Postoperative infection and natural killer cell function following blood transfusion in patients undergoing elective colorectal surgery. *Br J Surg* 1992; **79:** 513–16.
5. Francis DMA. Relationship between blood transfusion and tumour behaviour. *Br J Surg* 1991; **78:** 1420–8.
6. Office of Medical Applications of Research, National Institutes of Health. Platelet transfusion therapy. *JAMA* 1987; **257:** 1777.
7. Office of Medical Applications of Research, National Institutes of Health. Fresh frozen plasma: indications and risks. *JAMA* 1985; **253:** 551.
8. Coleman DH, Stevens AR. Rate of blood regeneration after blood loss. *Arch Int Med* 1953; **92:** 341–9.
9. Kay LA, Noble RS. Autologous blood transfusion. *Haem Rev* 1988; **2:** 305–26.
10. Goodnough LT. Preoperative autologous blood donation in orthopaedic surgery: its utilisation and efficacy and the ipact of erythropoeitin therapy. Presented at the Haemonetics Research Institute Symposium, Boston, USA, Sept 1989.
11. Erlenwein S, Keissewetter H, Jung F, Wentzel E, Vogel W, Dykmans J, Bach R, Hahman H, Scheiffer H, Bette L. Isovolaemic haemodilution in patients with ischaemic heart disease. In: *Hydroxyethyl Starch: A Current Overview,* Lawin P, Zander J, Weidler B (eds). Stuttgart: Thieme, 1992.
12. Royston D, Bidstrup BD, Taylor KM, Sapsford RD. Effect of aprotinin on the need for blood transfusions after repeat open heart surgery. *Lancet* 1987; **ii:** 1289–91.
13. Thompson JF, Roath OS, Francis JL, Webster JHH, Chant ADB. Aprotinin in peripheral vascular surgery. *Lancet* 1990; **335:** 911.
14. Lord RL, Roath OS, Thompson JF, Chant ADB, Francis JL. Effect of aprotinin on neutrophil function after major vascular surgery. *Br J Surg* 1992; **79:** 517–21.

13

Anaesthesia and postoperative care

CS Waldmann and C Verghese

Vascular surgery is a growing specialty and presents a particularly difficult challenge to the anaesthetist. In a recent prospective audit, hospital mortality in general surgery was 1.3% whilst that for vascular surgery was 6.2%.[1] Vascular patients are older, stay in hospital longer and have more intercurrent disease than general surgical patients.[2] In our own experience, an anaesthetic audit for the year 1991 showed that 60% of general surgical patients were ASA I, 34% were ASA II and only 6% were ASA III or worse (see Table 13.1). By contrast, the corresponding figures for vascular surgical patients were 27% ASA I, 33% ASA II and 40% ASA III–V.

The main causes of postoperative morbidity are cardiac and renal problems. Coronary artery disease is particularly common in this group of patients. This may create a hazard when the aorta is cross-clamped in major aortic procedures, but even patients undergoing distal reconstruction have a greater number of complications during and after anaesthesia.

Table 13.1 The American Society of Anesthesiologists' classification

ASA I	A normal healthy patient
ASA II	A patient with mild systemic disease
ASA III	A patient with severe systemic disease that limits activity but is not incapacitating
ASA IV	A patient with an incapacitating systemic disease that is a constant threat to life
ASA V	A moribund patient not expected to survive 24 hours with or without an operation

Preoperative risk assessment

Cardiac

Patients presenting for vascular reconstruction usually have widespread atherosclerosis and are likely to be hypertensive. In patients over 65 years of age, 40% have been shown to have a blood pressure greater than 150/100.[3] Occasionally patients may be taking old-fashioned antihypertensives such as methyldopa and reserpine.

Goldman *et al.*[4] described an index of cardiac risk (see Table 13.2) and demonstrated that the likelihood of postoperative cardiac problems occurring increased as the index rose.

In a study in our hospital using Detsky's modification[5] of Goldman's index, 93 patients were prospectively analysed. Angina was the only risk factor that was independently statistically significant in predicting postoperative cardiac problems.[6] However, as the cardiac risk score rose, so did the likelihood of postoperative cardiac problems. Even in the presence of a normal ECG and the absence of cardiac symptoms, significant myocardial disease may exist. In order to detect this asymptomatic but significant disease, the use of stress tests, ejection fraction studies and coronary angiography may be necessary.

Stress tests

These attempt to relate changes in coronary artery blood flow (induced by exercise or pharmacological dilatation) with subsequent myocardial ischaemia (measured by ECG) or ventricular perfusion or movement (measured by isotope scanning).

Exercise stress test (EST). Exercise testing reveals significant coronary artery disease in 30% of asymptomatic patients with a normal resting ECG[7] (Fig. 13.1). Perioperative myocardial infarction occurred in 37% of patients with a positive ischaemic response compared with 1.5% of those without. An important aspect is the absence of chest pain in 80% of those patients having ischaemic ECG changes during EST. However, the higher rate of false positives (40%) and false negatives (15%) means that EST is of doubtful value in predicting the need for coronary angiography.

Dipyridamole – thallium scanning (DT scan). While more expensive than EST, DT scanning is a valuable

Table 13.2 Risk factor scores for calculating the Goldman cardiac risk index

Risk factor	Points
Third heart sound or raised jugular venous pressure	11
Myocardial infarct within 6 months	10
More than 5 ventricular ectopic beats per minute	7
Rhythm other than sinus	7
Age greater than 70 years	5
Intraperitoneal, thoracic or aortic surgery	3
Emergency	4
Aortic stenosis	3
Poor general condition	3

The Goldman cardiac risk index

Class	Points	Nil or minor complications (%)	Life-threatening complications (%)	Cardiac death (%)
I	0–5	99	0.7	0.2
II	6–12	93	5	2
III	13–25	86	11	2
IV	25+	22	22	56

alternative. Known as the 'lazy man's stress test',[8] it is particularly useful in patients with claudication significant enough to prevent them using a treadmill. The scan requires the use of a coronary artery dilator (dipyridamole) linked to the radioisotope thallium and demonstrates areas of ischaemic myocardium. Boucher *et al.*[9] found that following a negative scan there were no untoward cardiac events during vascular operations, but in those patients with a positive scan there was a 50% incidence of postoperative cardiac symptoms. It has been suggested that all patients about to undergo vascular reconstruction might be screened by a DT scan, but this would be costly. An initial stratification of risk using clinical predictors might allow the number of DT scans to be halved.[10]

Ejection fraction (EF) measurements

Left ventricular ejection fraction can be measured noninvasively using echocardiography or by radioisotope scanning. We have been using a technique in which 0.03 ml/kg of a specifically prepared stannous

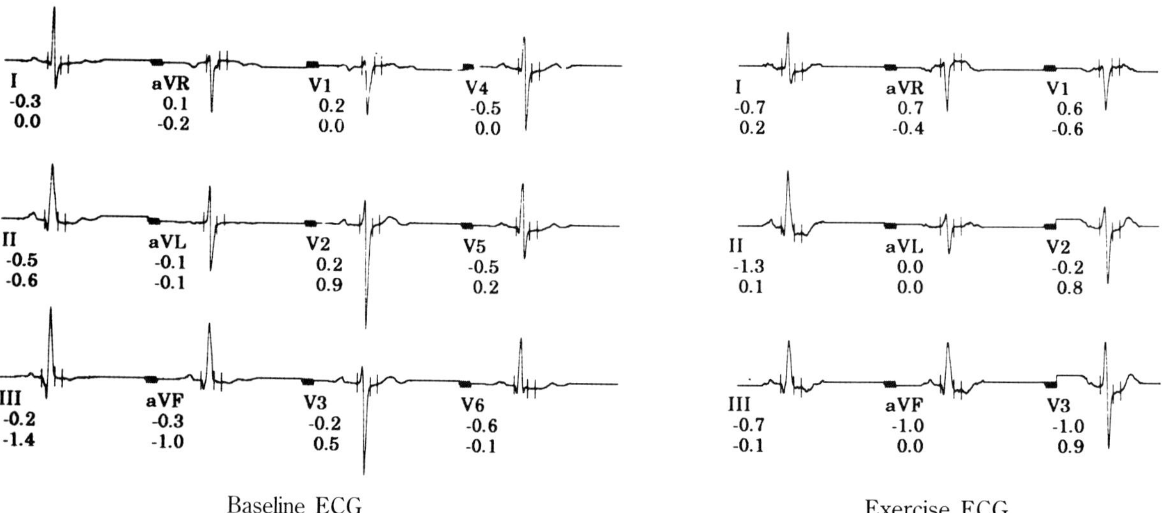

Fig. 13.1 Baseline and exercise ECG showing the development of widespread ST changes. The test had to be terminated owing to angina.

agent, which coats red cells, is injected intravenously. Thirty minutes later 600 MBq of technetium 99 m is given to tag to the tin. The ejection fraction is then assessed by a gamma camera gated to the ECG.

A preoperative EF of less than 40% is reported to be predictive of perioperative myocardial infarction and reinfarction.[11] An EF of less than 50% at rest, with abnormal myocardial contractility and/or less than a 5% EF increase following exercise, might indicate the need for coronary angiography.[12] A miniature probe system for continuous online monitoring of EF is now available for clinical use.[13]

Coronary angiography

In spite of the high incidence of coronary artery disease in patients with peripheral vascular disease, routine coronary angiography is not widely carried out. It should be restricted to those patients with severe, unstable symptoms.[14,15]

Respiratory function

Respiratory function deteriorates with age. Apart from a decreased responsiveness to carbon dioxide, which may be aggravated by opioids, anaesthetic agents and muscular relaxants, there is an increased potential for aspiration of stomach contents into the lungs. A decreased cough response has been demonstrated in the aged.[16] Average paO_2 has been shown to be reduced with age in a way that can be approximated by the formula[17]

$$paO_2 \text{ (mm/Hg)} = 100 - 0.54 \times \text{age}.$$

Vascular patients often have a history of heavy smoking and consequently poor respiratory function. An assessment of the patient's respiratory reserve may be made by accompanying the patient on a short walk, as well as looking at the chest X-ray, pulmonary function tests and baseline blood gas analysis.

Diabetes mellitus

The major risk factors for patients with diabetes mellitus (insulin and non-insulin dependent) are the associated end organ diseases: cardiovascular dysfunction, renal insufficiency, abnormalities in joints (limitation of head extension), poor wound healing and peripheral neuropathies. The combined presence of hypertension and diabetes is a strong indication of autonomic neuropathy and poor prognosis. A thorough assessment of end organ disease preoperatively along with perioperative management of blood glucose levels and intensive postoperative care of those with autonomic system abnormalities is currently thought to be the most appropriate management of these patients.[18]

Age

In a series of 108 878 anaesthetics with an overall mortality of 2.19%, there was a 6% mortality in those patients over 64 years of age.[19] Nevertheless, aortic reconstruction can be performed safely in older patients. Almost 20 years ago a series of 111 patients over 80 years of age was described with a mortality rate of only 2% following elective aortic aneurysm repair.[20] However, it is well established that increase in age is associated with an increased postoperative mortality following aneurysm resection.[21] Age and infirmity, nevertheless, are not synonymous. Age alone does not necessarily preclude anaesthesia for major aortic reconstruction. In a recent editorial[22] the term 'agism' was used to emphasize that perhaps society in general deprives people of services, including medical treatment, because of their age. Following successful aortic reconstruction even older patients can expect a life expectancy parallel to that of their peers.[23]

Preoperative management

The preoperative assessment of patients about to undergo major vascular operations should begin in the outpatient department when the diagnosis is confirmed. Preoperative and anaesthetic evaluation may not be adequate if they take place on the day prior to operation.

In our practice six units of blood are normally cross-matched prior to operation. There is now a growing tendency to use autologous blood by taking off two units at induction, haemodiluting the patient and then replacing the blood later, or by the use of cell-saving machines or a predonation scheme (see Chapter 12).

Management of coexisting disease

Diabetes

The preoperative assessment of a patient with diabetes should include an evaluation of the overall nutritional state. The adequacy of therapy for glucose control and previous responses to anaesthesia and operation can also be assessed. Fifty per cent of patients with diabetes and hypertension have autonomic neuropathy, compared with 10% when hypertension is absent. Patients with severe autonomic dysfunction are at an increased risk of gastroparesis and cardiorespiratory arrest. Signs of autonomic dysfunction such as early satiety, lack of sweating, impotence and a decreased response in pulse rate changes with deep inspiration or orthostatic manoeuvres (usually 15 beats/min but less than 5/min in autonomic dysfunction) are easily elicited. Measuring the degree of beat-to-beat variability in the preoperative ECG may also help to establish a diagnosis of autonomic dysfunction. Postural hypotension, resting tachycardia and noctural diarrhoea are other indicators.

Thus, a preoperative evaluation of glucose control, response to previous operation, a search for end-organ disease (particularly autonomic dysfunction), scheduling of the operation early in the day, coupled with close monitoring of blood glucose levels preoperatively and the monitoring of high-risk patients for 24 hours postoperatively, further reduce the morbidity and mortality in this group of patients.

Hypertension

Approximately 40% of patients presenting for vascular reconstruction have a history of hypertension. Anaesthesia in these patients is associated with sensitivity to most anaesthetic drugs and extreme lability of blood pressure. Hypertensive vascular patients are more likely to develop postoperative hypertension, but this does not appear to be a predictable risk factor. However, it should alert the anaesthetist to other problems such as electrolyte abnormalities, decreased intravascular volume and altered organ function. It is our practice to continue any beta-adrenoceptor blocking drugs up until the time of the operation.

Cardiac disease

Except in an emergency, the presence of congestive heart failure would necessitate deferral of operation. Arrhythmias may be present and need evaluating and control before operation. Rapid atrial fibrillation may require preoperative digitalization, and the presence of first and second degree heart blocks may require the insertion of a temporary pacing wire to cover the perioperative period. In the presence of an artificial heart valve, there should be discussion between surgeon, anaesthetist, microbiologist and haematologist regarding the type and duration of anticoagulation and antibiotic treatment. The presence of a permanent pacemaker must be noted. Some may be affected by diathermy and need to be switched to a fixed rate with a magnet. However, it is usually sufficient to place the diathermy plate as far from the pacemaker as possible, to use short bursts of diathermy and to monitor cardiac rhythm.

Renal problems

Acute renal failure is frequently reported following infrarenal aortic cross-clamping. Even with improvements in patient selection, anaesthetic management and surgical techniques, a 0.2–3% incidence of acute renal failure has recently been published, with a mortality of up to 25% despite aggressive management.[24] It has been suggested that preoperative renal ultrasound or IVP should be carried out to detect any ureteric obstruction or distortion produced by the aneurysm; to determine the excretory function of the two kidneys; and to ensure that horseshoe kidney will not be encountered unexpectedly.

Visit by the anaesthetist

This is a most important aspect of a patient's management and will familiarize the anaesthetist with any intercurrent medical and potential anaesthetic problems. Patients with coronary artery disease may be taking a number of drugs. Continuation of these drugs should be assessed on an individual basis.

The anaesthetist should ensure that blood is cross-matched, even when cell-saving techniques are used. The availability of an ITU bed should also be confirmed. The anaesthetist may also alter the timing of a preoperative dose of subcutaneous heparin so that it is administered after the epidural cannula is inserted if regional blockade is proposed. This minimizes the risk of epidural haematoma formation. Premedication with oral benzodiazepine, or parenteral opioid and an antisialogogue, is influenced by the personal choice of the anaesthetist. It is necessary to ensure the patient is not allergic to any anaesthetic drugs or antibiotics. We use cefuroxime 750 mg starting at induction of anaesthesia.

Visit by the intensive therapy nurse

The patient may benefit from being psychologically prepared for a stay on the ITU and a visit to the unit may be beneficial. In our hospital the ITU nurse routinely visits all patients likely to be admitted. In a recent study,[25] 20 patients about to undergo major operations, including aortic aneurysm resection, were visited by one of our nurses. The survey demonstrated that the visit and the supply of an information booklet about the ITU was useful. The patients commented that they would have preferred additional advice and time to absorb the details of the proposed operation.

Resuscitation of shocked patients

If rupture has occurred, resuscitation must be performed at the same time that the operation is started. Immediate stabilization may be obtained by the use of a compression suit applied for transfer from the emergency department to the operating theatre. It is regarded as unnecessary and often impossible to achieve a systolic blood pressure greater than 80 mm/Hg until the surgeon has control of bleeding.

Anaesthetic technique

Much of this chapter is concerned with problems associated with infrarenal aortic reconstruction. However, mention should be made of *carotid artery surgery*. Positioning involves elevating the shoulders and rotating the head away from the side of the operation. Extreme head rotation should be avoided since it may result in sharp angulation and compression of the vertebral artery. The proximity of the carotid sinus may be the reason why these patients are at particular risk of bradycardia. The choice of drugs for induction of general anaesthesia should be to maintain cerebral blood flow, but reduce cerebral metabolic oxygen consumption and produce minimal postoperative neuralgic effects. Excessive increased cerebral blood flow should be avoided in order to prevent cerebral haemorrhage and oedema formation. Barbituates may produce a 50% reduction in cerebral metabolic rate, but this advantage may be offset by arterial hypotension. For this reason ketamine has been recommended for anaesthetic induction and maintenance. Unlike regional anaesthesia, general anaesthesia does not lend itself easily to monitoring of the adequacy of regional cerebral perfusion. Internal carotid artery stump pressure is a useful measure of cerebral perfusion by the collateral circulation, as are somatosensory evoked potentials (see Chapter 19).

Monitoring for aortic reconstruction

Pulse oximetry and end-tidal carbon dioxide have only been available in most operating theatres and ITUs relatively recently. Along with monitoring of tidal volume and ventilator disconnect alarms, they are considered mandatory by the Association of Anaesthetists of Great Britain.

Pulse oximetry

Pulse oximetry is the measurement of arterial blood oxygen concentration by detection of light absorption by use of a finger probe. Subtracting the nonpulsatile component from the total signal gives a clinical measurement of arterial oxygenation.

ECG

The modified bipolar chest–manubrium configuration of leads (CM5) has the greatest likelihood of detecting ischaemia both intraoperatively and postoperatively.[26] CM5 involves the use of a right arm lead in the second right intercostal space, a left leg lead in the V5 position and a ground lead placed anywhere.

Arterial blood pressure

Use of an indwelling arterial cannula allows accurate beat-to-beat assessment of blood pressure. Appropriate intervention can then be made for any major changes that may occur at induction, intubation, skin incision, cross-clamping, unclamping or during the postoperative period. The cannula also allows for easy sampling of arterial blood.

Damage to the wall of the artery, resulting in aneurysm formation or complete occlusion with distal gangrene, is a complication of radial artery cannulation if the collateral circulation is inadequate. Allen's test[27] may demonstrate palmar reflow of blood but does not guarantee that ischaemic necrosis will not occur. Slogoff *et al.*[28] demonstrated, in a prospective study of 1699 cardiovascular surgical patients, that partial or complete occlusion of the radial artery occurred in more than 25% of patients after decannulation, yet no ischaemia or disability was demonstrated.

Generally, cannulation of the nondominant hand with a 20 g Teflon parallel-sided cannula is preferred. Brachial and axillary artery cannulation have also been described. The closer the intra-arterial cannula is to the aorta, the more useful the information displayed by the arterial wave trace on the monitor. The shape of the arterial waveform may be used for assessing ventricular contractility and stroke volume, and for a visual assessment of systemic resistance.

Central venous pressure

Monitoring central venous pressure (CVP) is of limited value in assessing the adequacy of blood volume. It is useful as long as the patient has adequate left ventricular function. Mangano noted a close, and clinically useful, correlation between CVP and PCWP (pulmonary capillary wedge pressure) changes induced by alterations in preload in patients with an EF > 0.5 presenting for coronary bypass grafting.[11] The triple-lumen catheters now in use are invaluable for drug administration, particularly of inotropes. Position of the monitoring lines and the endotracheal tube can be assessed in the ITU by chest X-ray.

Pulmonary artery pressure

Balloon-tipped pulmonary artery (Swan–Ganz) catheters are used as an indirect measurement of left atrial pressure and to measure cardiac output. Modern catheters have the facility for measuring cardiac output and derived parameters, such as cardiac index, systemic vascular resistance, oxygen delivery and oxygen consumption. They can also continuously monitor mixed venous saturations, and assess right ventricular ejection fraction.

In general, pulmonary artery wedge pressure (PAWP) is kept in the range 6–13 mm/Hg and is used as a guide to intravenous fluid therapy. Low readings indicate hypovolaemia and high readings indicate either fluid overload or myocardial ischaemia. A high reading (>15 mm/Hg) might reflect myocardial ischaemia in a hypovolaemic patient. ECG changes suggesting ischaemia (ST segment depression) occur after PAWP changes.

Some anaesthetists do not feel confident about the placement of Swan–Ganz catheters because of possible complications. Rao *et al.*[29] reported a series of 6245 pulmonary artery lines with an incidence of only 0.064% intrapulmonary haemorrhage. Other complications of PA catheter insertion include pneumothorax, intra-arterial cannulation, dysrythmias and knotting.

The presence of a low ejection fraction (<50%) is generally considered an indication for the use of left atrial pressure monitoring.

Blood sampling

Perioperative monitoring of arterial blood gases (including mixed venous oxygen saturation), haemoglobin and activated clotting time all give valuable information. Postoperatively, on the ITU, blood gases, electrolytes, full blood count, clotting and blood sugar levels are routinely monitored. Serial haemoglobin measurements give an early warning of persistent bleeding, particularly as the use of vasoactive drugs may mask the classical signs of hypovolaemia.

Temperature

Central and peripheral temperatures are easy to measure and give valuable information about peripheral tissue perfusion and adequacy of volume replacement. Hypothermia has a number of deleterious effects including severe vasoconstriction, hypertension and adverse effects on blood clotting. These can be avoided by the use of a heat–moisture exchanger to warm the inspired gases, warmed IV fluids, warm air mattresses and a space blanket when transferring the patient back to ITU.

Colonic pH

Significant intestinal ischaemia, particularly that involving the left colon, may occur in 2% of elective and 32% of emergency aortic cases.[30,31] Early detection of this complication may decrease the mortality associated with it. Ischaemic colitis occurs owing to inadvertent damage to the inferior mesenteric artery, trauma from clamping, or hypotension and poor perfusion. Mortality following intestinal ischaemia may be as high as 90%. Intramural pH (pHi) measured with intraluminal tonometry demonstrated that a pHi of less than 6.86 on the day of operation was a predictor of ischaemic colitis and death following aortic reconstruction.[32] If the pHi is low, aggressive therapy to improve gut perfusion and oxygenation should be instituted.

Urine output

An indwelling silastic urethral catheter is inserted following induction of anaesthesia. Alternatively, a suprapubic catheter may be used as there is some evidence that this reduces the risk of postoperative urethral stricture formation.[33]

Induction and maintenance

Elective operation

No single anaesthetic agent or technique is ideal for all patients presenting for aortic reconstruction. Some anaesthetists feel that induction should occur in the operating theatre, with a large-bore cannula and radial artery line already having been inserted under local anaesthesia. This ensures careful monitoring during induction and no disconnection from machine or monitoring equipment when transferring the patient from the induction room into theatre.

It avoids the possible risks of undetected hypoxia, hypertension or hypotension. Others prefer induction to take place in the anaesthetic room using non-invasive monitoring (ECG and pulse oximetry), and hence not subject the patient to the possible anxiety-provoking atmosphere of the operating theatre. Induction in the operating theatre is the choice for emergency cases and in cardiovascularly unstable patients.

A commonly accepted method of general anaesthesia alone is with high doses of opioid (e.g. fentanyl 50–100 μg/kg) with a benzodiazepine such as midazolam in conjunction with nitrous oxide, pancuronium and isoflurane. Others prefer general anaesthesia in conjunction with epidural anaesthesia using local anaesthesia supplemented with opioids peroperatively and continuing postoperatively with opioids alone. Both techniques prevent the surgically induced stress response. The latter technique allows early extubation if this is deemed appropriate.

Whichever method of anaesthesia is chosen, there should be minimal sympathetic response to laryngoscopy, nasogastric tube insertion, endotracheal intubation and bladder catheterization as demonstrated by ECG and blood pressure monitoring. The high-dose opioid method may necessitate overnight ventilation in the ITU and is preferable if there is an increased risk that a patient will need re-exploration for bleeding. If postoperative ventilation is envisaged then a plastic endotracheal tube with a high-volume low-pressure cuff of suitable length and diameter should be used. This type of cuff minimizes damage to the tracheal mucosa due to an interruption of capillary perfusion. Diffusion of nitrous oxide into the cuff can increase cuff pressure, which should therefore be monitored.

Emergency operation

In emergency cases, anaesthesia is modified according to the degree of urgency. An acutely painful aneurysm presenting without blood loss can be dealt with in the same way as an elective case.

The controlled and monitored nature of the elective case is replaced by immediate intubation and aortic compression. Induction of anaesthesia must allow for a slow circulation time. Etomidate, benzodiazepine, ketamine and fentanyl, in conjunction with pancuronium for muscle relaxation, are often used because they cause minimal depression of the cardiovascular system.

Anaesthesia always takes place in theatre with the surgeon scrubbed. The patient is prepared for the operation to start as soon as induction occurs. Because of the large amounts of blood that may be required, cell-saving systems are ideal. The blood infused should be warm. If old autologous blood is given, blood filters are used to prevent microaggregates depositing in the lungs, possibly resulting in adult respiratory distress syndrome. Fresh frozen plasma and platelets may also be required to correct any bleeding diathesis caused by the loss of large volumes of blood and the transfusion of coagulant-deficient stored blood.

Two large-bore cannulae will be needed. In the absence of good peripheral veins the central veins can be cannulated with the wide-bore introducers normally used for Swan–Ganz catheters. Once the aortic clamp has been applied and the patient's cardiovascular system stabilized, anaesthesia can be maintained as for elective cases.

Use of regional blockade

Despite the well-known and accepted advantages of regional anaesthesia alone or in combination with general anaesthesia, this technique has not been universally adopted. This is largely due to the lingering controversy surrounding the use of epidural anaesthesia in patients receiving anticoagulants. The main concern is of haematoma formation in the epidural space with the risk of serious disablement as a consequence. Since 1952 about 100 cases of epidural haematomata following epidural anaesthesia have been described in patients on full anticoagulation,[34] but none of these followed vascular operations. Safe placement of epidurals in 3164 patients who subsequently received anticoagulants has been documented.[35] A recent editorial by Wildsmith and McClure[36] suggests that for patients receiving subcutaneous heparin prophylaxis, the preoperative dose can either be omitted or given 4 hours prior to insertion of the epidural catheter. Alternatively, subcutaneous heparin can be given in the anaesthetic room after the block is performed. Peak heparin levels occur in the plasma about 2 hours after administration. These authors also advise removal of epidural catheters an hour before the next dose of prophylactic heparin.

A survey of Danish hospitals revealed one case of epidural haematoma when subcutaneous heparin was used for thromboprophylaxis.[37] Sensible use of regional techniques in conjunction with appropriate timing of subcutaneous heparin administration should prevent problems.

Fluid and blood replacement

Initially we use colloid and crystalloid to maintain cardiac output. This is followed by a mixture of red cells and colloid as whole blood is now generally unavailable. The increasing use of cell-saving systems reduces the need for homologous blood with all its attendant complications. Often, we haemodilute patients at induction, drawing off up to two pints of blood before heparinization of the patient. This can be retransfused towards the end of the operation following haemostasis. Because of the rapidity with which blood and colloid may need to be transfused all fluid should be warmed. The use of heparin and protamine should be closely monitored using activated clotting times. Protamine, if used to reverse the effect of heparin, may cause myocardial depression or an allergic response. Prolonged operation time and massive blood transfusion will inevitably require the cooperation of the haematologist to help organize blood, fresh frozen plasma and platelet transfusion. The use of other blood and blood products and correction of clotting is fully discussed in Chapter 12.

Aortic clamping and unclamping

Severe myocardial dysfunction following aortic cross-clamping may occur in patients with coronary artery disease.[38] In patients with aortic aneurysms systolic blood pressure and vascular resistance rise, and cardiac output and stroke volume fall slightly when the heart is healthy. In the presence of a diseased heart, the increased work-load may not be tolerated and a rise in pulmonary capillary wedge pressure (PCWP), ischaemic ECG changes and a reduced cardiac output may be seen. This can be prevented by vasodilator therapy. The cross-clamp has less effect in chronic aortic occlusive disease because of the presence of a collateral circulation.

Two dramatic changes occur at the time of unclamping of the aorta. Firstly, reperfusion of the lower limbs is associated with a washout of numerous ischaemic metabolites including lactate, levels of which may be elevated for some time. There is an associated rise in end-tidal carbon dioxide. In order to counteract the adverse effects of the released metabolites, a variety of therapies have been used. Sodium bicarbonate is now thought inappropriate because it worsens intracellular acidosis. The use of human albumin solutions has been suggested as a means of 'mopping up' free oxygen radicals. The second dramatic effect is that releasing the clamp may be followed by a dangerous reduction in blood pressure.

We find that adverse changes at the time of unclamping can be reduced by prior use of intravenous fluid therapy, glyceryl trinitrate, and by decreasing the concentration of anaesthetic that might add to myocardial depression. It is important to ensure that the surgeon warns the anaesthetist well in advance of removing the aortic cross-clamp.

Renal protection

Renal function must be protected during major vascular reconstruction as renal failure is associated with increased mortality.

Maintenance of renal perfusion can be achieved by adequate hydration, cardiac output, blood pressure and oxygenation. Urine output is still often used as the sole monitor of renal perfusion, although apparently adequate volumes of urine may be produced despite renal impairment (i.e. through nonoliguric renal failure). Inadvertent temporary clamping of the renal arteries is associated with a drastic fall in urine output.

'Renal' doses of dopamine (2 μg/kg/min) throughout the operation and for 24 hours postoperatively, and the use of mannitol at the time of clamping, are two methods widely used to encourage urine output. It has been demonstrated[39] that during aortic clamping, dopamine at 2 μg/kg/min causes a significant rise in sodium and potassium output, creatinine clearance and urine output. It was concluded that its use protects the kidney from the deleterious effects of clamping.

Dopexamine hydrochloride, a new synthetic catecholamine, which stimulates dopaminergic receptors of the D_1 and D_2 subtypes as well as B_2 receptors (unlike dopamine), has recently been used for renal protection in patients receiving orthotropic liver transplantation. It has been shown to be at least as effective as dopamine.[40] Because this drug can improve gut perfusion as well, it may in the future have a role to play in abdominal aortic reconstruction.

Postoperative management

Patients recovering from aortic vascular operations are at risk of developing cardiac, respiratory and renal failure in the immediate postoperative period. Close monitoring of intravascular volume status, temperature, respiratory and renal function is necessary, in addition to adequate analgesia and assessment of graft patency and lower-extremity blood flow.

Transfer from theatre to ITU

Ideally the ITU should be situated next to the vascular theatre. In our hospital there is a 300 m and two-floors journey between theatre and intensive care, so there are many inherent dangers during transfer. We have developed a trolley whereby patients can be monitored and treated appropriately during this journey as if they were in the ITU. Their lungs are ventilated using a portable ventilator (Draeger Oxylog). Intra-arterial BP, pulse oximetry and ECG are monitored using a battery-operated monitor (Propaq). The main problem in transfer is a rise of blood pressure. This we control by ensuring adequate analgesia and sedation and, if necessary, by giving small bolus doses of glyceryl trinitrate.

Use of intensive therapy or high-dependency units

Monitoring should not stop at the end of the operation but should continue until the patient is stable. Large-volume fluid shifts occur in the early postoperative period, and rewarming and vasodilatation may take place after moving the patient from the operating theatre with a subsequent drop in blood pressure. Inadequate attention to sedation and analgesia may result in high systolic blood pressures.

Surgeons vary in their approach to postoperative care after elective aortic reconstruction, some preferring to return patients to their own surgical ward, some to a high-dependency unit and some to the ITU. The fluctuating bed occupancy of a typical district general hospital ITU occassionally results in elective aortic cases being cancelled.

In our hospital there is no high-dependency unit and major vascular cases are routinely admitted to the intensive therapy unit for postoperative management. Campbell *et al.*[41] assessed the need for intensive care in the first 48 hours following aortic reconstruction in 45 patients. All but two patients had significant medical events (such as hypertension, hypotension, hypoxia, oliguria) requiring intervention.

Respiratory support

Following uncomplicated aortic reconstruction it may be possible to extubate the stable patient immediately if epidural analgesia is being used. However, following prolonged operation where the patient may be cold, and in the presence of large doses of systemic opioid, it may be preferable to leave the patient sedated, intubated and ventilated until it is certain he is cardiovascularly stable and not bleeding.

Blood pressure management

Hypertension is a common and potentially serious complication in the immediate postoperative period. This may be attributable to overzealous peroperative fluid replacement, hypothermia with consequent compensatory vasoconstriction, rebound hypertension and vascular hyper-reactivity. If, in spite of adequate analgesia and sedation, the BP remains elevated, we find a nitroglycerin infusion useful.

Hypotension is frequently related to hypovolaemia which may become apparent as the patient warms up. It can easily be corrected by a further fluid challenge under CVP and PA catheter control. Patients with poor LV function may become hypotensive as a result of poor cardiac output in spite of an adequate PCWP. They may require inotropic support, usually in the form of dobutamine, which can be titrated against the cardiac index as measured by thermodilution using the PA catheter. Prolonged hypotension may endanger coronary artery, cerebral, intestinal and renal blood flow.

Analgesia

Opioids

Patients who require mechanical ventilation overnight are generally sedated with propofol or midazolam in conjunction with an opioid such as morphine or alfentanil. Following extubation analgesia is continued using morphine. This can be administered intravenously using a patient-controlled device and can be continued when the patient is discharged to the ward.

Epidural

Postoperatively the patient can receive opioids via an epidural catheter. We often use diamorphine at a rate of 0.5 – 1 mg hourly. This can occasionally be associated with respiratory depression and pruritis, both of which are reversible with naloxone without any reduction in analgesia. The advantage of epidural opioids over local anaesthetic agents is the lack of motor blockade and hypotension.

Stress ulceration prophylaxis

We no longer encourage the prophylactic use of antacids or H_2 antagonists. It is felt that this practice increases the incidence of nosocomial pneumonia. We now use a solution of sucralfate administered 4-hourly via the nasogastric tube.

Antibiotics

In the absence of allergy we give cefuroxine 750 mg 8-hourly intravenously, starting at the time of induction. The antibiotic is continued either intravenously or orally until all monitoring lines, drips and the urinary catheter are removed.

Anticoagulation

Patients with normal coagulation receive 5000 units of heparin subcutaneously twice-daily. If an epidural catheter has been used we remove it at least 8 hours after the last dose of heparin.

Renal support

In the ITU, urine volumes are measured hourly and maintained at levels greater than 50 ml/hour by ensuring adequate blood pressure, CVP, PCWP and cardiac output. 'Renal-dose' dopamine is continued and aliquots of mannitol and boluses of frusemide are given if required. In the event of acute renal failure developing, it may be necessary to institute haemofiltration in the hope that acute tubular necrosis will resolve. The problems with haemofiltration are that the groin cannot be used for the shunt in the presence of a trouser graft, and the use of heparin may encourage bleeding from the suture lines.

Final remarks

Vascular surgery presents anaesthetists and intensivists with many problems. Over the last 20 years there has been a downward trend in mortality, particularly in that associated with elective operations. Emergency procedures are still associated with a very high mortality. However, emergency aortic operations and anaesthesia are still occasionally performed by trainee surgeons and anaesthetists without adequate supervision and vascular training.

Jenkins *et al*[42] claimed that aortic aneurysm repairs should only be performed in major centres by specialist vascular surgeons. In the CEPOD report of 1987,[43] deficiencies in the care of major aortic surgical patients are highlighted. The 1990 NCEPOD report[44] suggested an overall improvement in their management compared with the earlier report. The 1990 report surveyed 449 operations of which 254 were performed by a consultant surgeon, 74 cases by a senior registrar and 118 cases by other grades, and made two important points relating to this chapter. Firstly, there should be a thorough preoperative assessment undertaken by competent specialists; and secondly, there must be an adequate ITU/HDU service for the care of patients undergoing vascular reconstruction. In a recent survey by Vella *et al.*[45] on aortic reconstruction performed in a district general hospital, a consultant surgeon was involved in 72.5% of cases, and a consultant anaesthetist in 61.3%.

Perhaps until all cases are performed with consultant surgeons and consultant anaesthetists with specialized vascular interest in attendance, we should not draw too many conclusions from published mortality rates.

References

1. Browse DJ, Galland RB. An audit of hospital mortality: general compared with vascular surgery. *Ann Roy Coll Surg Eng* 1991; **73:** 121–4.
2. Jaffe V, Chadwick L, Tomkins M, Galland RB. General surgery with a special interest in vascular surgery: an audit of relative workload. *Ann Roy Coll Surg Eng* 1991; **73** (Suppl): 90–3.
3. Knight PR, Hantler CB. Anaesthesia and the geriatric patient: hypertension in the elderly. *Clin Anaesthesiol* 1986; **4:** 1003–23.
4. Goldman L, Cadera D, Nussbaum SR, *et al.* Multifactorial index of cardiac risk in non-cardiac surgical procedures. *N Engl J Med* 1977; **297:** 945.
5. Detsky AS, Abrams HB, Forbath W, Scott JR, Hilliard JR. Cardiac assessment for patients undergoing non-cardiac surgery. *Arch Intern Med* 1986; **146:** 2131–4.
6. Chadwick L, Galland RB. Preoperative clinical evaluation as a predictor of cardiac complications after infrarenal aortic reconstruction. *Br J Surg* 1991; **78:** 875–7.
7. Cutler BS, Wheeler HB, Paraska JA, Cardullo PA. Applicability and interpretation of electrocardiographic stress testing in patients with peripheral vascular disease. *Am J Surg* 1981; **141,** 501–6.
8. Leppo JA. Dipyridamole–thallium imaging: the lazy man's tress test. *J Nucl Med* 1989; **30:** 281–7.
9. Boucher CA, Brewster DC, Darling RC, *et al.* Determination of cardiac risk by dipyridamole–thallium:

imaging before peripheral vascular surgery. *N Engl J Med* 1985; **312:** 389–94.
10. Eagles KA, Coley CM, Newell JB, *et al.* Combining clinical and thallium data optimises preoperative assessment of cardiac risk before major vascular surgery. *Ann Intern Med* 1989; **110:** 859–66.
11. Mangano DT. Perioperative cardiac morbidity. *Anaesthesiology* 1990; **72:** 153–84.
12. Jain KM, Patil KD, Doctor NS, Peck SL. Preoperative cardiac screening before peripheral vascular operation. *Am Surg* 1985; **51:** 77–81.
13. Broadhurst P, Cashman P, Crawley J, Raftery E, Lahiri A. Clinical validation of a miniature nuclear probe system for continuous on-line monitoring of cardiac function and SF segment. *J Nucl Med* 1991; **32:** 37–43.
14. Brown OW, Hollier LH, Pairolero PC, Kazmier FJ, McCready RA. Abdominal aortic aneurysm and coronary artery disease. *Arch Surg* 1981; **116:** 1484–8.
15. Gouny P, Bertrand M, Coriat P, Kieffer E. Perioperative cardiac complications of surgical repair of infrarenal aortic aneurysms. *Ann Vasc Surg* 1989; **4:** 328–34.
16. Pontoppidan H, Beecher HK. Progressive loss of protective reflexes in the airway with the advance of age. *JAMA* 1960; **174:** 2209–13.
17. Kitamura H, Sava T, Kezono E. Post-operative hypoxaemia: the contribution of age to the maldistribution of ventilation. *Anaesthesiology* 1972; **36:** 244–52.
18. Olefsky JM. Endocrine and reproductive diseases. In: *Textbook of Medicine*, 13th edn, Cecil and Loeb (eds). Philadelphia: WB Saunders, 1985: 1320–41.
19. Farrow SC, Fawkes FGR, Lunn JR, *et al.* Epidemology in anaesthesia. II: Factors affecting mortality in hospital. *Br J Anaesth* 1982; **54:** 811–17.
20. O'Donnell TF, Darling RC, Linton RR. Is 80 years too old for aneurysurectomy? *Arch Surg* 1976; **111:** 1250–7.
21. Soreide O, Lillestol J, Christensen O, *et al.* Abdominal aortic aneurysms: survival analysis of four hundred and thirty-four patients. *Surgery* 1982; **91:** 188–93.
22. Smith R. The church on ageing. *Br Med J* 1990; **301:** 829–30.
23. Esseltyn CB, Humphries AN, Young JR, Beven EG, DeWolfe WG. Aneurysmectomy in the aged? *Surgery* 1970; **67:** 34.
24. Cunningham AJ. Anaesthesia for abdominal aortic surgery: a review. *Can J Anaesth* 1989; **36:** 426–44.
25. Derham C. An evaluation of the preoperative information given to patients by intensive care nurses. *Inten Care Nurs* 1991; **7:** 1–6.
26. Froelicher VF, Wolthius R, Keiser N, *et al.* A comparison of the bipolar exercise electrocardiographic leads to lead V5. *Chest* 1976; **70:** 611–16.
27. Allen EV. Thromboangitis obliterans. Method of diagnosing chronic occlusive arterial lesions distal to the wrist with illustrative cases. *Am J Med Sci* 1929; **178:** 237–44.
28. Slogoff S, Keats AS, Arlund C. On the safety of radical artery cannulation. *Anaesthesiology* 1983; **59:** 42–7.
29. Rao TLK, Gorski DW, Shah KB. Safety of pulmonary artery catheterisation. Exhibition at International Anaesthetic Research Society, New Orleans, 1983.
30. Bandyk DF, Florence MG, Johansen KH. Colon ischaemia accompanying ruptured abdominal aneurysm. *J Surg Res* 1981; **30:** 297–303.
31. Wakefield TW, Whitehorse WM, Wu SC, *et al.* Abdominal aortic aneurysm rupture: statistical analysis of factors affecting outcome of surgical treatment. *Surgery* 1982; **91:** 586–95.
32. Fiddian-Green RG, Amelin PM, Herrman JB, Arous E, Cutler BS, Schiedler M, Wheeler HB, Baker S. Prediction of the development of sigmoid ischaemia on the day of aortic operations. *Arch Surg* 1986; **121:** 654–60.
33. Dineen MD, Wetter LA, May ARL. Urethral strictures and aortic surgery: suprapubic rather than urethral catheters. *Eur J Vasc Surg* 1990; **4:** 535–8.
34. Beck H, Brasson F, Doehn M, Barse H, Dziaozka A, Schulte AM, Esch J. Epidural catheters of the multiorifice type: dangers and complications. *Acta Anaesth Scand* 1986; **30:** 549–55.
35. Rao TKL, El-Elt AA. Anticoagulation following placement of epidural and subarachnoid catheters: an evaluation of neurologic sequelae. *Anaesthesiology* 1981; **55:** 618–20.
36. Wildsmith JAW, McClure JH. Editorial: Anticoagulants and central nerve blockade. *Anaesthesia* 1991; **46:** 613–14.
37. Wille-Jorgensen P, Jorgensen LN, Rasmussen LS. Lumbar regional anaesthesia and prophylactic anticoagulant therapy. *Anaesthesia* 1991; **46:** 623–7.
38. Attia RR, Murphy JD, Snider M, *et al.* Myocardial ischaemia due to infrarenal aortic cross-clamping during aortic surgery in patients with severe coronary artery disease. *Circulation* 1976; **53:** 961–5.
39. Salem MG, Crooke JW, McLoughlin GA, Middle JG, Taylor WH. The effect of dopamine on renal function during aortic cross-clamping. *Ann Roy Coll Surg Eng* 1988; **70:** 9–12.
40. Gray PA, Bodenham AR, Park GR. A comparison of dopexamine and dopamine to prevent renal impairment in patients undergoing orthotopic liver transplantation. *Anaesthesia* 1991; **46:** 638–41.
41. Campbell WB, Ballard PK, Goodman DA. Intensive care after abdominal aortic surgery. *Eur J Vasc Surg* 1991; **5:** 665–8.
42. Jenkins AMcL, Ruckley CV, Nolan B. Ruptured abdominal aortic aneurysm. *Br J Surg* 1986; **73:** 395–8.

43. Buck N, Devlin HB, Lunn JN. *Report of the Confidential Enquiry into Perioperative Deaths.* London: Nuffield Provincial Hospitals Trust, 1987.
44. Campling EA, Devlin HB, Hoile RW, Lunn JN. *Report of the National Confidential Enquiry into Perioperative Deaths 1990.* Published April 1992 by the National Confidential Enquiry into Perioperative Deaths.
45. Vella V, Duthie G, Shandall A, Shute K. Aortic aneurysms – who should do them? *Ann Roy Coll Surg Eng* 1990; **72:** 215–17.

14

Complications of major vascular operations

RJ Corson, AT Edwards and CN McCollum

By its very nature vascular surgery is prone to complications. Patients with vascular disease tend to be older and have a higher incidence of concomitant cardiac disease. Over 85% of a vascular surgeon's operative work-load may be classified as major whereas only 18% of general surgical operations fall into this category.

Publication of the CEPOD report, and the increasing interest in surgical audit, have heightened awareness amongst surgeons of the value of auditing their complications. This should encourage them to identify problems in their practice which might need attention. Many aspects of vascular operations – in particular femoropopliteal bypass, aortic reconstruction and carotid endarterectomy – have been the subjects of large nationally funded multicentre studies which have looked at the efficacy of these procedures and have provided a baseline against which all surgeons can compare their results.

The practice of vascular surgery has progressed rapidly in recent years and is now a major speciality in its own right. Undoubtedly this development should be encouraged. Concentrating the majority of vascular operations in the hands of experienced and appropriately trained surgeons will lead to a further improvement in results. The recommendation of the Vascular Surgical Society of Great Britain and Ireland is that hospitals undertaking vascular operations should have at least two trained surgeons with a major interest to provide the continuous level of care expected in the 1990s.

General complications

Cardiac

The most important cause of postoperative morbidity and mortality following major vascular reconstruction is myocardial ischaemia which is responsible for 40–70% of the mortality associated with major aortic operations. This is not surprising as atherosclerosis is a generalized disease; indeed, 93% of all patients undergoing aneurysm repair have abnormal coronary angiograms.[1]

History and examination remain the best indicators of risk, with 'clinical scoring' consistently performing better than any other investigation. History, physical examination, and a standard 12-lead ECG can be used to calculate the risk of postoperative cardiac disease using the Goldman classification (see Table 13.2). Although this gives an indication of the importance of previous clinical events and has a clear value in research, it is not routinely used in clinical practice.

Other cardiac investigations, such as exercise ECG screening which is severely hampered by coexisting claudication, are of limited value. Although a normal ejection fraction (EF) on echocardiography is a good prognostic indicator, the specificity is poor as patients with low ejection fractions often escape problems.[2] Twenty-four hour ambulatory ECG assessment has recently been advocated, but the routine use of this investigation in all patients cannot yet be justified.[3]

Having decided to operate, recent studies have clearly shown that maximizing preoperative cardiac haemodynamics improves outcome.[4] This may be done in the anaesthetic induction room or in the intensive-care unit on the night prior to surgery.

Carotid (stroke)

Carotid stenoses are found in 6–16% of patients undergoing abdominal aortic operations, but the incidence of stroke in elective aortic reconstruction is less than 2%, with a mortality from stroke of less than 1%.[5]

As yet there are no clear guidelines, but asymptomatic patients probably do not require carotid investigation. Patients with transient cerebral ischaemia, amaurosis fugax or recent stroke should be investigated by Doppler spectral analysis and duplex

Doppler so that carotid stenoses of greater than 70% may be considered for prophylactic operations, either before or with the aortic reconstruction.

Graft infection

Fortunately this is now rare owing to the routine use of antibiotic prophylaxis, but infection does occur in the groin wound in at least 5% of patients. Fortunately only a small proportion of these infections involve the graft. As with most procedures where a prostheses is implanted, any focus of infection should be cleared preoperatively if possible. True graft infection usually necessitates complete removal of the graft and revascularization of the lower extremities, either by an extra-anatomic reconstruction such as an axillobifemoral graft or by replacement with either autogenous artery, vein or rifampicin-soaked gelatin-impregnated Dacron.[6] Graft infection is usually due to contamination at the time of the original operation.

False aneurysms

These may occur at any arterial anastomosis but are more frequent at the femoral anastomosis. They may occur secondary to infection, suture line disruption or technical failure. Hypertension which is a feature in over 60% of patients may also play a part. False aneurysms are usually asymptomatic but may be painful or promote distal emboli, so we feel that those greater than 3 cm diameter should be repaired. This is usually by excision or by inlay of an additional short length of prosthetic graft between the previous graft and the host artery under the cover of perioperative antibiotics.

Lymph leakage

This is most likely to occur in the groin but can occur anywhere along the length of subcutaneous prosthetic grafts. The danger is of secondary infection. Large collections should be aspirated percutaneously using meticulous aseptic technique. Most lymph leaks settle with conservative treatment within two weeks, but re-exploration and ligature of any obvious vessels is occasionally necessary. Methylene blue, injected subcutaneously between the toes, a few hours before reoperation may aid the identification of lymphatic vessels.

Aortic surgery

The results of surgery for aneurysmal and occlusive disease of the abdominal aorta have improved greatly since Dubost's first successful repair in 1952, owing to improvements in surgical technique, patient selection and hospital care. Postoperative complications may be related to the extent of the operation, cross-clamp time, problems of haemostasis and the experience of the surgeon. Indeed, as Kerstein and Sweeny have emphasized: 'there are no new complications or new technical misadventures in the repair of aortic aneurysms, only new surgeons'.[7] At present the accepted mortality following aortic surgery is quoted as being around 5%, but certain patients carry a much greater risk due to extensive disease and concomitant pathology.[8] Adequate preoperative assessment is essential to minimize and/or avoid postoperative complications.

Pulmonary complications

Pulmonary complications and respiratory failure are leading causes of morbidity in all varieties of surgery. The risk factors include a history of pulmonary disease, smoking, age, obesity, length of operation, and operative blood loss. Stopping smoking for at least one month reduces the risk, although Smith *et al.* claim that stopping smoking 5–7 days preoperatively is just as effective.[9] Peak expiratory flow and arterial blood gas measurements are accepted investigations Forced mid-expiratory flow measured in millilitres per second is the most predictive of the simple tests as it may reflect the capacity to cough and clear secretions.[10]

Preoperative preparation and postoperative physiotherapy remain the mainstays for reducing pulmonary complications. In those at risk, a 48-hour period of intensive physiotherapy and bronchodilator therapy is indicated as this has been shown to reduce postoperative complications.

Postoperative epidural analgesia has been shown to cause less suppression of normal pulmonary reflexes, such as coughing and hypoxic drive.[11] It is routinely used in our practice.

Renal complications

Acute renal failure following aortic reconstruction increased the mortality rate from 1% to over 10% in some series.[12] The single most important risk factor is preoperative renal insufficiency with an elevated serum creatinine, found in 5–10% of patients undergoing elective operation.[13] Adequate preoperative and postoperative hydration significantly diminish this risk. If it proves necessary to occlude the renal blood flow for more than a few minutes, renal function can be protected by infusion, directly into the renal artery, of cold (4°C) crystalloid solution with mannitol.[12]

Haemostasis

One consideration prior to elective operation is the need for homologous blood transfusion, where despite improvements in surgical technique the average blood transfusion requirement continues to be 4–6 units.[14] Stored blood carries a risk of impaired coagulation, infection such as post-transfusion hepatitis, immunosuppression, and impaired oxygen transport.[15–17]

Various techniques have been developed to reduce transfusion requirements. The most appropriate by virtue of simplicity for routine clinical practice are preoperative simple haemodilution and red cell salvage techniques.[18] In preoperative haemodilution, sufficient blood is taken from the patient following induction of anaesthesia to reduce the haemoglobin to around 11 g/dl. This fresh blood is stored in theatre at room temperature until wound closure, or if required because of uncontrolled haemorrhage. Of the red cell salvage methods, simple collection into a heparinized resevoir is the easiest; but the coagulation system is still activated and may lead to subclinical diffuse intravascular coagulation. To combat this, systems which centrifuge and remove activated cells and clotting factors from whole blood have been developed. These machines wash and centrifuge salvaged blood, removing any operative debris, activated clotting factors, free haemoglobin and heparin. The resulting red cell suspension may then be reinfused relatively safely.

These methods should be made available particularly for ruptured aneurysms or inflammatory aneurysms and when an aortocaval fistula is expected. Deihl and his colleagues have clearly shown that the incidence of cardiac, pulmonary and renal complications is associated with multiple transfusions.[15]

Thrombosis/embolism

Occlusion of aortic or iliac grafts is rare and is almost always due to technical problems, often at the distal anastomosis. These may include an intimal flap or kinking of an overlong graft in the retroperitoneal tunnel. Limb thrombosis may also occur owing to debris being dislodged during mobilization or suturing, or to intraluminal thrombus formed at operation. This can be avoided by gentle handling of the vessels, by adequate heparinization of the occluded vessels, and by a careful flushing and back-bleeding procedure on removal of the clamps. In this way the use of Fogarty catheters may be minimized.

Intestinal infarction/ischaemic colitis

This relatively unusual complication is rare following bypass for occlusive disease, but it may follow aneurysm repair where transmucosal infarction of the left colon requires resection in 2–5% of ruptured aneurysms but in fewer than 1% of elective repairs.[19] Arterial insufficiency due to loss of the inferior mesenteric and internal iliac arteries is by far the most common cause, but vasospasm associated with the shock of rupture or major operation undoubtedly contributes in most cases. In the absence of symptomatic ischaemia, the mesenteric arteries generally do not need to be repaired unless reconstruction in a difficult aneurysm requires exclusion of both internal iliac arteries. In these circumstances a widely patent inferior mesenteric artery with a small patch of aorta should be implanted into the graft. Lesser degrees of mucosal ischaemia have also been detected in the rectosigmoid region by colonoscopy and biopsy in 10% of elective repairs and in 60% of patients with rupture.[19,20]

During repair of the AAA, the inferior mesenteric arterial orifice should be closed by internal suture, as the ascending and descending branches form an important collateral link. In the postoperative period, ischaemic colitis is often masked by wound pain. Colitis should be suspected if the patient develops signs of sepsis at approximately 3–6 days, with pyrexia, abdominal pain, a raised white cell count, metabolic acidosis, jaundice and often diarrhoea which may be blood-stained. Early diagnosis is essential, but plain abdominal X-rays are of little help until free gas below the diaphragm follows perforation. However, sigmoidoscopy or colonoscopy are useful in the earlier investigation of the distal colon. In the absence of perforation, initial treatment is supportive, with bowel rest, intravenous fluids and antibiotics. Severe peritonitis due to infarction or perforation requires resection with formation of a stoma. Occasionally, if the initial event settles, ischaemia may lead to stricture formation.

Spinal cord ischaemia

This occurs during repair of a thoracoabdomonal aneurysm in up to 20% of cases and in a ruptured abdominal aortic aneurysm in 3% of cases.[21] When it occurs the deficit is most commonly T_{10} to L_2

due to disruption in flow or an inadequate artery of Adamkiewicz, which is the major source of supply to the lower anterior spinal artery. In thoracoabdominal surgery spinal arteries may need to be implanted, but in abdominal aneurysm repair adequate perfusion of the spinal cord is best ensured by avoiding systemic hypotension.

Sexual dysfunction

The presence of impotence should be established in the preoperative history, and may indicate distal aortic, common or internal iliac disease. If the para-aortic and superior hypogastric nerve plexi are preserved, then iliac revascularization will restore sexual function in 30–50% of cases.[22] For those with no preoperative history, the patient is at risk of impotence if both common iliac vessels are ligated during graft placement. More frequently, damage to the parasympathetic nerve supply will result in absent ejaculation, which following adequate explanation is rarely seen by the patient as a major problem.

Surgical shock

Removal of the aortic clamp and reperfusion of the pelvic viscera and lower limbs inevitably causes a fall in blood pressure owing to the release of stored metabolites. This can be minimized by ensuring adequate volume replacement during the operation and immediately prior to cross-clamp release. The clamp should be removed slowly and blood flow through the graft controlled by the surgeon's other hand over 3–5 minutes until haemodynamic stability is restored.

The administration of agents to minimize this reperfusion-induced effect (such as the oxygen free radical scavenger mannitol) has recently been advocated and shown to reduce post-reperfusion organ dysfunction.[23]

The approach

The transperitoneal approach through a transverse incision is now used by many surgeons as it allows access to both renal and iliac vessels and any concomitant pathology. It is also less painful than a midline incision and may be associated with fewer pulmonary complications.[24]

However, when there have been previous abdominal operations, the retroperitoneal approach avoids bowel injury and may reduce postoperative ileus.[25] It is also the approach of choice in patients known to have a horseshoe kidney.

Technical tips

Trauma to the inferior vena cava, left renal vein and gonadal vessels may be largely avoided by careful blunt dissection and avoiding passing instruments around the arteries. Arterial bleeding from the origin of the lumbar and inferior mesenteric vessels should be controlled from within the lumen of the aorta itself. A properly constructed arterial anastomosis should be virtually dry (except for suture holes in PTFE grafts), but any bleeding can be controlled by horizontal mattress sutures with attached patches of grafts if necessary. The patient who continues to bleed or rebleeds in the postoperative period should be immediately returned to theatre so that haemostasis may be properly secured.

Ruptured aortic aneurysm

The incidence of rupture is rising with the increased prevalence of aortic aneurysms in the elderly. The diagnosis depends upon a high index of suspicion in predominantly elderly men who present with symptoms of acute onset of abdominal/back pain or collapse. Any patient with evidence of a palpable mass and past history of aneurysmal disease should be treated as a rupture until the diagnosis is confirmed at laparotomy. Unlike the elective situation, preoperative selection is difficult; but if the patient has had a good quality of life prior to rupture he or she merits immediate operation. This should be performed by an experienced vascular surgeon.

Profound hypotension may occur following induction of anaesthesia, which should therefore be delayed until the surgeon is gowned and the abdomen drapped. Although the surgeon must work quickly, care should be taken to avoid accidental injury to the intestine and its mesentry. Pancreatitis may develop early, or acalculous cholecystitis late, following rupture and may be an occult cause of multiple organ failure. Assessment of the abdomen postoperatively in these patients is notoriously difficult; clinical examination being limited by a painful wound or worse in a sedated, ventilated patient. Ultrasonography can be helpful in detecting the presence of intra-abdominal collections but is imprecise in defining pancreatic and intestinal pathology, particularly colonic infarction. CT or ^{111}In-labelled leucocyte scanning is more accurate in defining occult sepsis but may not be practical in the unstable ventilated patient with multiple organ failure.

Postoperative care

In a study of the role of intensive care in aortic surgery, 80% of patients required intervention for a significant medical condition such as hypertension, hypotension, oliguria, hypoxia, and chest complications.[26] This demonstrated the need for close medical supervision, especially as 60% had more than one complication which was not predictable on preoperative history and examination. Whether this supervision requires admission to an intensive-care unit or a surgical high-dependence area is less important than the level of nursing and medical care which is essential in the early postoperative phase.

Aortoenteric/aortocaval fistula

The graft may occasionally erode into the gut, particularly the third and fourth parts of the duodenum where it is in close proximity to the fixed small bowel. This may be avoided by ensuring retroperitoneal cover for the prosthesis, using omentum if necessary. When an aortoenteric fistula does occur the average time to presentation is quoted as 33 months from the time of the original operation.[27] However, the presentation may vary. The patient may experience minimal discomfort and chronic gastrointestinal haemorrhage associated with anaemia. Often these small 'warning bleeds' precede the most dramatic of presentations (i.e. exsanginating haemorrhage). Diagnosis requires a high index of suspicion in a patient with abdominal pain following previous aortic reconstruction. In shocked patients with evidence of an upper GI haemorrhage, endoscopic examination is essential to exclude peptic ulceration which remains a common cause of bleeding in such patients. The endoscopist should, if possible, examine the third and fourth parts of the duodenum. CT imaging occasionally demonstrates the graft eroding through bowel wall into the lumen. Usually the graft must be removed and replaced initially by an orthotopic rifampicin-soaked gelatin-impregnated graft. In the absence of gross infection, others have advocated the more conservative approach of separation and suture of the aortic and enteric defects.

Aortocaval fistulae are a significant problem whereby patients present with profound hypotension associated with tachycardia and high-output cardiac failure. A harsh machine-like murmur may be heard in the abdomen on auscultation. Three-quarters are associated with a ruptured AAA, 20% are due to trauma and 10% to infection.[27] Once more, cell-salvage equipment will prove useful to recover rapid blood loss on opening the aneurysm sac until venous bleeding can be controlled. The aorta should be opened and the fistula compressed within the sac which controls bleeding while the vein wall is sutured. The profound hypotension sometimes associated with this condition may lead to renal failure.

Suprarenal aneurysmal disease

This is associated with a greater morbidity and mortality due to the extent of the operation and proximal cross-clamping leading to ischaemia and reperfusion of a large part of the body, including vital organs. Renal, pulmonary and coagulation failure are all common, with myocardial infarction and ischaemic paraplegia as the main causes of death. Various methods have been proposed to reduce renal ischaemia, such as cold perfusion of the renal vessels with cooled Ringers' lactate containing mannitol. The infusion of antioxidants such as mannitol has also been proposed to reduce organ damage following ischaemia reperfusion. This is not the province of the occasional vascular surgeon, and requires the facilities of a vascular surgery centre.

Carotid surgery

Carotid endarterectomy is currently undergoing a revival following the publication of the results of European and North American stroke intervention studies demonstrating that carotid endarterectomy reduced subsequent stroke in symptomatic patients with >70% stenoses of the relevant carotid artery.[28,29] It should be emphasized that the trial participants were experienced surgeons who performed this operation regularly. However, a worrying report from the UK revealed that a significant proportion of endarterectomies in this country are still being performed by 'occasional' carotid surgeons. Experienced carotid surgeons should achieve an operative mortality of no more than 1% with perioperative stroke in less than 3%; figures which compare very favourably with the natural history of symptomatic carotid stenoses. The principal complications of carotid endarterectomy are perioperative stroke and myocardial ischaemia, both of which are potentially fatal.

Investigation

Conventional arteriography in patients with carotid disease is hazardous and may produce temporary or permanent neurological deficits, usually mild, in 2.4% of patients. Digital subtraction angiography reduces this risk, but the quality of images (especially in intravenous studies) may be poor. The advent of noninvasive colour-flow duplex ultrasonography has revolutionized the investigation of carotid disease, and our practice is now to operate without recourse to arteriography where the duplex image is of adequate quality to issue a confident report.

The operation

Adequate exposure of the carotid artery is essential, but mobilization must be gentle to prevent dislodgement of platelet emboli and embolization of atherosclerotic material or platelet thrombus.

Cerebral protection

Cerebral ischaemia and permanent central neurological damage during the operation may be avoided by preventing platelet emboli and monitoring adequate cerebral perfusion during clamping of the internal carotid. Carefully cleaning the endarterectomized surface under magnification and flushing the artery before removal of clamps reduce thrombosis and embolism.

Some method of assessing the adequacy of cerebral perfusion during carotid clamping is now essential. This has been done by assessing the stump pressure following external and common carotid clamping. If the stump pressure falls rapidly or is nonpulsatile, a shunt should be used. Transcranial Doppler assessment of the middle cerebral artery blood flow offers greater security as it can be used to select which patients need a shunt and may monitor for shunt kinking. Direct and noninvasive measurement of intracerebral oxygen saturation using near-infrared light spectroscopy is now achievable. Thus carotid endarterectomy has become very much safer with the surgeon reassured that he need not hurry as the quality of cerebral perfusion can now be monitored continuously.

Nerve injury

The incidence of cranial nerve palsy is reported to be as high as 7% following carotid endarterectomy. Minor changes in voice quality or difficulties swallowing are often blamed on the endotracheal tube or anaesthetist.

The hypoglossal nerve must always be identified and preserved as it passes between the external and internal carotid arteries. The ansal branch of the hypoglossal nerve usually needs to be sacrificed but causes little or no recognizable deficit. The vagus nerve lies within the carotid sheath and is prone to damage along with its recurrent laryngeal and superior laryngeal branch. Rarely the glossopharyngeal nerve or the cervical branch of the facial nerve may be damaged.

Vasomotor instability

Some surgeons routinely divide the carotid sinus nerve early in the course of the operation to avoid wide fluctuations in blood pressure and occasional hypotension and bradycardia when the receptors are newly exposed following endarterectomy.

We minimize the amount of dissection around the carotid nerve and now have few problems with unstable blood pressure. Local anaesthetic injected around the carotid sinus may reduce fluctuations in arterial pressure, but it is difficult to see how this will influence postoperative hypotension in susceptible patients.

Thrombosis

Thrombosis is a serious complication that occurs only occasionally in the immediate postoperative period. The endarterectomized segment is highly thrombogenic and liable to thrombosis, especially during periods of hypotension (which should be avoided). Full systemic heparinization, careful cleaning of the endarterectomized surface under magnification, and antiplatelet therapy all help to prevent occlusion. Narrowing at the arteriotomy may be avoided by inserting a patch of reversed vein or Dacron whenever the internal carotid is small. Intimal retention sutures using 7/0 materials, both proximally and distally, should be used freely to avoid intimal flaps.

Carotid restenosis

Symptomatic carotid restenosis occurs in only 2–3% of patients, but follow-up with duplex scanning reveals restenosis of more than 50% in 10–15% of patients. Occasionally these may be clamp injuries or excessive narrowing of the arterial lumen by primary closure; but most are due to intimal hyperplasia that may be mediated by platelet adhesion causing local release of growth factors. As a result many surgeons always use a patch and platelet inhibitory drugs postoperativley.

Not all recurrent stenoses require operation and most surgeons would confine intervention to those with symptomatic stenoses of more than 75%. The operation is technically more difficult owing to periarterial scarring, but in skilled hands the risk of cranial nerve injury should not be high. In the case of recurrent atherosclerosis a further endarterectomy may be possible. Stenoses due to myointimal hyperplasia are usually best repaired by reversed vein or a prosthetic graft.

Femorodistal reconstructions

New techniques, such as *in situ* vein grafting, venous cuffs and the introduction of suitable alternatives to autogenous vein, have encouraged ever more distal reconstructions to the calf vessels. As a result there has been a decline in primary amputation with most patients in vascular centres being offered at least one attempt at reconstruction. As these reconstructions are often performed on the elderly with severe distal disease, it is not surprising that vascular surgeons are devoting increasing time to the treatment of these grafts when they fail.

Patient selection

All patients should undergo investigation to determine the sites of all haemodynamically significant lesions, the adequacy of the in flow, and the state of the runoff. Occasionally, unexplained or unexpected graft failure may herald a thrombotic tendency such as polycythaemia, thrombocythaemia, antithrombin III deficiency, defects of fibrinolysis, heparin-induced thrombosis, anti-cardiolipin antibodies, or more frequently a previously unrecognized malignancy which may be diagnosed months later but which is usually disseminated.

Graft failure

Graft occlusion may precipitate either an acutely ischaemic limb or the recurrence of the preoperative symptoms if the collaterals are adequate; indeed, graft failure may be detected only at routine clinical follow-up.

Patency is influenced by the availability of vein, the distal anastomosis and the severity of proximal and distal disease. Reconstructions above the knee do well, with 5-year patency rates of 70–80%.[30] The choice of arterial conduit above the knee is not critical as long as antiplatelet therapy is given for prosthetic grafts. For reconstructions below the knee, patency depends much more on the availability of autologous vein. When prosthetic material is used, thrombosis within 12 months will occur in 40–60% of reconstructions to the distal popliteal and in even higher proportions of bypasses to calf vessels.[30]

There does appear to be some benefit from Miller venous cuffs or Taylor venous patches, but these have yet to be adequately investigated. The use of adjuvant arteriovenous fistulae is tenuous.

Early failure (under 30 days)

Failures within the first month are predominantly due to technical problems or graft thrombosis. Poorly constructed anastomoses may cause narrowing or intimal flaps, which should be detected by intraoperative completion angiography or other outflow investigation. Where the outflow is poor, particularly when prosthetic material is used, infusion of PGE1 or a prostacyclin analogue, low-dose heparin and postoperative platelet inhibitory drug therapy may protect patency.[31]

Late failure

The importance of vein graft stenoses, which appear to develop within weeks, has only recently been appreciated. These appear to be progressive and an adequate surveillance programme will detect stenosis in 15% of grafts.

Although transluminal angioplasty may be attempted, the restenosis rate is relatively high and we favour vein patch angioplasty under local anaesthesia. In prosthetic grafts, continued platelet deposition along the graft will lead to progressive narrowing and intimal hyperplasia at the distal anastomoses. These processes appear not unlike accelerated atherosclerosis and can be inhibited by antiplatelet agents.

Leg swelling

Leg swelling is very common in distal reconstruction and is associated with a higher incidence of wound complications. It is rarely due to deep vein thrombosis and was originally thought to be due to lymphatic obstruction. It is now apparent that this swelling is due to increased endothelial permeability following the ischaemia–reperfusion injury promoted by arterial reconstruction. This capillary leak can be prevented by the prophylactic use of a free radical scavenger such as intraoperative mannitol, or the xanthine oxidase inhibitor, allopurinol.

References

1. Hertzer NR, Bevan EG, Youmg JR, O'Hara PJ, Ruschhaupt WF, Groar RA. Coronary artery disease in peripheral vascular patients: a classification of 1000 coronary angiograms and results of surgical management. *Ann Surg* 1984; **199:** 223.
2. McCann RL, Wolfe WG. Resection of abdominal aortic aneurysm in patients with low ejection fractions. *J Vasc Surg* 1989; **10:** 240–4.
3. Golden MA, Whittemore AD, Donaldson MC, Mannick JA. Selective evaluation and management of coronary artery disease in patients undergoing repair of abdominal aortic aneurysms. *Ann Surg* 1990; **212:** 415–23.
4. Berlauk JF, Abrams JH, Gilmour IJ, O'Conner R, Knighton DR, Cerra FB. Preoperative optimization of cardiovascular hemodynamics improves outcome in peripheral vascular surgery. *Ann Surg* 1991; **214:** 289–99.
5. Crawford ES, Saleh SA, Babb JW, Glaeser DH, Vaccaro PS, Silvers A. Infrarenal abdominal aortic aneurysm: factors influencing survival after operation performed over a 25-year period. *Ann Surg* 1981; **193:** 699–708.
6. Strachan CJ, Newsome SW, Ashton TR. The clinical use of an antibiotic bonded graft. *Eur J Vasc Surg* 1991; **5:** 627–32.
7. Kerstein M, Sweeney TF. Abdominal aortic aneurysms. In: *Aortic Aneurysms: Surgical Therapy*, Campbell CD (ed). New York: Futura, 1981: 139.
8. Campbell WB. Mortality statistics for elective aortic aneurysms. *Eur J Vasc Surg* 1991; **5:** 111–13.
9. Smith PK, Fuchs JCA, Sabiston DC. Surgical management of aortic aneurysms in patients with severe pulmonary insufficiency. *Surg Gynae Obst* 1980; **151:** 407–11.
10. Stein M, Cassara EL. Pre-operative evaluation and therapy for surgery patients. *JAMA* 1970; **211:** 789–90.
11. Diebel LM, Lange P, Schneider F, *et al.* Cardiopulmonary complications after major surgery: a role for epidural analgesia? *Surgery* 1987; **102:** 660–6.
12. Abbott WM. Acute renal failure complicating vascular surgery. In: *Complications in Vascular Surgery*, Bernhard VM, Towne JB (eds). New York: Grune & Stratton, 1980: 363–77.
13. Cohen JR, Mannick JA, Couch NP, Whittemore AD. Abdominal aortic aneurysm repair in patients with perioperative renal failure. *J Vasc Surg* 1986; **3:** 867.
14. Abu Rahma AF, Robinson PA, Boland JP *et al.* Elective resection of 332 abdominal aortic aneurysms in a southern West Virginia community during a recent five-year period. *Surgery* 1991; **109:** 244–51.
15. Diehl JT, Cali RF, Hertzer NR, Beven EG. Complications of abdominal aortic reconstruction. *Ann Surg* 1983; **197:** 49–56.
16. Clarke PJ, Tarin D. Effect of per-operative blood transfusion on tumour metastases. *Br J Surg* 1987; **74:** 520–2.
17. Blair SD, Janvrin SB, McCollum CN, Greenhalgh RM. Effect of early blood transfusion on gastrointestinal haemorrhage. *Br J Surg* 1986; **73:** 783–5.
18. Corson RJ, O'Dwyer ST, McCollum CN. Avoiding blood loss in major surgery: haemodilution and other methods. *Haem Rev Commun* 1992; **7:** 47–53.
19. Hermreck AS. Prevention and management of surgical complications during repair of abdominal aortic aneurysms. *Surg Clin N Am* 1989; **69:** 869–94.
20. Hagihara PF, Ernst CB, Griffen WO. Incidence of ischemic colitis following abdominal aortic reconstruction. *Surg Gynae Obst* 1979; **149:** 571–3.
21. Szilagyi DE, Hageman JH, Smith RF, *et al.* Spinal cord damage in surgery of the abdominal aorta. *Surgery* 1978; **83:** 38.
22. Flannigan DP, Schuler JJ, Keifer T, *et al.* Elimination of iatrogenic impotence and improvement of sexual function after aortiliac reconstruction. *Arch Surg* 1982; **117:** 544.
23. Paterson IS, Klausner JM, Goldman G, *et al.* Pulmonary edema after aneurysm surgery is modified by mannitol. *Ann Surg* 1989; **210:** 796–801.
24. Greenall MJ, Evans M, Pollock AV. Midline or transverse laparotomy? A random controlled clinical trial. II: Influence on postoperative pulmonary complications. *Br J Surg* 1980; **67:** 191–4.
25. Sicard GA, Allen BT, Munn JS, Anderson CB. Retroperitoneal versus transperitoneal approach for repair of abdominal aortic aneurysms. *Surg Clin N Am* 1989; **69:** 795–806.
26. Campbell WB, Ballard PK, Goodman DA. Intensive care after abdominal aortic surgery. *Eur J Vasc Surg* 1991; **5:** 65–8.
27. Cunningham C, Goldstone J. Management of aortoenteric and aortocaval fistulae. In: *The Cause and Management of Aneurysms*, Greenhalgh RM, Mannick JA, Powell JT (eds). London: WB Saunders, 1990: 461–77.
28. North American Symptomatic Carotid Endarterectomy Trial collaborators. Beneficial effect of carotid endarterectomy in symptomatic patients with high-grade stenosis. *N Engl J Med* 1991; **325:** 443–53.
29. European Carotid Surgery Trialists' collaborative group. MRC European Carotid Surgery Trial: Interim results for symptomatic patients with severe (70–99%) or with mild (0–29%) carotid stenosis. *Lancet* 1991; **337:** 1235–43.
30. McCollum CN, Alexander CE, Kechinton GF, Frank PJ, Greenhalgh RM. PTFE or human umbilical vein for femoropopliteal bypass: a multicentre trial. *Eur J Vasc Surg* 1991; **5:** 435–43.
31. McCollum CN, Alexander C, Kenchington G, Franks PJ, Greenhalgh RM. Antiplatelet drugs in femoropopliteal vein bypass: a multicentre trial. *J Vasc Surg* 1991; **13:** 150–61.

15

Percutaneous techniques

Michael R Rees

Percutaneous therapeutic techniques for peripheral arterial disease were initiated by Dotter and Judkins in 1963.[1] They passed a 12Fr catheter over an 0.44-inch wire to dilate a femoral artery stenosis in a lady facing amputation. This technique, based on passing sequentially larger catheters into an artery to dilate the vessel, was only used in a very limited fashion and was restricted by the large sizes of catheter required to obtain dilatation. The term 'transluminal angioplasty' was first used to describe the method which has now been more commonly called the Dotter technique, although balloon angioplasty was first described by Andreus Gruentzig in 1974.[2] The development of an expandable balloon solved the problem of dilating a large vessel through a small arterial puncture site. Gruentzig's original balloon was based on a 7Fr shaft. However, balloons are now routinely used for dilatation of peripheral vessels with a 5Fr shaft, and catheters are now available for coronary and small peripheral vessel angioplasty with a balloon size of 4 mm on a 1.4Fr shaft. Balloon angioplasty initially developed slowly but has now become an accepted method of treating vascular disease.

Percutaneous transcatheter techniques have rapidly expanded over the last decade to include thrombolysis, atherectomy, embolisation, laser therapy, and one of the more recent but perhaps most significant developments, the vascular stent. Intravascular imaging has also become possible, initially with percutaneous angioscopy and more recently using small-diameter ultrasound probes to image vessels with both two-and-three dimensional ultrasound. The combination of a variety of transcatheter therapies and endovascular imaging provides a powerful array of techniques for the diagnosis and treatment of vascular disease by the percutaneous approach.

The percutaneous approach

Most transcatheter therapeutic techniques achieve arterial entry by means of a modification of the Seldinger technique which was first described in 1953.[3] In this method a needle puncture is made into an artery, through which a wire is introduced. Following placement of the wire a catheter is threaded over it. Catheters up to and including 19Fr size have been introduced intra-arterially by this technique, although most techniques are based on 5–9Fr diameter devices. The combination of a pre-shaped catheter and selective guide wire can reach any significant vessel.

Catheters and guide wires have become very sophisticated, with a wide variety of sizes and materials being available. Wires range from those which are very stiff and which can support bulky devices, to those which are very small and flexible to access small vessels. Latterly very slippery hydrophilic wires have become available which can pass through very tortuous and even occluded vessels. Wire sizes are available from 0.038-inch to 0.010-inch diameter. Usually the artery is first accessed using a larger wire, with the smaller wires being used to enter smaller vessels and branches. Wires can be pre-shaped, as in a J-shaped tip wire, to reduce trauma to the vessel, or can be made so that the tip of the wire can be shaped by the operator to a specified curve for a particular purpose.

What is the role of angioplasty?

Balloon angioplasty has become a widely used method of treatment particularly in the USA and many European countries. It is effective, relatively simple in straightforward cases and reduces the trauma to the patient and length of stay compared with a corresponding surgical approach (Figs. 15.1–15.3). It has a high level of primary success (over 90% in most sites in stenotic disease) with a

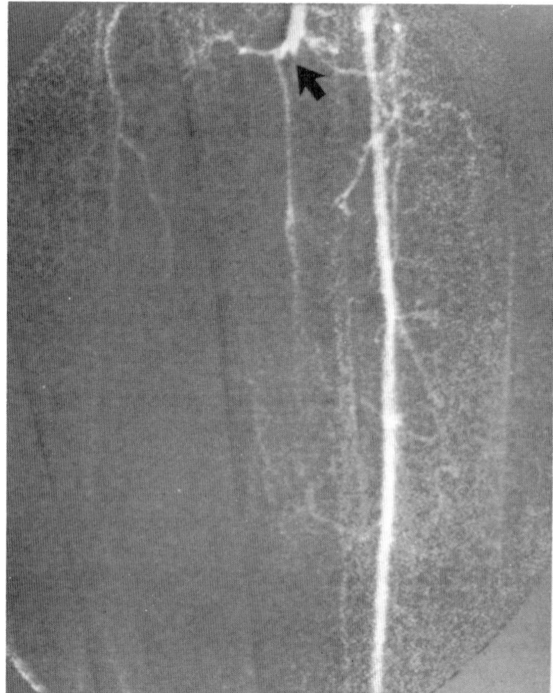

Fig. 15.1 Occlusion of the tibioperoneal trunk.

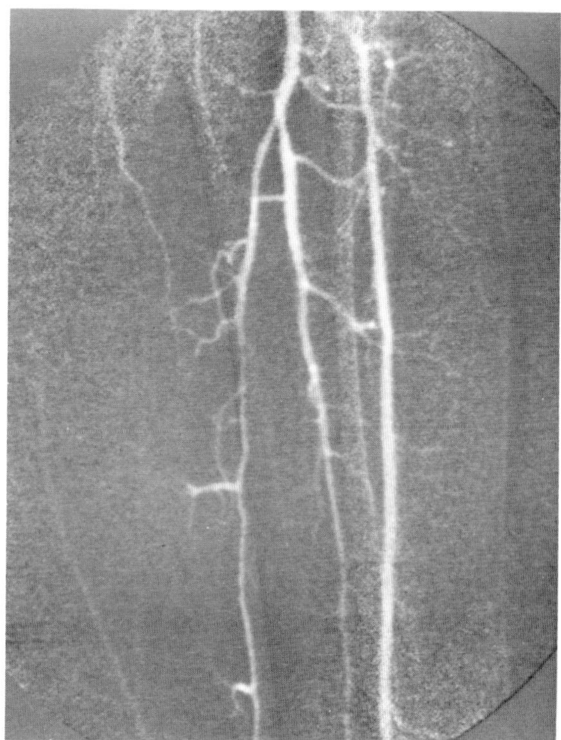

Fig. 15.3 Final angiogram showing three-vessel runoff.

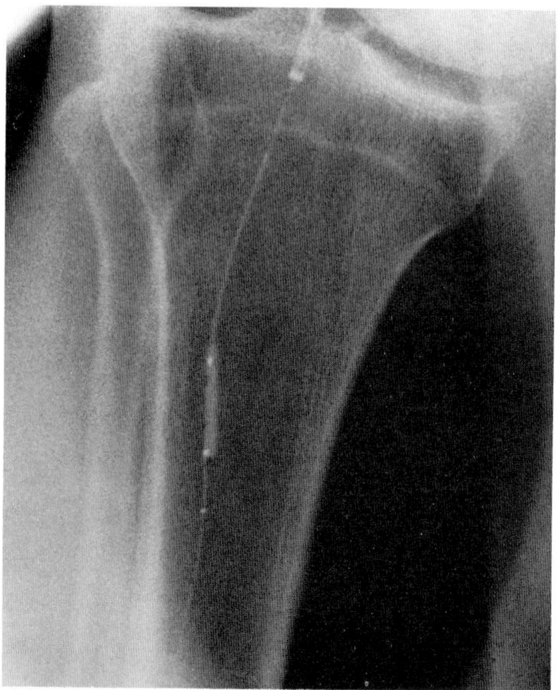

Fig. 15.2 Passage of a 3mm balloon through the occlusion over a 0.0014-inch (35 micron) guide wire. The balloon is guided via a guiding catheter.

correspondingly low level of serious complications. Balloon angioplasty rates for peripheral disease in the UK are relatively low. This is due to many factors, perhaps the most important of which is the relatively conservative approach of UK doctors who view claudication as an essentially benign disease. Also, patients are reluctant to visit their GPs with symptoms of claudication. Recent surveys have shown that despite peripheral vascular disease affecting 8% of the population aged 55–74 years,[4] as few as 10% of symptomatic patients consult their doctors. These trends result in patients presenting with relatively advanced disease, which may not be amenable to angioplasty.

Perhaps the answer is to treat early-stage disease as happens in other countries. However, in order for this to be acceptable it should be established that angioplasty does not result in short-term improvement with longer-term deterioration as some workers have suggested. In a recent study[5] of 101 limbs treated by angioplasty, 16% showed a reduction in limb blood flow after 6 months compared with the pre-angioplasty level. However, in 53 patients the contralateral limb, although diseased, was not treated; 25% of these limbs also showed a reduction in limb blood flow. This would indicate that any deterioration in limb blood flow is unlikely to be due to angioplasty alone and is probably due to a combination of other factors.

Complications of peripheral angioplasty are low. The most significant include haematoma and pseudoaneurysm formation at the puncture site, dissection of the artery, and distal embolisation. These occur in about 5% of cases with approximately one-third requiring surgical intervention.[6,7]

The most significant problem affecting the use of angioplasty is the phenomenon of re-stenosis (Fig. 15.4). Re-stenosis affects all vessels that have been treated by angioplasty. Some vessels have higher re-stenosis rates than others: coronary artery re-stenosis occurs in 30–40% of cases, with iliac 10–25%[8] and femoral 15–50%, depending on the type of disease treated. Long and occluded lesions have a higher re-stenosis rate than short stenoses. Various procedures and drug regimens have been investigated to reduce re-stenosis rate, with no consistent outcome. However, it does appear that some types of intravascular stents may be helpful. Similar claims have been made for atherectomy procedures but the evidence for this is less clear. Many drugs are being investigated to reduce re-stenosis, but only high-dose cytotoxic drugs and local radiotherapy have been shown experimentally to reduce re-stenosis. There are currently trials of many drugs that may have an impact in this area, including lipid lowering agents, ACE inhibitors and low-dose heparin. Heparin appears to affect re-stenosis by reducing the rate of post-angioplasty thrombosis, and continued heparin therapy after angioplasty may play a role in reducing recurrent disease.

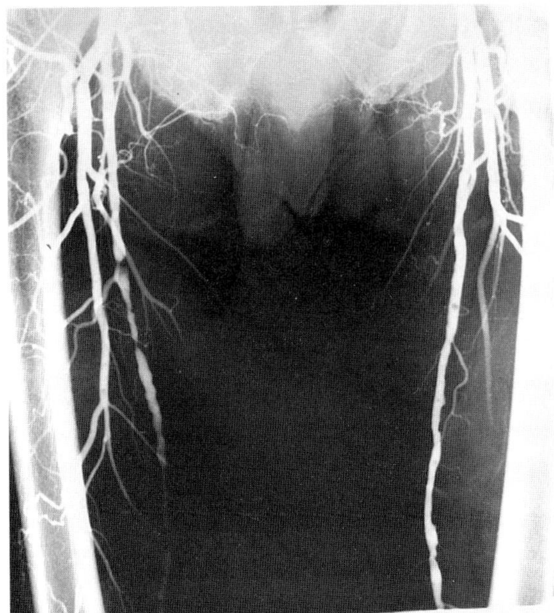

Fig. 15.4 Diffuse re-stenosis of right superficial femoral artery following angioplasty.

Balloon angioplasty

The original hypothesis for the mechanism of action of balloon angioplasty was that it compressed atheromatous plaque into the wall of the artery. However, histological studies and more recently intravascular ultrasound and angioscopy[9] have demonstrated that it acts by splitting the intima and media and by disrupting plaque. This involves splitting of the vessel wall in nondiseased as well as in diseased areas. The factors which determine a successful angioplasty are therefore complex.

Successful angioplasty should cause enough disruption of the vessel to obtain a patent lumen without resulting in extensive damage which would produce dissection or flow-limiting intimal tears. The degree of dilatation should produce good flow in the vessel without creating a very thrombogenic surface or conditions which would create low flow or excessive turbulence. There is also a relationship between the degree of vessel damage and re-stenosis. Re-stenosis is primarily a result of intimal hyperplasia. The triggering mechanisms for what is essentially an aggressive healing response are unclear but probably include excessive vessel disruption and formation of thrombus. The long-term results are better in large-diameter arteries, despite technically good results now being achieved in smaller peripheral vessels.

There is a wide variety of balloon technology available, which includes balloons of various sizes from 1.5 mm to 30 mm. Balloon materials which are compliant will mould to the contour of the vessel and increase in diameter with increasing pressure. Noncompliant balloons are designed to withstand high pressures (up to 20 atmospheres). Angioplasty balloons now have very low profiles to enable them to be passed across tight lesions, and are coated with materials that make them very slippery.

Technically, therefore, angioplasty can be applied to most sites affected by atherosclerosis. The applicability of angioplasty in any given circumstance will depend on a combination of factors and not just the angiographic appearance. These factors include the site of the lesion, its length, the suitability of the patient for operation, and consideration of the surgical alternatives. In general, focal stenotic disease in the femoral, iliac or renal arteries are best treated by angioplasty, and long occlusions in the femoral and iliac vessels best treated by operation. The availability of thrombolysis, however, has blurred these guidelines and it is now possible to adopt a combined percutaneous approach of thrombolysis and angioplasty for even long chronic occlusions with some success.

Other devices

A variety of devices and techniques have been developed to replace or enhance balloon angioplasty and to extend the indications for percutaneous vascular intervention. These fall into three distinct groups: (a) devices for treatment of occlusions (lasers, the Kensey catheter); (b) devices to remove plaque (lasers, atherectomy devices, the Rotablator); (c) devices to maintain vessel patency (stents, hot balloons, the laser balloon).

Devices for treatment of occlusions

Lasers

When first reports of the use of lasers in the treatment of vascular disease were published it was assumed that this method would enhance and perhaps eventually replace angioplasty.[10] Following initial enthusiasm, the use of lasers rose rapidly with a number of different systems (e.g. hot-tip, Nd-YAG/sapphire, pulsed dye, pulsed YAG). None of these has produced consistent results, particularly in reducing the rates of re-stenosis, and many have produced results inferior to those of comparable surgical and conventional angioplasty techniques.[11]

The two primary uses of lasers were (a) to reopen occluded vessels by creating a new passageway through the occlusion which could be followed by balloon angioplasty, and (b) to ablate plaque.

The success of recanalization is very technique-dependent and a variety of guidance methods have been developed to overcome the problem of steering the device through the occlusion. These include spectroscopy,[12] ultrasound[13] and angioscopy.[14]

The major problem with laser systems is to find one which will ablate plaque without causing damage to surrounding tissue. Thermal damage from continuous wave lasers can be very extensive.[15] Pulsed lasers may have a smaller effect on surrounding tissues but there are considerable technical problems in delivering laser energy over a wide enough surface area to effect ablation. Much of the effects of these laser systems may be simply mechanical, producing a Dotter effect in the vessel. Lasers still may play a role in certain circumstances, such as the ablation of calcified tissue and treatment of intimal hyperplasia. However, as yet the final place of lasers in the treatment of peripheral disease is not established.

Mechanical devices

Soon after the initial work with lasers was published the Kensey catheter was introduced.[16] This is a mechanical device for the treatment of arterial occlusions (Figs 15.5 and 15.6). It employs a blunt, rapidly rotating cam together with a fluid jet which creates a vortex at the tip of the catheter. The plaque is pulverized to small particles by a combination of mechanical energy and the action of the fluid jets. These particles are dissipated into the bloodstream.[17] Experimentally the device had been shown to leave normal arterial tissue undamaged, whilst selectively acting on the harder, less compliant plaque.

The clinical use of this catheter is limited by the high number of perforations and dissections in severely diseased vessels where the arterial wall is calcified and is therefore less compliant. Follow-up results also proved disappointing. It has a potential role as a method of local delivery of drugs or thrombolytic agents. Prior to its widespread testing in humans, experimental evidence gave a mixed picture as to the likelihood of particles being created which would embolise downstream. In practice, with this and other mechanical systems the problem of embolisation does not appear to be clinically significant, but the longer-term effects of microembolisation have not been studied.

Lower speed rotational devices such as the Rotacs system have also been used fairly extensively. These are designed not to ablate plaque but to provide some mechanical energy and torque to a flexible olive-tipped wire which finds the path of least resistance through an occluded vessel. There is good evidence to show that they are effective in creating a channel through an occluded vessel to allow for additional therapy such as balloon angioplasty. The frequency of dissections and perforations with this type of device is low.[18]

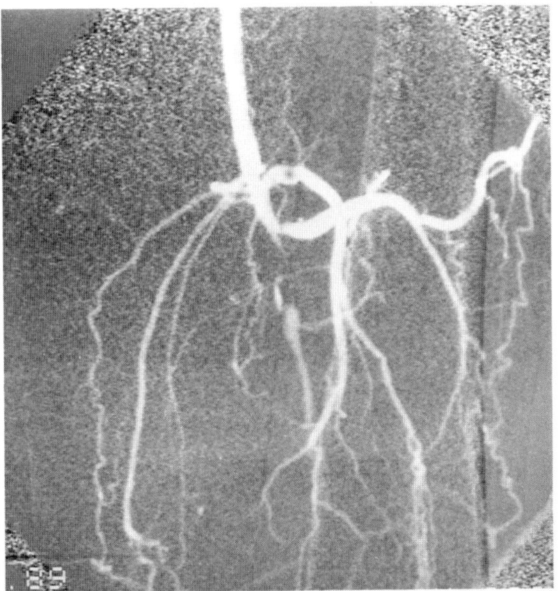

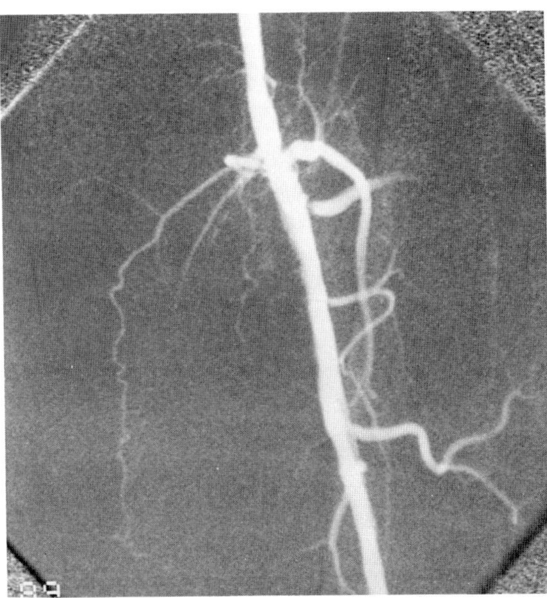

Fig. 15.5 (Left) An occlusion of the superficial femoral artery at its origin. The same occlusion is shown on the right following recanalization with a mechanical device (Kensey catheter) and subsequent balloon angioplasty.

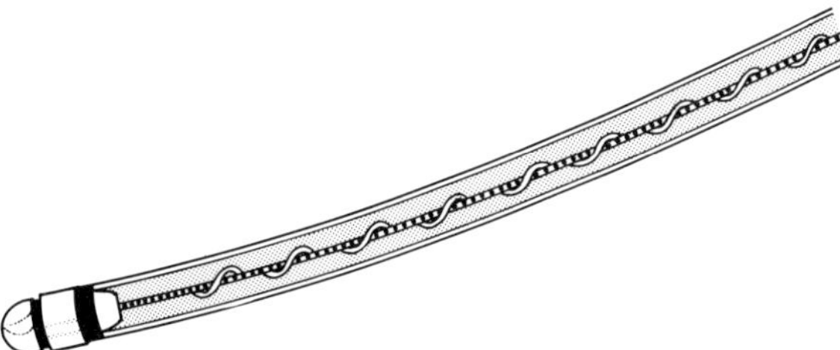

Fig. 15.6 The Kensey catheter, showing its internal drive shaft (coiled appearance) and blunt distal cam.

Hydrophyllic wires

One of the main reasons why the use of lasers and mechanical devices has decreased is the introduction of hydrophyllic guide wires. These become very slippery when wet and can be passed through a high percentage of occlusions, taking the path of least resistance through the vessel. They are simple to use and have a very low complication rate. One of their most significant disadvantages is that there may be a subintimal passage of the wire through the occlusion, although this can in part be prevented by careful guidance. There is some debate whether there is any disadvantage to a subintimal passage and subsequent dilatation. Most authors feel that this is undesirable but a significant minority have promoted the benefits of this method.[19]

Atherectomy

The aim of atherectomy devices is to remove plaque by cutting the atheromatous material while leaving normal intima undamaged. Several different devices have been evaluated. The most commonly used is the Simpson atherectomy device,[20] which has a small cutting blade housed in a capsule at the distal end of a flexible catheter. This produces a small longitudinal cut in the vessel. The cutting blade is apposed to the vessel wall by a low-pressure balloon which is placed on the opposite side of the capsule to the cutting blade. To be effective the catheter must be rotated in the vessel through several different positions and a cut made at each position. Early reports indicated that this method might produce a reduction in re-stenosis rates, but later research has revealed that the re-stenosis rates are at least as high as that of conventional angioplasty. The main advantages of this technique are that it is useful in treating eccentric lesions and very hard fibrous lesions which do not dilate easily with a balloon. It may also be of use in the treatment of dissections.

A new development is an atherectomy device which can effect a circular cut in a vessel. This device, termed the Fischell pullback atherectomy device, cuts with the aid of external compression of the artery by an inflatable pressure cuff which compresses the vessel on to the cutting blade of the device. The device is first passed through the lesion over a guide wire, the housing of the blade is extended, exposing the blade which is passed through the lesion. The blade, driven by a low torque motor, rotates at 300 rpm. The resected material is collected in the catheter housing as the catheter is pulled back through the lesion.[21] This is the first device for peripheral use that can be used as a precise cutting tool. The depth and amount of cut can be controlled by catheter selection, degree of external compression and number of passes. Unlike other atherectomy devices, the amount of material removed is usually substantial.[22] Further follow-up data are required to determine if this device has any effect on the degree of re-stenosis.

Devices to maintain vessel patency

Intravascular stents

The development of intravascular stents may be the most significant advance in percutaneous vascular therapy since the introduction of balloon angioplasty. The concept is to provide support to the vessel following angioplasty. There are several stents in clinical use and undergoing evaluation. All current stents are metallic, the most common materials being stainless steel, nitinol and tantalum (Figs 15.7–15.11).

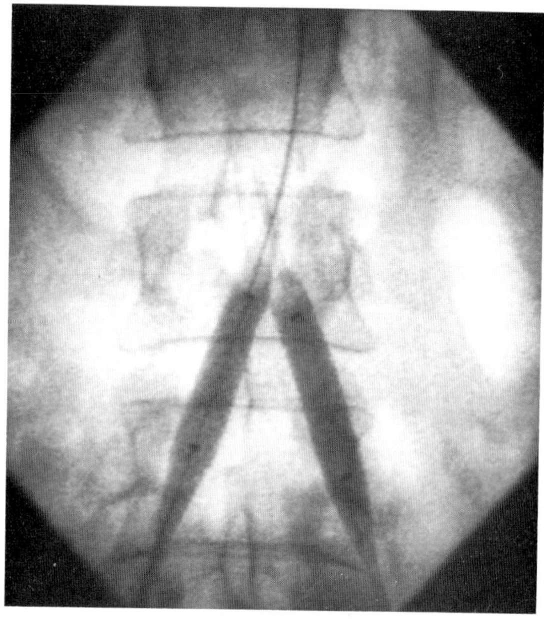

Fig. 15.7 Kissing balloon angioplasty of the aorta and common iliac vessels.

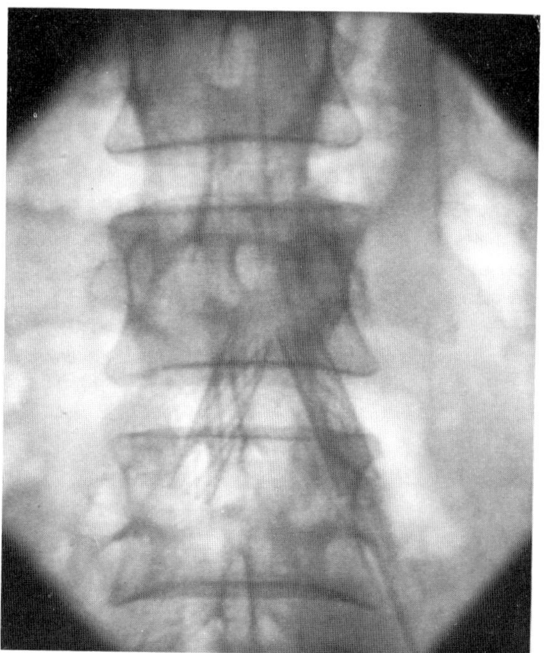

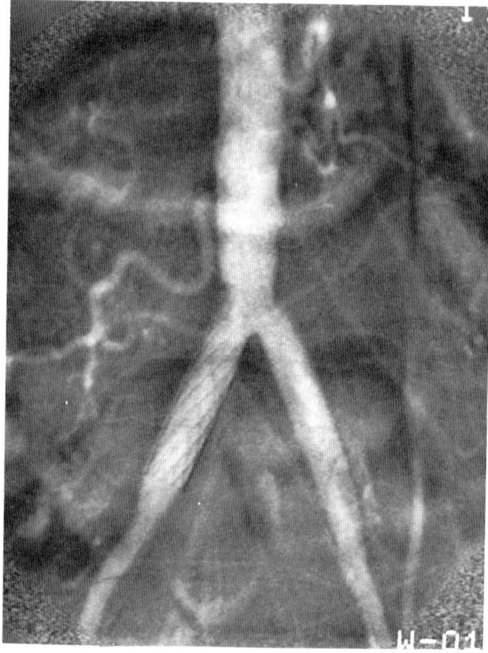

Fig. 15.8 (Left) Placement of bilateral Palmaz stents (plain radiograph). The right picture shows the final angiographic appearance with stents *in situ*.

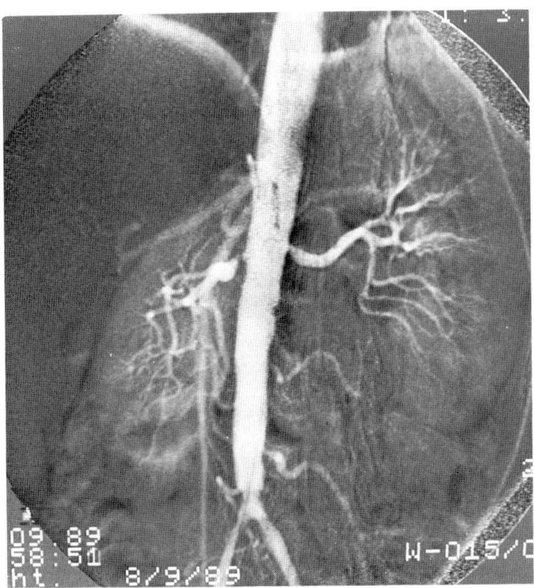

Fig. 15.9 Angiogram showing bilateral renal stenoses and severe disease at the aorto-iliac junction.

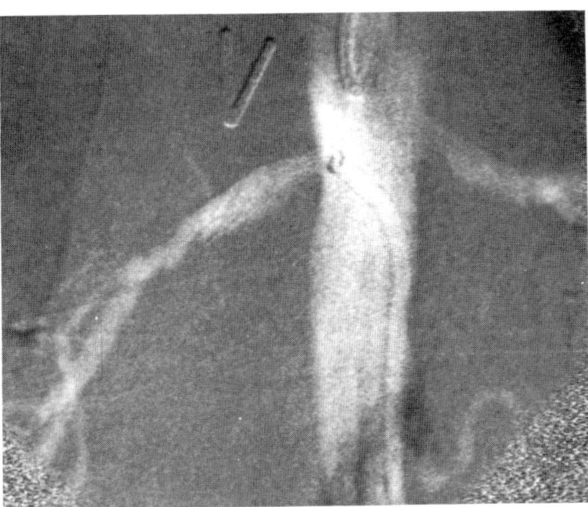

Fig. 15.10 The same patient as in Fig. 15.9 following bilateral renal artery angioplasty and placement of a Palmaz stent in the right renal artery.

The most widely used stent at present is the Palmaz stent. This is a balloon-expandable stent made from stainless steel. It expands to form a lattice-like structure within the artery. This stent has been placed in iliac, renal, femoral, tibial, coronary and carotid arteries, as well as in the abdominal aorta and patent ductus arteriosus. It has also been used extensively in the venous system. Another widely used stent is the wallstent, which is self-expanding, also made of stainless steel, mounted on a specially designed introducer. On releasing the stent, it expands to a predetermined size. Other stents such as the Wictor and the Gianturco–Rubin are balloon-mounted wire coil stents. The Strecker is also a wire stent but has a woven pattern and is constructed from tantalum.

The major indications for stent placement are for a significant dissection following angioplasty, particularly if this is flow-limiting, and following recanalization of an occlusion, particularly a chronic occlusion. A more controversial indication is to reduce further re-stenosis in a patient who has already developed re-stenosis.

The use of stents does seem to have reduced the incidence of acute occlusion following angioplasty. There is accumulating evidence that patients with postangioplasty dissections or with recanalized occlusions have an improved patency rate following stent placement. The evidence for stents reducing the rate of re-stenosis under other circumstances is incomplete.[23]

There is some evidence that not all stents have the same patency rates. The wallstent has a significant early closure rate in small vessels, and the Strecker stent has a significant re-stenosis rate due to intimal hyperplasia. At the moment the Palmaz stent has the lowest re-stenosis and occlusion rate. However, its application is limited by its comparative rigidity. It cannot therefore be used in areas where the vessel will be subject to stress (e.g. over a joint). In coronary arteries stress due to movement has been partially overcome by the introduction of an articulation between two halves of the stent (the Schatz modification). This modified stent has also been used in renal arteries. However, re-stenosis can occur at the area of articulation where the stent circumference is incomplete. Re-stenosis can also occur at the ends of a stent where its arms may penetrate the intima.

The increasing use of stents has extended the indications for angioplasty.[24] It is now possible to treat distal stenotic and occlusive aortoiliac disease by a combination of angioplasty and stenting, this type of disease having been previously a surgical preserve.

Early use of stents is being reported in the carotid circulation with some success. However, it is likely that the use of stents in this vessel will be limited to areas where the artery is protected by the jaw or skull.

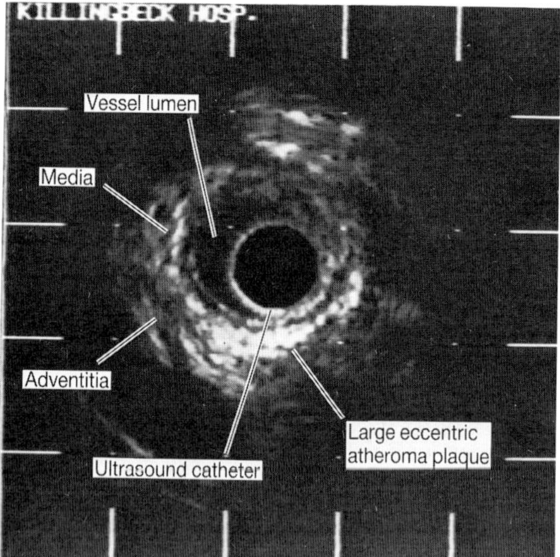

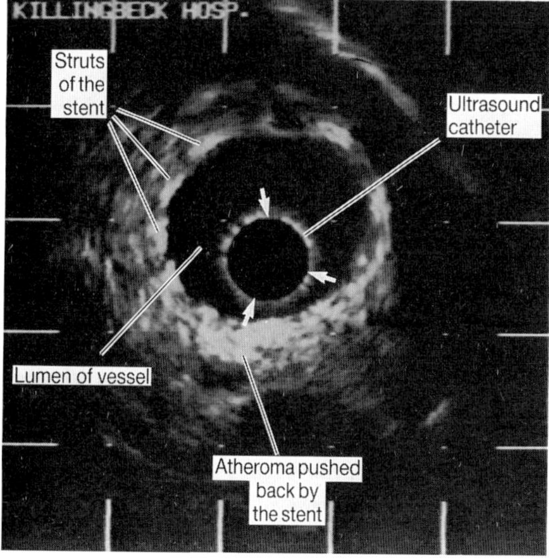

Fig. 15.11 The top picture shows an intravascular ultrasound image of the iliac artery before stent placement. The round shadow in the centre of the lumen is the intravascular ultrasound catheter. Underneath is the intravascular ultrasound image of the artery after stent placement.

Thrombolysis

The ability to restore patency for a recently thrombosed vessel without operation is clearly desirable. Experience with catheter-based local thrombolysis has demonstrated that patency can be successfully achieved in most acute arterial occlusions. The treatment may be prolonged, requiring the placement of arterial catheters in the treated vessel for hours, and in some cases days.

A variety of new catheters have been developed to allow for prolonged infusion. These can be divided into two types: (a) small-diameter hollow wires having a variable length of distal catheter with infusion holes, and (b) small-diameter catheters with either a double or triple lumen to allow for guidewire infusion and flush ports. Both of these catheter types are typically small-diameter, the infusion wires have a diameter of 0.035–0.038 inches and the infusion catheters are 3–5 Fr.

The doses of thrombolytic drug used should ideally not produce systemic effects. For example, rtPA is infused at a rate no greater than 1–2 mg/hour, and urokinase at 20 000–60 000 iv/hour. As with any long-term catheter placement the patient should be heparinized to achieve an activated clotting time 2–3 times normal.

More controversial is the use of thrombolysis in cases of chronic occlusion. Some workers have achieved encouraging results,[25] success being based on the supposition that even in chronic occlusions, there is a central core of the occluded artery that consists of thrombus that is still susceptible to thrombolysis. The use of rtPA which is more effective on formed thrombus may be preferable in these circumstances.

Intra-arterial imaging

Angioscopy

Angioscopy is the imaging of the lumen of a vessel by a fibreoptic endoscope. A clear field of view is obtained by flushing the vessel with crystalloid. This technique is becoming established at operation because it is easier to obtain a clear field of view with surgical control of the artery. New methods of perfusion of the vessel by peristaltic pumping, which can be intermittent, or imaging catheters which have low-pressure balloons to occlude completely or partially a vessel, have enabled angioscopy to become a reliable percutaneous technique.[26] The clinical role of percutaneous peripheral angioscopy has not been established. Nevertheless, the appearance of the endothelium before and after intervention provides new information on the mode of action and effectiveness of percutaneous techniques.[27] In particular, valuable information is being gained on the action of the newer atherectomy devices. There is certainly

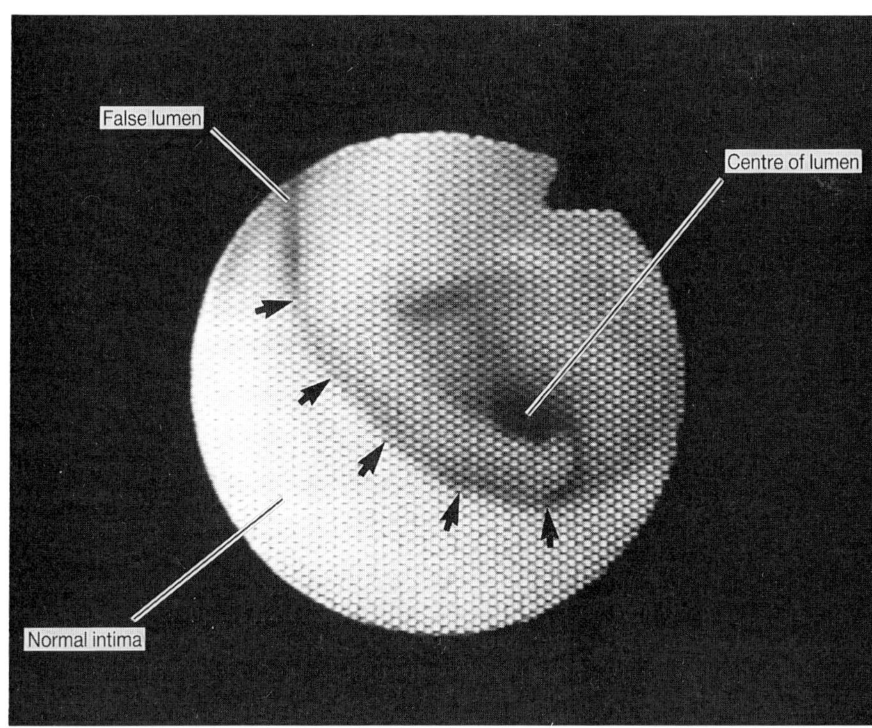

Fig. 15.12 Angioscopic image of an artery showing a dissection following angioplasty. The large dissection flap is outlined by the arrows.

the potential of carrying out interventional techniques under angioscopic guidance in the future.

Intravascular ultrasound

Although developed after angioscopy, this has rapidly become a more accepted and widespread technique for percutaneous use. Ultrasound avoids the need to obtain a clear or bloodless field before an artery can be imaged. Typically, the catheter consists of an ultrasound probe which is guided down the vessel over a fine guidewire. There is a channel to flush the device to maintain an ultrasound window between the probe and the vessel. Ultrasound devices are being used to diagnose the extent and nature of dissections particularly to help distinguish the true and false lumen. They are also useful in diagnosing the extent of stenotic disease and in monitoring the results of therapy. Ultrasound is proving particularly useful in the deployment of stents and to determine the end point of vascular interventions.[28] Current ultrasound catheters are 4–8 Fr in size and usually need to be delivered into the artery via a guiding catheter.

References

1. Dotter CT, Judkins MP. Transluminal treatment of arteriosclerotic obstruction: description of a new technique and preliminary report of its application. *Circulation* 1964; **30:** 654.
2. Gruentzig A, Kumpe DA. Technique of percutaneous transluminal angioplasty with the Gruntzig balloon catheter. *AJR* 1979; **132:** 547.
3. Seldinger SI. Catheter replacement of the needle in percutaneous arteriography: a new technique. *Acta Radiol* 1953; **39:** 368.
4. Fowkes FG, Housley E, Cawood EH, Macintyre CC, Ruckley CV, Prescott RJ. Edinburgh Artery Study: prevalence of asymptomatic and symptomatic peripheral arterial disease in the general population. *Int J Epidem* 1991; **20:** 384–92.
5. Thorley PJ, Sheard K, Rees MR. The use of isotope limb blood flow in the assessment of peripheral angioplasty. *Br J Radiol* 1991; **64** (Suppl): 18.
6. Katzen BT. Percutaneous transluminal angioplasty for arterial disease of the lower extremities. *AJR* 1984; **142:** 23.
7. Gardiner GA, Meyerovitz MF, Stokes KR, *et al.* Complications of transluminal angioplasty. *Radiology* 1986; **159:** 201.
8. Wilson AR, Fuchs JCA. Percutaneous transluminal angioplasty: the radiologist's contribution to the treatment of vascular disease. *Surg Clin N Am* 1984; **64:** 121.

9. Rees MR, Gehani AA, Ashley S, Davies A. Percutaneous video angioscopy in peripheral vascular disease. *Clin Radiol* 1989; **40:** 347.
10. Cumberland DC, Sanborn TI, Taylot DI, *et al.* Percutaneous laser thermal angioplasty: initial clinical results with a laser probe in total peripheral artery occlusions. *Lancet* 1986; **1:** 2457–9.
11. Ashley S, Brooks SG, Gehani AA, Thorley P, Parkin A, Kester RC, Rees MR. Isotope limb blood flow measurement in patients undergoing peripheral laser angioplasty. *J Biomed Eng* 1991; **13:** 221–4.
12. Geschwind H, Dubois-Rande JL, Shafton E, Boissignac G, Wexman M. Percutaneous pulsed laser-assisted balloon angioplasty guided by spectroscopy. *Am Heart J* 1989; **117:** 1147–52.
13. White RA, Kopchok GE, Tabbara MR, Cavaye DM, Cornier F. Intravascular ultrasound guided holmium: YAG laser recanalisation of occluded arteries. *Lasers Surg Med* 1992; **12:** 239–45.
14. White GH, White RA, Colman PD, Kopchok GE. Experimental and clinical applications of angioscopic guidance for laser angioplasty. *Am J Surg* 1989; **158:** 495–500.
15. Rosenthal E, Montarello JK, Palmer T, Curry PV. Coronary artery thermal damage during percutaneous hot tip laser assisted angioplasty. *Am J Cardiol* 1989; **64:** 116–20.
16. Zeitler E, Kensey K. First own results with dynamic angioplasty with the Kensey catheter. *Ann Radiol* 1988; **31:** 77–81.
17. Gehani AA, Sheard K, Ashley S, Brooks S, Kester RC, Rees MR. Dynamic angioplasty of total arterial occlusions. *Br J Surg* 1990; **77:** 1139–41.
18. Vallbracht C, Liermann DD, Prignitz I, Beinborn W, Roth FJ, Kollath J, Landgraf H, Kaltenbach M. Low-speed rotational angioplasty in chronic peripheral artery occlusions: experience in 83 patients. Work in progress. *Radiology* 1989; **172:** 327–33.
19. Bolia A, Miles KA, Brennan J, Bell PR. Percutaneous transluminal angioplasty of occlusions of the femoral and popliteal arteries by subintimal dissection. *Cardiovasc Interven Radiol* 1990; **13:** 357–63.
20. Simpson JB. Percutaneous removal of atheromatous plaques in peripheral arteries. *Lancet* 1988; **1:** 384–6.
21. Fischell TA, Fischell RE, White RJ, Chapolini R. Ex-vivo results using a new pullback atherectomy catheter (PAC). *Catheter Cardiovasc Diag* 1990; **21:** 287–9.
22. Sivananthan UM, Browne TF, Rees MR. Treatment with the Pullback Atherectomy catheter: assessment with angioscopy and intravascular ultrasound. *Radiology* 1992; **185**(P): 162.
23. Sapoval MR, Long AL, Raynaud AC, Beyssen BM, Fiessinger JN, Gaux JC. Femoropopliteal stent placement: long-term results. *Radiology* 1992; **184:** 883–9.
24. Katzen BT, Becker GJ. Intravascular stents: status of development and clinical application. *Surg Clin N Am* 1992; **72:** 941–57.
25. Barr H, Lancashire MJ, Torrie EP, Galland RB. Intra-arterial thrombolytic therapy in the management of acute and chronic limb ischaemia. *Br J Surg* 1991; **78:** 284–7.
26. Diethrich EB, Yoffe B, Kiessling JJ, Santiago O, Bahadir I, Stern LA, Lavine D. Angioscopy in endovascular surgery: recent technical advances to enhance intervention selection and failure analysis. *Angiology* 1992; **43:** 1–10.
27. Siegel RJ, Chae JS, Forrester JS, Ruiz CC. Angiography, angioscopy and ultrasound imaging before and after percutaneous balloon angioplasty. *Am Heart J* 1990; **120:** 1086–90.
28. Dake MD. Intravascular ultrasound. *Curr Opin Radiol* 1991; **3:** 181–7.

16

Investigation and management of Raynaud's phenomenon

Jill JF Belch

It is now over 130 years since Maurice Raynaud first described the syndrome that bears his name.[1] He defined it as episodic digital ischaemia provoked by cold and emotion. It is classically manifest by pallor of the affected part followed by cyanosis and rubor. The pallor reflects vasospasm in the digital vessels (Fig 16.1); the cyanosis arises from deoxygenation of the static venous blood; and the rubor results from reactive hyperaemia following the return of blood flow.

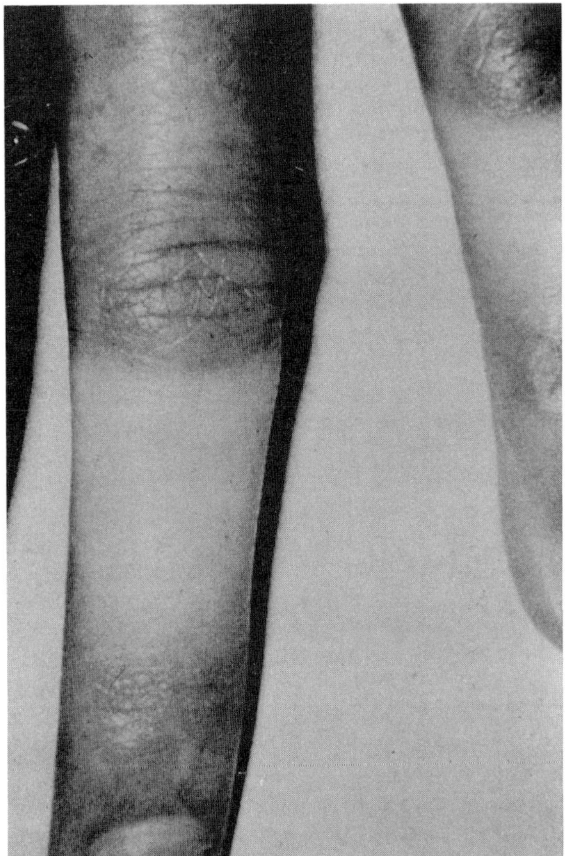

Fig. 16.1 The vasospasm of Raynaud's phenomenon.

Raynaud's phenomenon (RP) is nine times more common in women than in men and has an overall prevalence in the population of approximately 10%, although it may affect as many as 20–30% of women in the younger age groups. There is also a familial predisposition which is more marked if the age of onset is less than 30 years.[2]

RP can be a benign condition but, if severe, can cause digital ulceration and gangrene. Until recently little was known about the true aetiology and extent of the disorder. This lack of knowledge has led to difficulties in the treatment and prediction of prognosis in RP. It is now known that Raynaud's original definition requires significant modification. For example, the full triphasic colour change is not now thought to be essential for the diagnosis of RP as a history of cold-induced digital blanching with subsequent reactive hyperaemia can still reflect significant vasospasm. Furthermore, stimuli other than cold and emotion can provoke an attack; for example, hormones,[3] trauma and chemicals, including those in tobacco smoke.[4] Furthermore, advances have recently been made in the understanding of the extent of RP, its aetiology, progression and treatment and these are reviewed below.

The systemic nature of vasospasm

Raynaud's phenomenon is recognized clinically by the characteristic colour changes in the fingers and toes. Similar findings are also observed in the earlobes and the tip of the nose. Recently, 'systemic' vasospasm has been reported. RP has been associated with cerebral artery spasm, migraine headaches and coronary artery spasm,[5] where myocardial perfusion measurement in patients undergoing a cold pressor test showed that the majority of severely affected RP patients had a reversible cold-induced perfusion defect. It has been suggested that the myocardial contraction band necrosis seen in RP associated with connective tissue disorders (CTDs) may be due to RP of the intramural vessels of the heart. Vasospasm in the lung has been reported in RP following a reduction in the lungs' diffusing capacity after the induction of digital vasospasm by a cold challenge.[6] Again, in RP with CTD this pulmonary vasospasm may contribute to the development of pulmonary fibrosis. Furthermore it has been estimated that between 50% and 75% of patients with RP and the CTD systemic sclerosis have symptoms relating to their oesophagus. In about half, physical abnormalities such as stricture and achalasia are present; but in the rest, and in other patients with RP and oesophageal symptoms, no abnormality can be detected by endoscopy, manometry, pH testing or barium swallow. Recently, oesophageal vasospasm has been detected: a cold challenge to the oesophagus produced a delay in the rewarming time in patients with RP.[7]

With this evidence of vasospasm in the heart, lung and oesophagus, it is interesting to speculate that abnormalities of the vasculature may exist throughout the entire patient. These abnormalities may contribute to the wide spectrum of symptoms seen in RP such as hypertension, infertility, pre-eclampsia, and impotence.

Phenomenon, syndrome or disease?

One of the major problems for clinicians in this area of medicine has been the inconsistent terminology used to describe Raynaud's attacks. RP is the general term used to describe cold-related digital vasospasm. It is subdivided according to the presence or absence of an associated disorder: Raynaud's syndrome (RS) if there is, and primary Raynaud's disease (RD) if there is not. This European classification is not, however, accepted globally. In the USA and Australasia, syndrome and phenomenon tend to be used interchangeably making assessment of the literature difficult. A further complication has been identified from long-term studies which have shown that RP may be the precursor of systemic illness by over 20 years.[8] Whilst the majority of patients presenting to their own general practitioner have primary RD, recently developed sensitive laboratory procedures have shown that more than half of the patients referred to hospital have an associated systemic disease, (i.e. RS). Table 16.1 lists some of

Table 16.1 Conditions associated with Raynaud's syndrome (percentage incidence of RS for each disease)

Immunological	**Drugs**
Systemic sclerosis (90%)	Ergotamines and other migraine therapies
Systemic lupus erythematosus (10–44%)	Beta-blockers
Mixed connective tissue disease (85%)	Cytotoxic drugs
Dermatomyositis/ polymyositis (20%)	Cyclosporin
Rheumatoid arthritis (10–15%)	**Others**
Cryoglobulinaemia (10%)	Malignancy
Sjogren's syndrome (33%)	Endocrine (e.g. hypothyroidism)
Occupational	Uraemia
Vinyl chloride disease	Hepatitis B
Vibration white finger disease	Reflex sympathetic dystrophy
Ammunition workers (outside work)	Arteriovenous fistula
Frozen food packers	
Obstructive	
Thoracic outlet syndrome (e.g. cervical rib)	
Atherosclerosis (especially thrombangiitis obliterans)	

the more important conditions associated with RS, the best recognized of these being the CTDs and RS of occupational origin.

RS is found in the majority of patients with systemic sclerosis (SSc) and mixed connective tissue disease (MCTD) and also in patients with systemic lupus erythematosus (SLE), polymyositis and dermatomyositis, and Sjogren's syndrome.[2] RS occurs in rheumatoid arthritis (RA) and hyperviscosity syndromes in a percentage similar to that seen in the normal population (10%); however, the symptoms tend to be more severe.

RP of occupational origin can also occur in workers exposed to polyvinyl chloride (PVC) and vasospasm can occur in ammunition workers outside their place of work when the vasodilatory effects of the nitrates are removed. The most common form of occupational RS is Vibration White Finger disease (VWF). As it's name suggests, VWF occurs in workers exposed to vibrating machines such as chainsaws, pneumatic drills and buffs. It is estimated that 40–90% of all workers using vibrating equipment have RS, although the symptoms may resolve in 25% of cases if a job change is effected early in the course of the disease; i.e. before grade II on the Taylor Pelmear Scale of Classification.[9] Clinicians previously thought that the symptoms in this form of RP affected only the hands, but VWF has recently been described as affecting both fingers and toes.

Long-term exposure to cold in the absence of vibration can also be associated with the development of RP and is said to occur in 14% of men working outdoors. Furthermore, about half of the workers who fillet frozen fish and frequently rewarm their fingers develop RP.[10] Rewarming produces larger differences in temperature and thus more tissue damage, which probably contributes to the higher frequency seen in this latter group of workers.

Many other conditions are associated with RS and the challenge in dealing with this condition is not in making the diagnosis of vasospasm but rather in differentiating between primary Raynaud's disease and secondary Raynaud's syndrome and, possibly most importantly, detecting early those who may progress to develop such an underlying condition.

RP as a precursor of connective tissue disease

The conditions that are most frequently associated with RP are the CTDs (Table 16.1). One of the earliest studies of disease progression was carried out by Gifford and Hines.[11] In a study of 6229 patients with RP over 28 years of age they found progression to a CTD in 24%. Another early study[12] suggested a figure of 50%. Both of these studies, however, were published prior to 1950 and since then there has been an increasing awareness that RS may be much more common than previously thought. At present the frequency with which secondary conditions are recognized varies widely with reported studies and may depend in part on the development of the RP at the time seen, the thoroughness with which a search for an associated disorder is undertaken, and clinical referral patterns. The latter is clearly illustrated in a recent review.[13] In 1976, the authors reported an 81% incidence of RS in their population of 100 RP patients. By 1988 the study population had grown to 615 patients but the percentage of those with RS had fallen to 46%. The authors commented that in the early years of their study the patients were only referred if severely symptomatic. As the authors' interest in RP became more widely known more patients with mild symptoms were referred.

The early detection of a CTD in a patient with RP can be difficult, but recently more clearly defined abnormalities have been described which have strong links with disease progression and are important when investigating the patient with RP.

Investigation of Raynaud's phenomenon

Diagnostic techniques

In the majority of cases the diagnosis of RP can be made from the clinical history. Blanching is necessary for this diagnosis and those patients who do not exhibit blanching but merely report cyanosis after exposure to cold have acrocyanosis. This is a closely related disorder but the site of spasm is usually in the post-capillary venules. Thus, a history of digital blanching on exposure to cold, plus or minus cyanosis or rubor, in the absence of clinical evidence of obstructive vascular disease allows the diagnosis of RP to be made. It is only rarely that objective measures of blood flow are needed; for example, when the patient is unable to give a clear history, or in the presence of occlusive vascular disease when the contribution of vasospasm to the clinical problem needs to be determined.

There are many different techniques used to measure blood flow to the digits, but satisfactory standards of measurement have not yet been adequately established owing to their variation in healthy individuals, especially after a cold challenge. In clinical practice measurement of digital systolic pressure following local cooling of the hand in cool water at a temperature of approximately 15°C is widely used due to its simplicity. A drop in the pressure of more than 30 mmHg is usually significant. This technique, however, will give a significant number of false negatives unless the following precautions are observed. The patient must be warm and vasodilated before the first pressures are recorded. Superficially this appears obvious, but many patients who had cold hands at the start of the test have been told they do not have RP when no further pressure drop has been detected after cold challenge. Obviously, if vasoconstriction is already present only a small fall can occur after the cold challenge. The starting digital pressures must be as near brachial pressure as can be achieved. The best way to obtain this is by leaving the patient to acclimatize in the laboratory for 30 minutes. If in doubt, the rubber-gloved hand can be rewarmed in water of about 34°C. Poor flow prior to the start of the test can also occur at the time of ovulation in women.[3] Assessments should be avoided mid-cycle in pre-menopausal women. Failure to detect a pressure drop can also occur because of excessive vasodilatation. The most common source of error here is to see the patient at the clinic, start treatment, for example, with calcium channel antagonists, and complete a card for later vascular laboratory assessment. Some patients respond so well to treatment that a significant drop in pressure cannot be obtained whilst on this treatment. All vasoactive drug treatment should be stopped 24 hours prior to testing should such testing be necessary. Additionally, if the patient comes in from a warm environment the body itself is warm and this protects the patient against developing vasospasm if digital cooling is used in isolation. We routinely proceed to body cooling if this appears to be a problem. Unfortunately this facility is not available everywhere, but avoiding testing on hot days will help. Occasionally the patient will present to the laboratory with hot burning hands, a vasospastic attack having occurred during transit, and the patient then being in the reactive hyperaemic phase. Tests carried out in this phase will also fail to produce a significant pressure drop. Ideally patients should not have had a vasospastic attack on the day of the test. In practice this is difficult to achieve, and allowing 2–3 hours to elapse between events may be sufficient.

Other techniques used to assess blood flow can also be applied to the Raynaud's hand. Strain guage plethysmography is one such test. In this method, a finger cup with a small tubular outlet serves as the plethysmograph and encloses the terminal phalange of the finger. This is connected to a pressure transducer to measure changes in fingertip volume on a recorder. A cuff is then placed proximal to the finger cup to produce venous occlusion, the fingertip swells and the size to which it swells is proportional to the arterial inflow and the accumulation of blood in the fingertip is measured. The initial slope of the curve is assumed to represent arterial inflow. The disadvantages of this test are that considerable skill on the part of the operator is required; and, since measurement is discontinuous, it cannot assess changes in flow. Thus in fingers with fibrosed subcutaneous tissue as in the CTDs there is little vascular space to fill so that flows are difficult to measure. Conversely, the technique is also inadequate for measuring high blood flows as the finger fills so quickly that the slope of the curve is difficulty to quantify.

Radioisotope clearance methods, where the patient is given an injection of a radioactive preparation over the area of measurement, can also be used. The emitted radiation is measured by a detector focused on the injected spot. The radioactive tracer will be washed out by blood flow leading to an exponential decline of the radioactivity intensity which can be transformed into an estimate of blood perfusion. The method is costly, however, and a variable injection depth and tissue damage caused by the injection are potential sources of error. It cannot be adequately used with a cold challenge unless a different digit is used, and the procedure is by necessity invasive.

Thermography uses skin temperature as an indication of finger blood flow. However, skin temperature is dependent not only on blood flow but also on arterial and venous blood temperature. Although thermography is noninvasive, it is unreliable in unskilled hands. Furthermore, the equipment is expensive and requires a temperature-controlled environment for optimum results.

Laser Doppler flowmetry has become popular for evaluating skin microcirculation. The nature of the signal detected is related almost exclusively to the number and velocity of moving red blood cells. It is noninvasive, and measurement occurs directly and continuously with a short response time. This makes it ideally suited for measuring changes in microcirculatory flow. The same precautions apply to this technique as to the simple pressure estimation, however, and furthermore the results can be difficult to interpret as the depth of penetration of the laser light means that the results will include some contribution from the arterial venous anastomotic blood flow. Additionally, a temperature-controlled environment is required.

Each of the above techniques, apart from the first, require sophisticated equipment. Although they can be usefully employed in RP, there are numerous drawbacks. Unless one is involved in clinical trials where accurate assessment of flow is required, measurement of the digital systolic pressures before and after cold challenge is usually sufficient.

Assessment

Once the diagnosis of RP is confirmed an aetiological programme is required. As RP is a common condition such a programme should be simple, noninvasive and relatively cheap and sensitive. A detailed history is essential. Those with an obvious associated disorder will be easily detected, but difficulties arise in diagnosing early CTD or predicting those likely to progress to CTD. There are three areas which can prove useful in early disease: (a) clinical features, (b) microscopic nailfold examination, and (c) laboratory tests.

Clinical features

The occurrence of certain clinical features may suggest a higher likelihood of disease progression (Table 16.2). The American Rheumatism Association criteria for the various CTDs have high specificity but low sensitivity for the diseases. Thus patients who present with isolated features of CTD will not fulfil the ARA criteria. Nevertheless these RP patients are more likely to develop a CTD than those without such a symptom.[8] Of these the most specific is digital ulceration. In the absence of trauma or some other unusual occurrence, digital ulceration is strongly linked to later CTD development; so too are sclerodactyly and pitting scars over the pulps of the fingers. Thus, isolated features of CTD occurring in association with RP should raise clinical suspicion.

The age of onset of RP may also be important. RP is a frequent finding in young women in their teens and twenties and most have primary RD. Those presenting first in their 30s and 40s are at risk of developing RS.[14] Eighty per cent of patients with RP onset at age of 60 years or above will have an associated disorder, though in this older age-group the majority of cases are secondary to atherosclerosis.[15] Conversely, RP occurring in very young children, though rare, is usually due to an underlying CTD.

Other suspicious symptoms which perhaps should alert the clinician are the recurrence of chilblains in an adult, the occurrence of severe attacks persisting throughout the summer months, and an asymmetrical colour change with few digits involved initially can also suggest RS versus RD. It is also of interest that those patients who do develop systemic sclerosis are much more likely to develop limited SSc (calcinosis, Raynaud's, eosophagitis, sclerodactyly, telangiectasia – CREST) if the history of the preceding RP spans many years. Those presenting with SSc within one year of onset of RP tend to have diffuse SSc (previously called progressive systemic sclerosis).[16] Questions relating to the patient's occupation or exposure will often, particularly in men, allow a diagnosis of VWF to be made. Drug history is equally important and it should be noted that even the cardioselective beta-blockers produce a degree of peripheral vasoconstriction.

A physical examination is also useful. The presence of obstructive vascular disease can be gauged and signs of associated autoimmune conditions such as thyroid disease, vitiligo, etc. noted. Particular attention should be paid to the microscopic examination of the nailfolds.

Table 16.2 Symptoms, signs and investigations suggestive of progression to Raynaud's syndrome

Clinical	Laboratory
Any feature of CTD	Detection of antibodies
Digital ulceration	Raised ESR
Older age of onset	Elevated fVIIIvWFAg
Young children	**Nailfold microscopy**
Recurrence of chilblains as adult	Abnormal vessels
Asymmetrical attacks	
Vasospasm all year round	

Nailford microscopy

Direct observation of the capillaries in human skin date back to the early 1900s. Recent refinements have permitted photographic recordings of the rows of horizontal capillary loops at the nailfold just prior to the cuticle, but less sophisticated apparatus allows a clinician to examine the nailfold vessels as part of his/her routine clinical work-up. Using a simple ophthalmoscope at the highest power the nailfold can be visualized. Normally no vessels can be seen but patients with RP likely to progress have abnormally dilated nailfold capillary loops (Fig. 16.2). It should be noted, however, that these abnormal vessels can appear after trauma and in other microangiopathic states such as diabetes mellitus. Nevertheless, it is one of the more sensitive indices for disease progression. It has been suggested that when nailfold capillary microscopy and serum antibody determinations are combined they can detect more than 90% of patients destined to have SSc.[17]

Laboratory tests

Laboratory tests should include routine blood biochemistry, including thyroid function as hypothyroidism produces RP. Other autoimmune diseases can occur simultaneously in the same patient. A full blood count may show a normochromic normocytic anaemia of a chronic disorder in RS, or an iron deficiency anaemia in a young woman augmenting the symptoms of primary RD. The ESR is usually normal in RD but it may be elevated in RS. Urinalysis will help detect early renal disease in CTD or diabetes, and

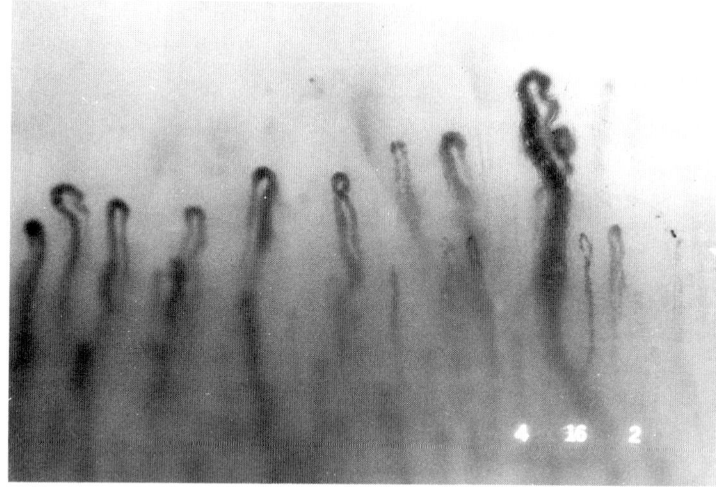

Fig. 16.2 Nailfold microscopy showing abnormal vessels. (Courtesy Dr Francis Lefford, Department of Anatomy and Developmental Biology, University College, University of London.)

a chest X-ray will determine whether a bony cervical rib is present (see Chapter 23) or basal lung fibrosis which is seen in early CTD.

Improvements in the techniques of antinuclear antibody determination have substantially increased the usefulness of this approach in RP. Whilst the mild patient presenting to a general practitioner does not require testing, those patients severe enough to require consideration for hospital referral should have them carried out. When confronted with the immunopathology request form some clinicians are faced with a wide variety of tests to chose from, whilst other forms have a blank box which requires completion. Both can be problematical for the uninformed. The basic tests for RP of suspected immunopathological origin are: rheumatoid factor titre for detection of RA; antinuclear antibody for SLE (anti-DNA antibody is usually automatically carried out in most laboratories if the antinuclear antibody is positive); anticentromere antibody for limited SSc (CREST), and antitopoisomerase antibody (formally scleroderma 70 antibody) for diffuse SSc.[18] Whilst none of the above are entirely specific, nor indeed fully sensitive, they provide a good framework for the early diagnosis of the rheumatic disorders and could form the basis of a discussion with the immunopathologist at a later date. The presence of these antibodies early on in the RP suggests that later progression to RS will occur.[19]

Another test that may be useful is a measure of the endothelial product and blood coagulation factor VIII von Willebrand factor antigen (previously factor VIII related antigen). Factor VIII von Willebrand factor antigen (fVIIIvWFAg) is released in large quantities by a damaged endothelium. In RD it is usually normal but it is elevated in RS[20] and it may also have a predictive value in its evolution,[21] though this still requires further evaluation in larger studies.

Cryoglobulinaemia, where cold-precipitated proteins are detected, is a very rare disorder, as is cryofibrinogenaemia. Although both allow the precipitation of large molecules in the cool digital circulation, and thus can cause RP, they should not be tested for during the initial screen. These disorders occur only infrequently and the tests require special sample preparation at the time of blood letting. It should be considered in a patient with severe RP where all other tests have proven negative.

Thus it can be seen that the diagnosis of a Raynaud's phenomenon attack should not be difficult, whereas the investigations for associated disorders can be more complex. The importance of early detection of an underlying disorder cannot be overstated. The diagnosis of a CTD has implications for future screening and follow-up. The diagnosis of an occupational disorder may have important financial consequences for the patient in terms of compensation awards. A change in occupation may ameliorate the disease and possibly prevent progression. Further lifestyle changes directed by the careful evaluation of the RP patient can also provide a significant benefit; for example, the withdrawal of betablockade, some antimigraine drugs, or modification of diet in early diabetes.

Once the patient has been assessed as outlined above, the majority of hospital referred patients require some form of drug treatment. In order to direct such treatment, however, it is important to understand some of the aetiological considerations of RP.

Aetiology of vasospasm

Several factors are considered to have aetiological importance in RP. They fall into three broad categories: (a) neurogenic mechanisms, (b) blood and blood vessel wall interactions, and (c) abnormalities of the immunological responses.

Neurogenic mechanisms

Two major theories have been presented to explain the vasospasm seen in RP. Maurice Raynaud believed that hyper-reactivity of the sympathetic nervous system caused an increase in vasoconstrictor responses to cold.[1] Lewis[22] hypothesized a 'local fault' in which precapillary resistance vessels were hypersensitive to local cooling. Most work has focused on the peripheral sympathetic nervous system. The alpha-adrenergic receptor sensitivity and/or density is increased in RP. Other studies have shown a pathophysiological role for the beta-presynaptic receptors with an increase in the responsiveness in the nerve endings in the RS peripheral vessels.[23]

The role of the central sympathetic system is, however, less clear. Local vibration of one hand induces vasoconstriction of the other which is abolished by a proximal nerve blockade. This suggests the existence of a central sympathetic vasoconstrictive mechanism. In support of this concept is the fact that the central sympathetic vasoconstriction induced by body cooling is necessary to produce vasospasm which may occur even in the absence of local digital cooling. However, other work does not support this concept. Infusions affecting alpha- and beta-adrenergic receptors in RD patients do not show any abnormalities in the responses to reflex cooling or indirect heating.[24] Thus, although not clearly defined, abnormalities of the nervous system may exist in RP. Conversely, although early work suggested an autonomic dysfunction in RS, later studies could not substantiate it.[25]

An intriguing finding is one relating to a potential dysfunction of a calcitonin gene-related peptide (CGRP) dependent neurovascular axis. CGRP is a potent vasodilator, and pilot work suggests that the quantity of CGRP-containing neurones in the digital skin of patients with RP may be decreased when compared with normal subjects.[26]

Blood and blood vessel wall interactions

Abnormal blood vessel tone does not, however, explain all the features of RP. Flow in the microcirculation is critically dependent on the intactness of the endothelium and the properties of the cellular and liquid elements of blood.

The endothelium is a functioning organ releasing important chemicals, one of which is prostacyclin (PGI_2), a potent antiplatelet agent and vasodilator. Although prostacyclin may be elevated in the early stages of disease, in the later stages PGI_2 stimulating factor may be decreased, facilitating platelet aggregation and vasoconstriction. Endothelin, another endothelial product, has the opposite effect, causing vasoconstriction. Elevated baseline plasma levels of endothelin have been reported in RP which are further increased by cold challenge.[27] As discussed earlier, fVIIIvWFAg is released from the damaged endothelium and its release can have prothrombotic effects[20] by its participation both in the coagulation cascade and in platelet aggregation. Other manifestations of endothelial dysfunction have also been detected in RP, such as decreased tissue plasminogen activator and increased plasminogen activator inhibitor levels, thus producing a net defect in the lysis of fibrin.[28]

The blood cells may also be abnormal in RP. The platelet is more aggregable, releasing increased amounts of the vasoconstrictor and platelet aggregant thromboxane A_2 (TxA_2) and other platelet release products. The RBC appears less deformable in RP generally, and cold temperatures will increase the red blood cell stiffness as will the acidosis present in cold ulcerated fingers.[29] Hard red cells can occlude the microcirculation and thus augment a vasospastic attack. An important role has also been claimed for the white blood cell in maintaining flow in the small vessels. Polymorphonuclear leucocyte activation with increased release of prothrombotic free radicals and increased cell aggregation has been reported in RP, and this might also contribute to the decreased flow seen in this disorder.[30]

It should be noted that RD patients do not show the abnormalities listed above while the majority of RS patients do. Thus, whilst these changes are likely to be a consequence of the RP rather than a cause, they may augment the symptoms of vasospasm.

Inflammatory and immune responses

More conventionally the white blood cell has been considered to be important as the producer and modifier of the inflammatory and immune responses. The endothelium is also involved in these processes by the production of its vasoactive agents, growth factors and growth inhibitors. Disordered immune/inflammatory responses occur in the majority of severe cases of RS via their association with the CTDs, but also in VWF which has no clear immune/inflammatory basis.[30] TNF and lymphotoxin, thymocyte/macrophage and T cell derived proteins, along with immune complex deposition in the vessel wall, are likely to be involved in the vascular damage seen in RS.[31]

Management of Raynaud's phenomenon

Most of the cellular abnormalities reported above are likely to be a consequence of the disease rather than a cause. Nevertheless, this may be therapeutically important as adherent and hard cells and viscous plasma may contribute to impaired blood flow and their correction may produce clinical improvement.

Supportive measures

Much can be done for patients with mild disease without recourse to drugs. Stopping smoking can be beneficial, as can changes in occupation and the withdrawal of drugs known to be associated with RP. Although the contraceptive pill has been linked anecdotally to the development of RP, this has never been conclusively proven in epidemiological studies. It is current practice to stop the contraceptive pill only if there is a clear link with the development of the disease. Likewise, RP is not a contraindication for hormone replacement therapy at the time of menopause. Treatment using selftraining biofeedback techniques has sometimes been successful but requires well-motivated patients. Many patients are apprehensive about their disease, reassurance is often required, and information regarding both their disease and the self-help group, The Raynaud's and Scleroderma Association (Alsager, Cheshire), is often gratefully received.

It is also important to advise patients how to protect themselves from the cold. Achieving this without becoming a hermit is difficult, but practical solutions do exist. Electrically heated gloves and socks are the perfect solution for some patients. A rechargeable battery fixed on a belt provides up to 3 hours of warmth, and the wires can be concealed beneath the clothing to give a normal appearance. Unfortunately they are sometimes difficult to obtain owing to Health Board budget restraints, and infrequently irritation of ulcers by the added heat has been noted. Chemical handwarmers obtained from local sports shops (or more cheaply from the above Association) provide a satisfactory alternative source of heat. 'Comfort shoes' obtained from surgical appliance departments can also be useful. The padded soles keep the feet warm and relieve the pressure on the toes which can result in vasospasm.

Sympathectomy

Upper-limb sympathectomy gives a high relapse rate and an especially poor response in RS.[32] It is, therefore, no longer indicated for RP in the upper limb. It should be noted, however, that the more selective sympathectomy operation has not yet been assessed in RP.

By contrast, sympathectomy still has an important role in the treatment of RP affecting the feet. This discrepancy is not understood, but sympathectomy of the lower limbs can produce rewarding results.

The surgeon may still contribute to the management of upper-limb Raynaud's by removal of infected nails which allows healing of severe long-term ulceration. In SSc the tightness of the skin over the fingertip also contributes to the decreased blood flow. Operations to remove part of the terminal phalanx and so relieve pressure may also be useful. Occasionally the ischaemia becomes so severe that amputation is necessary, but this is required increasingly infrequently.

Plasma exchange

The beneficial effect of plasma exchange may result from the alteration of platelet, white cell cell and red cell functions. Blood viscosity is lowered, and immune complexes are removed.[33] However, this form of treatment produces only limited success, is time-consuming and expensive. It is not a cure, requiring repetition at a later date. Consequently, plasma exchange is reserved for patients with severe intractable ulceration, and at the present time the prostaglandins are replacing this function.

Drug treatment of Raynaud's phenomenon

The drugs most commonly used in the treatment of RP are shown in Table 16.3 and a treatment protocol is outlined in Fig. 16.3.

Calcium channel antagonists

Many studies have been carried out on the use of calcium channel antagonists in RP, and nifedipine has

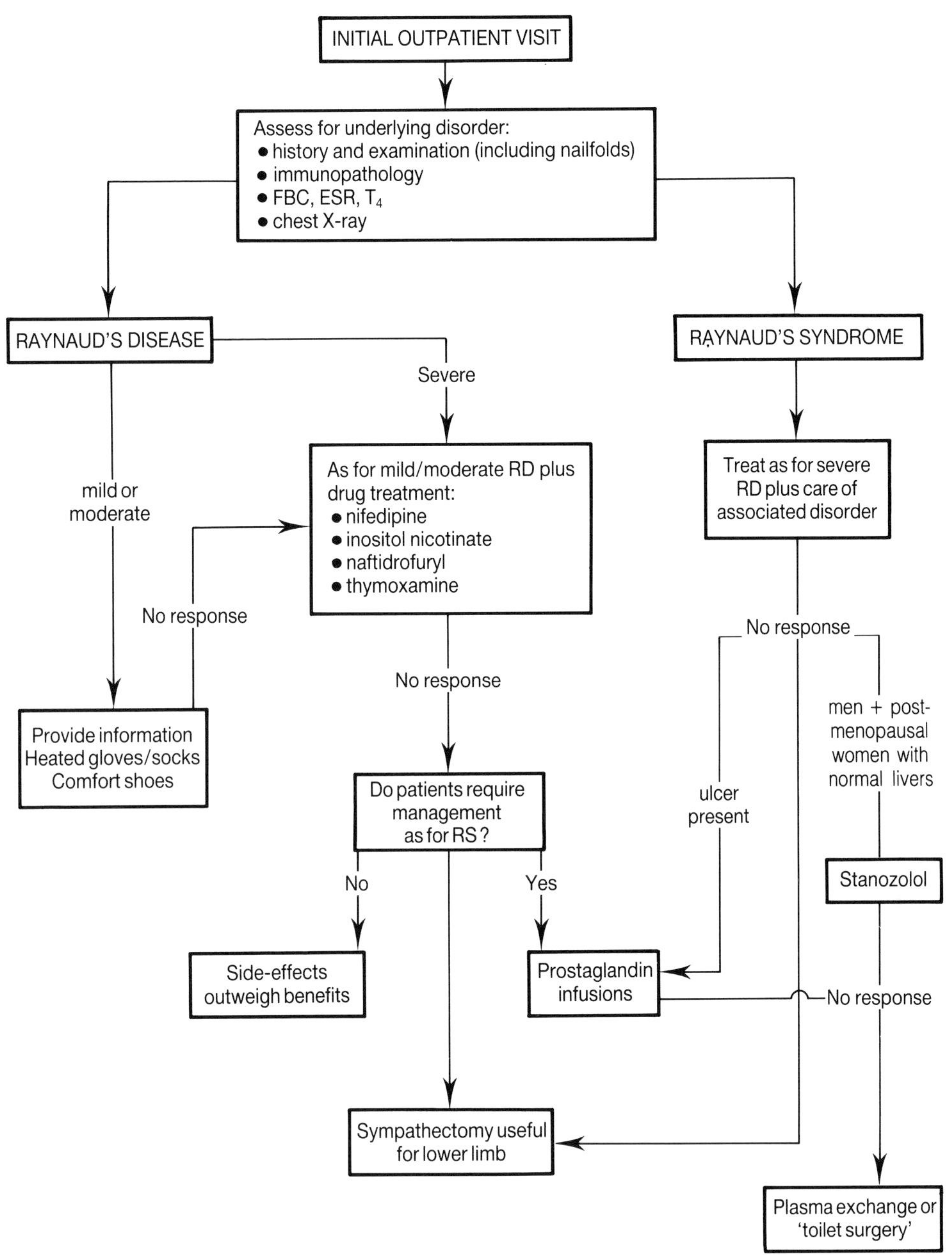

Fig. 16.3 A treatment flowchart for Raynaud's phenomenon.

now become the 'gold standard' of Raynaud's treatment.[34] Its mechanism of action in RP is predominantly vasodilatory, but it also has an antiplatelet and possibly other antithrombotic effects. Its use is, however, limited by vasodilatory side-effects to which the RP patient appears very susceptible. These include headaches, dizziness, flushing and ankle swelling. To attenuate these the patient should use the retard preparation commencing at 10 mg twice a day, increasing to three times a day; then after 2 weeks increasing to 20 mg twice a day, increasing to three times a day if required. The side-effects often disappear with continued treatment, so unless these are intolerable the patient should per-

Table 16.3 Drugs and dosages commonly used in RP

Drug	Dosage
Nifedipine retard	10 mg twice a day, increasing to three times; then 20 mg twice a day increasing to three times
Inositol nicotinate	500 mg three times a day, increasing to Hexopal Forte 750 mg twice a day
Naftidrofuryl	100 mg three times a day, increasing to 200 mg three times a day
Thymoxamine	40 mg four times a day, increasing to 80 mg four times a day; discontinue after 2 weeks if no response
Prostacyclin	Start infusion at 1 ng/kg/min; increase by 1 ng/kg/min every one hour to approximately 5 ng/kg/min or side-effects; 6–8 hour duration of infusion given 3–5 times
Epogam	12 caps/day for 3-month trial
Stanozolol	5 mg twice a day; monitor liver enzymes; restrict use to men or post-menopausal women

severe for 7–10 days before discontinuing the therapy. It has not, however, been passed for use in pregnancy and the patient must be advised to avoid pregnancy when this drug is prescribed.

If the side-effects of nifedipine require its discontinuation, two options are possible. The first is to use nifedipine capsules (not the retard tablets) as a rescue medication during a severe spasm attack. The tablet can be crushed by the teeth and placed below the tongue. Thus, the drug is not taken frequently enough to produce constant side-effects. The second option is to use another calcium channel antagonist with less vasodilatory effects. Both diltiazem and isradipine[35] may be useful and diltiazem is available in a slow release preparation. In contrast, verapamil has been found to be ineffective.

Vasodilators

The use of vasodilators in RP remains a little controversial as most studies have been uncontrolled. Four compounds do merit consideration however. Encouraging results in mild to moderate vasospasm have been obtained with inositol nicotinate (hexopal).[36] The drug may take up to 3 months to produce an effect and should therefore be given for at least this period of time. Similarly the use of naftidrofuryl (praxilene)[37] may produce benefit over the same time period, as may oxopentifylline (trental).[38] Thymoxamine (opilon) the selective α_1-blocker[39] may be tried initially for a period of two weeks. A trial of these treatments given in sufficient dosages for a sufficient period of time may be worthwhile. Simple vasodilators are often ineffective however particularly in severe disease such as is seen in hospital practice with the limiting factor being the development of side-effects at high dosage.

Prostaglandins

Prostaglandins (PGs) are the metabolic products of essential fatty acids (EFAs) and their discovery has opened up new therapeutic approaches to RP. PGE_1 and PGI_2 both have potent vasodilatory and anti-platelet properties whereas TXA_2 has opposite actions. It is possible to manipulate the balance of these chemicals in favour of antithrombotic and vasodilatory effects. PGE_1 treatment has to be given intravenously through a central line, with an incremental dosage regimen up to a maximum of 7.5 ng/kg/min.[40] Although 10 ng/kg/min was used in earlier studies, vasodilatory side-effects persuaded later workers to lower the dose. Most studies suggest a benefit from a 72-hour IV infusion of PGE_1 in RS, but it is probably unhelpful in RD.

PGI_2 also requires IV administration, though this can be through a peripheral vein.[41] A careful watch over the drip site should be kept to avoid the pronounced inflammatory response seen after infusion into the tissues. The PGI_2 treatment differs in that it is best given using a 6–8 hour 3 dose intermittent regimen over 3 days or 3 weeks. Infusion can be given for a longer time if ulceration is severe. The dose is also incremental, increasing from 1 ng/kg/min to a maximum of 5–7.5 ng/kg/min. The dosage should be titrated to side-effects. The intermittent regimen described above appears to prevent tachyphylaxis of platelets and rebound platelet aggregation after discontinuing the drip.

The beneficial effects of these PG infusions may last beyond the infusion time. In most studies the 6-week assessment continued to show a clinical and objective improvement in the RP symptoms. In our experience the effect can persist from between one week to 6 months when repetition of the infusion is required. As yet neither of the above are licensed as a treatment for RP. Nor is iloprost, a PGI_2 analogue which may also be beneficial in RP.[42] Whereas both E_1 and I_2 are unstable, iloprost is not and this makes it easier to handle, despite still requiring IV administration. All three PGs probably mediate some of their beneficial effect partly through vasodilation and modification of platelet behaviour. They may also have anti-white-cell effects and promote fibrinolysis. Despite their efficacy as a treatment, the PGs remain a second-line therapy because of their mode of administration. Orally active analogues are now being assessed, as is transdermal administration. These compounds are, however, in the early stages of development.

Other approaches to manipulating the body's own production of vasodilatory prostaglandins are being evaluated. Evening primrose oil is rich in gamma-linolenic acid (GLA) which is metabolized to dihomo-gamma-linolenic acid (DGLA), and fish oil is rich in eicosapentanoic acid (EPA) and decosahexanoic acid (DHA). DGLA, EPA and DHA are precursors of vasodilatory prostaglandins, and so dietary supplementation with these may stimulate endogenous production of such PGs. Few studies have investigated such treatments, however,[43,44] and both need to be given in full dose for at least 3 months before being deemed ineffective (viz. Epogam 12 capsules a day and Maxepa 10 capsules a day). Disappointingly, only a mild response has been detected and, as with the PGs, RP is not a licensed indication for their use. The other alternative for the patient is to purchase the compounds from a health foodstore but this proves to be very expensive.

Specific inhibition of the enzyme thromboxane synthetase results in a decrease in TxA_2 formation and should promote vasodilatation and platelet disaggregation. Nevertheless, studies of such compounds proved to be ineffective. Recent developments looking at a combination of thromboxane synthetase inhibition and thromboxane receptor site blockade may be more promising.

Fibrinolytic agents and others affecting blood rheology

The administration of low-molecular-weight dextran or ancrod, a defibrinating agent, have been reported to alleviate RP. However, both require parenteral administration, and the need to monitor blood coagulation and the development of antibodies to ancrod inhibits its application. Likewise, troxerutin (Paroven), a red cell deformability agent, has been shown to be useful in one small study. However, no convincing studies have been carried out recently using any of the three above agents.

Results obtained with stanozolol (Stromba), an anabolic steroid that increases fibrinolysis, are possibly more persuasive.[45] The drug is given in a dose of 5 mg twice a day and the beneficial effects can take up to 3 months to become apparent. Side-effects can be severe, however, and include virilization and elevation of liver enzymes. Use of this agent is now rarely employed and then only in males and post-menopausal women who have normal liver function tests.

Drugs for the future

The vasoactive compound serotonin has been shown to be increased in RS, possibly reflecting increased platelet aggregation and perhaps contributing to the vasoconstriction. Ketanserin, a serotonin antagonist with slight $alpha_1$ – adrenergic antagonistic effects, may be useful. This was recently demonstrated in a large multicentre study involving 222 patients with both RD and RS.[46] Unfortunately, owing to the multicentre nature of the study, objective tests of blood flow could not be measured. However, symptomatic benefit occurred which may mark this as a drug for the future treatment of RP.

A number of other vasoactive compounds are under scrutiny as potential treatments for RP. The better evaluation and understanding of the pathophysiology of RP has led to a better selection of treatments for study and significant advances in the treatment of RP continue to be made.

Conclusions

RP is a common condition affecting 10–20% of the female population. Until recently its diagnosis and treatment were both unsatisfactory. With a careful clinical history and examination and with selection of specific blood tests, it is now possible to diagnose RP correctly and to assess the likelihood of progression. Although a cure is not yet available, many patients with RP can achieve a satisfactory amelioration of their symptoms using a combination of drug therapy and non-drug aids. Nevertheless, it should be remembered that the final prognosis of RS is determined by that of the underlying disorder which must be detected, monitored and treated independently of the vasospastic symptoms.

Recommended further reading

1. Coffman JD. *Raynaud's Phenomenon*. Oxford: Oxford University Press, 1989.
2. Edwards JM, Porter JM. Associated disease in patients with Raynaud's syndrome. *Vasc Med Rev* 1990; **1**: 51–8.

References

1. Raynaud M. De l'asphyxre et de la gangrene symetriques des extremities. Paris, 1862 (translated by Thomas Barlow, London: New Sydenham Society, 1988).
2. Porter JM, Bardona EJ, Baur GM, Wesche DH, Andrasch RH, Rosch J. The clinical significance of Raynaud's syndrome. *Surgery* 1976; **80:** 756–64.
3. Lafferty K, De Trafford JC, Potter C, Robert VC, Cotton LT. Reflex vascular responses in the finger to contralateral thermal stimuli during the normal menstrual cycle: a hormonal basis to Raynaud's phenomenon? *Clin Sci* 1985; **68:** 10–15.
4. Goodfield MJD, Hume A, Rowell NR. The acute effects of cigarette smoking on cutaneous blood flow in smoking and non-smoking subjects with and without Raynaud's phenomenon. *Br J Rheum* 1990; **29:** 89–91.
5. Kahan A, Devaux JY, Amor B, *et al.* Nifedipine and thallium-201 myocardial perfusion in progressive systemic sclerosis. *N Engl J Med* 1986; **314:** 1397–402.
6. Baron M, Feiglin D, Hyland R, Urowitz MB, Shiff B. Gallium lung scans in progressive systemic sclerosis. *Arth Rheum* 1983; **26:** 967–74.
7. Belch JJF, Land D, Park RHR, McKillop JH, McKenzie JF. Decreased oesophageal blood flow in patients with Raynaud's phenomenon. *Br J Rheum* 1988; **27:** 426–30.
8. Belch JJF. Raynaud's phenomenon: its relevance to scleroderma. *Ann Rheum Dis* 1991; **50:** 839–45.
9. Taylor W. The hand–arm vibration syndrome, secondary Raynaud's phenomenon of occupational origin. *Proc Roy Coll Phys Edin* 1989; **19:** 7–14.
10. Mackiewica SJ, Piskorz M. Cold injury in frozen food handlers. *J Cardiovasc Surg* 1977; **18:** 151–4.
11. Gifford RW, Hines EA. Raynaud's disease among young women and girls. *Circulation* 1957; **16:** 1012–21.
12. Porter JM, Rivers SP, Anderson CJ, Baur GM. Evaluation and management of patients with Raynaud's syndrome. *Am J Surg* 1981; **142:** 183–9.
13. Edwards JM, Porter JM. Associated disease in patient with Raynaud's syndrome. *Vasc Med Rev* 1990; **1:** 51–8.
14. Kallenberg CGM. Early detection of connective tissue disease in patients with Raynaud's phenomenon. *Rheum Dis Clin N Am* 1990; **16:** 11–30.
15. Friedman EI, Taylor LM, Porter JM. Late-onset Raynaud's syndrome: diagnostic and therapeutic considerations. *Geriatrics* 1988; **43:** 59–70.
16. Kallenberg CGM, Wouda AA, The TH. Systemic involvement and immunological findings in patients presenting with Raynaud's phenomenon. *Am J Med* 1980; **69:** 675–80.
17. Fitzgerald O, Hess EV, O'Connor GT, Spencer-Green G. Prospective study of the evolution of Raynaud's phenomenon. *Am J Med* 1988; **84:** 718–26.
18. Cruz M, Mejia G, Lavalle C, Cortes JJ, Reyes PA. Antinuclear antibodies in scleroderma, mixed connective tissue disease and primary Raynaud's phenomenon. *Clin Rheum* 1988; **7:** 80–6.
19. Kallenberg CGM, Wouda AA, Hoet MA, van Venrooij WJ. Development of connective tissue disease in patients presenting with Raynaud's phenomenon: a six-year follow up with emphasis on the predictive value of antinuclear antibodies as detected by immunoblotting. *Ann Rheum Dis* 1988; **47:** 634–41.
20. Belch JJF, Zoma A, Richards I, Forbes CD, Sturrock RD. Vascular damage and factor VIII related antigen in the rheumatic diseases. *Rheum Int* 1987; **7:** 107–11.
21. Lau CS, McLaren M, Belch JJF. Factor VIII von Willebrand factor antigen levels correlate with symptom severity in patients with Raynaud's phenomenon. *Br J Rheum* 1991; **30:** 433–6.
22. Lewis T. The pathological changes in the arteries supplying the fingers in warm-handed people and in cases of so-called Raynaud's disease. *Clin Sci* 1938; **3:** 288–311.
23. Peacock JH. Vasodilatation in the human hand: observations on primary Raynaud's disease and acrocyanosis of the upper extremities. *Clin Sci* 1957; **17:** 575–86.
24. Fagius J, Blumberg H. Sympathetic outflow to the hand in patient with Raynaud's phenomenon. *Cardiovasc Res* 1985; **19:** 249–53.
25. Suarez-Almazor ME, Bruera E, Russell AS. Normal cardiovascular autonomic function in patients with systemic sclerosis (CREST variant). *Ann Rheum Dis* 1988; **47:** 672–4.
26. Bunker CB, Terenghi G, Springall DR, Polak JM, Dowd PM. Deficiency of calcitonin gene-related peptide in Raynaud's phenomenon. *Lancet* 1990; **336:** 1530–3.
27. Zamora MR, O'Brien RF, Rutherford RB, Weill JV. Serum endothelium-1 concentrations and cold provocation in primary Raynaud's phenomenon. *Lancet* 1990; **336:** 1144–7.
28. Belch JJF, Drury J, Flannigan P, *et al.* Abnormal biochemical and cellular parameters in the blood of patients with Raynaud's phenomenon. *Scot Med J* 1987; **32:** 12–14.
29. Belch JJF, McLaren M, Anderson J, *et al.* Increased prostacyclin metabolites and decreased red cell deformability in patients with systemic sclerosis and Raynaud's syndrome. *Prostag Leukotr Med* 1985; **17:** 1–9.
30. Lau CS, O'Dowd A, Belch JJF. White blood cell activation in Raynaud's phenomenon of systemic sclerosis and vibration-induced white finger syndrome. *Ann Rheum Dis* 1992; **51:** 249–52.
31. Kahaleh MB, Smith EA, Soma Y, Leroy EC. Effect of lymphotoxin and tumour necrosis factor on endo-

thelia and connective tissue cell growth and function. *Clin Immunol Immunopath* 1988; **49:** 261–72.

32. Hansteen V. Medical treatment in Raynaud's disease. *Acta Chir Scand* 1976; **465:** 87–91.
33. Zahavi J, Hamilton WAP, O'Reilly MJG, Leyton J, Cotton LT, Kakkar VV. Plasma exchange and platelet function in Raynaud's phenomenon. *Thromb Res* 1980; **19:** 85–93.
34. Finch MB, Copeland S, Passmore AP, Johnston GD. A double-blind cross-over study of nifedipine retard in patients with Raynaud's phenomenon. *Clin Rheum* 1988; **7:** 359–65.
35. Kahan A, Amor B, Menkes CJ. A randomised double-blind trial of diltiazem in the treatment of Raynaud's phenomenon. *Ann Rheum Dis* 1985; **44:** 30–3.
36. Sunderland GT, Belch JJF, Sturrock RD, Forbes CD, McKay AJ. A double-blind randomised placebo controlled trial of Hexopal in primary Raynaud's disease. *Clin Rheum* 1988; **7:** 46–9.
37. Nilsen KH. Effects of naftidrofuryl on microcirculatory cold sensitivity in Raynaud's phenomenon. *Br Med J* 1979; **1:** 10–21.
38. Neirotti M, Longo F, Molaschi M, *et al.* Functional vascular disorders: treatment with pentoxifylline. *Angiology* 1987; **38:** 575–80.
39. Grigg MJ, Nicolaides AN, Papadakis K, Wolfe JH. The efficacy of thymoxamine in Raynaud's phenomenon. *Eur J Vasc Surg* 1989; **3:** 309–13.
40. Clifford PC, Martin MFR, Sheddon EJ, Kirby JD, Baird RN, Dieppe PA. Treatment of vasospastic disease with prostaglandin E_1. *Br Med J* 1980; **281:** 1031–4.
41. Belch JJF, Drury JK, Capell H, *et al.* Intermittent epoprostenol (prostacyclin) infusion in patients with Raynaud's syndrome: a double-blind controlled trial. *Lancet* 1983; **8320:** 313–15.
42. Yardumian DA, Isenberg DA, Rustin M, *et al.* Successful treatment of Raynaud's syndrome with iloprost, a chemically stable prostacyclin analogue. *Br J Rheum* 1988; **27:** 220–6.
43. Belch JJF, Shaw B, O'Dowd A, *et al.* Evening primrose oil (Efamol) in the treatment of Raynaud's phenomenon: a double blind study. *Thromb Haemost* 1985; **54:** 490–4.
44. DiGiacomo RA, Kremer JM, Shah DM. Fish-oil dietary supplementation in patients with Raynaud's phenomenon: a double-blind, controlled, prospective study. *Am J Med* 1989; **86:** 158–64.
45. Jarrett PEM, Browse M, Browse NL. Treatment of Raynaud's phenomenon by fibrinolytic enhancement. *Br Med J* 1978; **ii:** 523–5.
46. Coffmann JD, Clement DL, Creager MA, *et al.* International study of ketanserin in Raynaud's phenomenon. *Am J Med* 1989; **87:** 264–8.

17

The foot in diabetes mellitus

Shukri K Shami and John H Scurr

The prevalence of diabetes mellitus (DM) in western populations is estimated at 2–4%. Good control of the blood sugar is important in avoiding complications, which include nephropathy, retinopathy, neuropathy, and macro- and micro-angiopathy. This control can only be achieved if both the patient and treating physician are highly motivated. However, some of the complications of diabetes seem to occur in spite of good control of the blood sugar.

The 'diabetic foot' is one of the most debilitating complications of DM and occurs in both insulin-dependent diabetes mellitus (IDDM) and non-insulin dependent diabetes. In Britain, it is said to account for more days spent in hospital than all the other complications of diabetes.[1] The risk of major amputation is 15 times higher in the patient with diabetes than in the general population.[2] It is estimated that the cost of foot complications in diabetes amounts to a staggering $500 million a year in the USA.[3] This chapter describes the causes, investigations, prevention and treatment of the 'diabetic foot'.

Definition

The 'diabetic foot syndrome' is a term used to describe infection, ulceration and gangrene that occurs in the feet of people with diabetes. The presentation of the diabetic foot ranges from a punched-out ulcer under a metatarsal head with minimal infection, to a swollen gangrenous lesser toe with no ulceration (Figs 17.1 and 17.2). Sometimes only cellulitis and lymphangitis are present with no apparent predisposing cause. Correct management of these cases ensures a reduction in morbidity and mortality, and with a modern multidisciplinary approach major amputations can be avoided in the majority of cases.[4]

Aetiology

Foot complications in diabetes are a result of peripheral arterial disease (PAD), peripheral neuropathy, or a combination of both. The precipitating cause of ulceration and it's pathogenesis are multifactorial and include abnormal stresses (vertical and shear), penetrating injuries, minor trauma, thermal injury, skin fissuring, and infection. Neuropathic ulcers have a much better prognosis than ischaemic ulcers. Traditionally, 'small vessel disease' or microangiopathy has been blamed as a cause of ulceration. This has led to pessimism on the part of the treating physicians as nothing could be done about it. There is no doubt that the microcirculation is compromised in

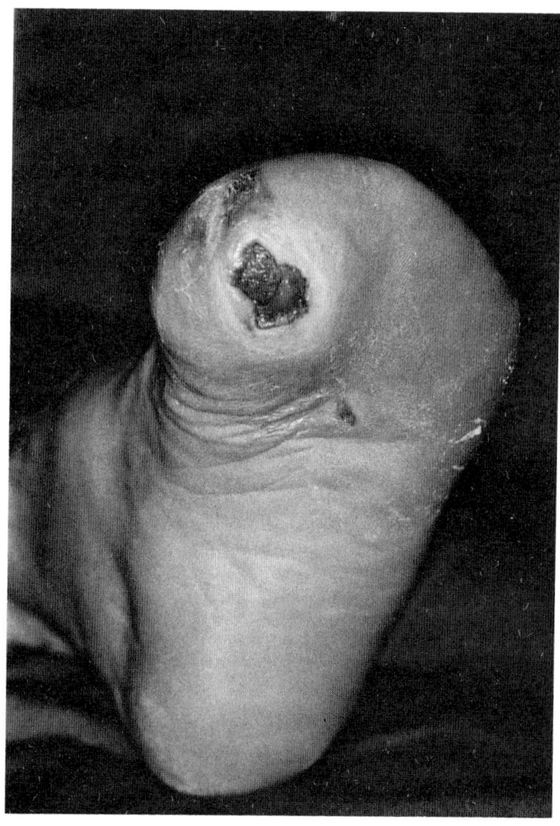

Fig. 17.1 Punched out ulcer under metatarsal head. There have been previous toe amputations.

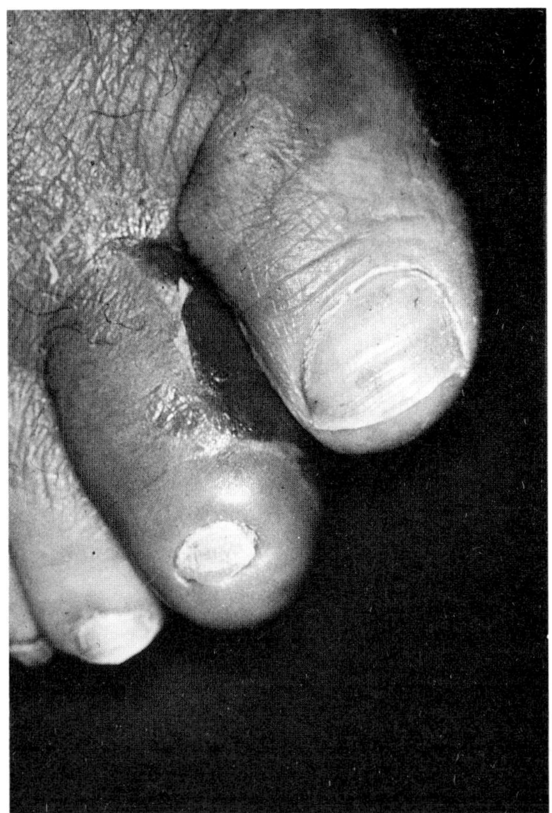

Fig. 17.2 Gangrenous second toe.

diabetes, but the importance of microangiopathy in the pathogenesis of the diabetic foot is still unresolved, and many authorities believe that it has no bearing on the condition. Fig. 17.3 shows the interplay of the factors involved in the pathogenesis of the diabetic foot.

Classification

Classifications are useful in order to develop therapeutic algorithms and for research communications. Numerous classifications of diabetic ulceration have been put forward, including those proposed by Oakley,[5] Wagner,[6] Gibbons,[7] Coleman[8] and Frykberg.[9] The Wagner classification (Table 17.1) is one of the most commonly used. We use a simpler classification based on management, and divide diabetic ulcers into neuropathic, ischaemic and neuroischaemic (or mixed) ulcers. Each type accounts for about a third of the ulcers seen and can be further

Table 17.1 The Wagner classification of diabetic foot lesions

Grade	Description
0	Intact skin
1	Superficial ulcer
2	Deep ulcer (tendon, bone, or joint exposed)
3	Deep ulcer with abscess or osteomyelitis
4	Gangrene of the forefoot
5	Gangrene of the whole foot

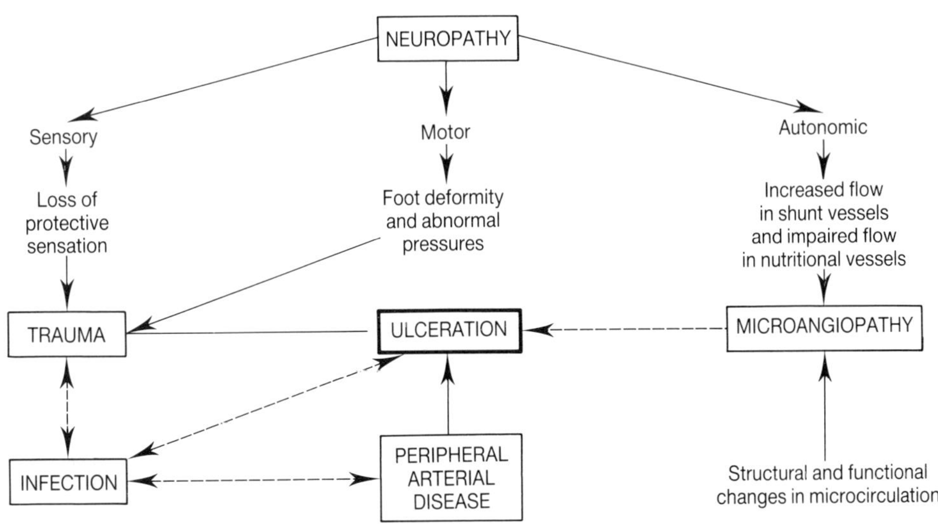

Fig. 17.3 The interplay of factors involved in the pathogenesis of the diabetic foot.

classified as 'simple' or 'complicated'. A 'simple' ulcer is one where infection is superficial and necrosis is minimal, compared with a 'complicated' ulcer, where there is infection and extensive tissue necrosis.

Pathogenesis

Peripheral neuropathy

Peripheral neuropathy is present in about 10% of patients with diabetes[10] and can affect both somatic and autonomic nerves. About a third of diabetic patients with neuropathy will suffer from foot ulceration.[11] Neuropathy can also occur through causes unrelated to the diabetes, such as spinal stenosis and tumours, amyloidosis and immunological disorders.

The cause of diabetic peripheral neuropathy is not known. Several mechanisms for its development have been proposed. It has been shown that neuropathy due to compression,[12,13] local anaesthetics,[14,15] neurotoxins,[16] and a galactose diet[17] is associated with increased endoneurial tissue pressure (ETP) which causes reduced blood flow in the vasa nervosum and axonal ischaemia.[12,13,18] The development of peripheral neuropathy in diabetes may be the result of ETP due to the accumulation of osmotically active sorbitol in nerves. Sorbitol is produced by increased metabolism of glucose through the polyol pathway by the enzyme aldose-reductase as a result of chronic hyperglycaemia. Other mechanisms for the development of neuropathy include decreased nerve myoinositol, reduced Na^+/K^+ ATP-ase activity, microangiopathy, genetic and environmental factors. Peripheral neuropathy in diabetics is mostly of the glove and stocking variety. The feet are affected to a greater extent than the hands, as the parts of the axons that are most vulnerable to dysfunction are those furthest away from the cell body. The neuropathy is often patchy and can selectively affect certain modalities of motor function and sensation while sparing others. Neuropathy predisposes to ulceration by a number of mechanisms.

Sensory neuropathy

This may be painful or painless; patients with painless neuropathy have diminished sensation and loss of 'protective' pain. This results in minor foot injuries occurring without being noticed. These injuries may be sustained by ill-fitting footwear, penetrating injury by stepping on a sharp object, or thermal injury (either hot or cold). Poor eyesight due to retinopathy can make it more difficult to discover these injuries, and so resulting lesions can become infected and deteriorate markedly before they are discovered.

Sensory neuropathy also results in diminished mechanical sensation which may allow patients to tolerate ill-fitting shoes, and diminished postural and joint position sensation which may interfere with normal gait and function of the foot.

Motor neuropathy

Motor neuropathy causes weakness of the intrinsic muscles of the foot and brings about an imbalance between the long flexors and extensors of the toes. This results in a characteristic deformity of the foot with a high medial arch (pes cavus), clawing of the toes and subluxation of the metatarso-phalangeal joints. This reduces the weight-bearing area of the foot. Since pressure is equal to force divided by the surface area on which the force is applied, a reduction in the weight-bearing area of the foot results in an increase in pressure on the areas remaining in contact with the ground. These high pressures are usually applied to the skin overlying the metatarsal heads and heel, in turn causing hyperkeratosis and callus formation. This makes the skin less pliable and flexible, and shear forces between the skin and underlying bone occur which may result in cavitation and bleeding under the skin. This cavity gets larger before it 'button-holes' out on to the skin and the full extent of the ulcer is only realized when the callus and skin overlying the cavity is removed. This is compounded by a loss of subcutaneous 'fat pads' between the skin and the metatarsal heads.

Autonomic neuropathy

Autonomic neuropathy affects the foot in two ways. The first is by loss of the sympathetic regulation of the microcirculation. Loss of the venoarteriolar reflex (vasoconstriction in response to a rise in venous pressure) results in increased capillary pressure on standing, leading to oedema formation and hyalinization of the capillaries. Loss of sympathetic tone also results in opening up of 'shunt vessels'. These are communications between arterioles and venules in the subpapillary dermal plexus. They are heavily innervated by the sympathetic system, and have an important role to play in thermoregulation. It is thought that people with diabetes have hot feet because of the opening of these shunt vessels as a result of sympathetic neuropathy. This was thought to deprive the skin of its nutritional blood supply by a 'steal syndrome', where the blood preferentially went through these shunt vessels rather than the papillary nutrient capillaries. Doubt has been cast on this theory,[19] and it is no longer generally accepted. Opening of shunt vessels, however, may lead to increased bone blood flow resulting in osteopenia and predisposing to bone destruction.[20]

Secondly, autonomic neuropathy predisposes to ulceration through loss of sudomotor function (sweating). This makes the skin dry and less supple, making it easier to traumatize and transmit shear forces to deeper layers. It also allows fissuring of the skin, facilitating the entry of micro-organisms, which may result in cellulitis or abscess formation.

Peripheral arterial disease

People with diabetes are more prone to cardiovascular and peripheral arterial disease than the general population. Intermittent claudication is 2–3 times commoner,[21] and diabetic patients with intermittent claudication are at least twice as likely to have rest pain and six times as likely to have gangrene as non-diabetics.[22] Atherosclerosis in diabetic patients particularly affects medium-sized vessels such as the peroneal and tibial arteries, with some sparing of larger vessels. A palpable popliteal pulse with absent ankle pulses is far commoner in diabetics than non-diabetics.[23] The foot vessels are also often spared,[24] making distal arterial reconstruction possible in these patients. It is important to remember that Doppler pressures in these patients can be misleadingly high owing to medial calcification and incompressibility of vessels. The importance of investigating the vascular system in patients with foot ulceration to determine whether there is a surgically correctable deficiency cannot be overstressed. The European concensus document[25] has stipulated that no person with diabetes should have an amputation without having angiography.

The reasons for diabetic patients being more prone to arterial disease is not certain, but is probably due to the following factors.

Hyperglycaemia

The Framingham study[21] has shown hyperglycaemia to be an independent risk factor in atherogenesis. The mechanism of action is not clear but may be abnormal glycosylation of vessel walls. Nonenzymic glycosylation of proteins, including albumin, follows exposure to hyperglycaemia. Initially ketoamine formation by the reaction of glucose with amino groups in the protein molecule is reversible when the hyperglycaemia is relieved. However, a nonreversible configuration of the ketoamines can form over time by rearrangement of the molecule. There is increased adherence of activated monocytes and macrophages to these advanced glycosylation end-products.[26] Such products tend to accumulate on long-lived proteins such as collagen and basement membrane. Furthermore, it has been shown that monocytes from poorly controlled IDDM patients are more adhesive.[27] This leads to increased adherence of monocytes and macrophages to the vessel wall in diabetes.[28] This could result in the local accumulation of vasoactive substances, increased proliferation of endothelium due to the release of growth factors, and damage to the vessel wall by free radicals.

Free radicals and white cells

Free radicals (superoxides, hydroxyl radicals and peroxides) are produced by macrophages and monocytes upon activation. They have been shown to cause tissue destruction, including vascular damage,[29] and may precipitate the initial microvascular damage.[30] Increased levels of free radical activity are seen in both type I and type II diabetes.[31,32] There is some evidence that people with diabetes are less able to prevent oxidative damage by free radicals owing to reduced levels of ascorbic acid, a free radical scavenger.[33]

Blood lipid abnormalities

Blood cholesterol and triglycerides (LDL and VLDL) are high in patients with diabetes and this may be important in atherogenesis. By contrast, HDLs, which are said to have a protective role in atherogenesis, have been found to be lower in some diabetics than non-diabetics,[34] but this may not apply to all groups of diabetic patients.

Hypertension

There is conflicting evidence on the prevalence of hypertension and its importance in atherogenesis in diabetes. On balance, it is likely to be a contributory, though not very important, factor resulting in vascular disease.

Other factors

Hyperinsulinaemia, rheological factors, growth factors, reduced physical activity, obesity and genetic factors have all been put forward as reasons for increased atherogenesis in these patients, but they remain to be proven. Smoking is a major risk factor for the development of atheromatous disease, but there is no evidence to show that smoking is more prevalent in this group.

Microangiopathy

Much has been written about 'small vessel disease' and its importance in diabetes. At one point it was thought to be one of the most important factors in the pathogenesis of foot ulceration. The term 'small vessel disease' is too vague and should not be used. A better term is 'microangiopathy', which should be used to describe the functional defect seen in the skin microcirculation in people with diabetes, together with the associated histological changes of thickening of the basement membrane of small arterioles and capillaries.

There is no doubt that there is a microcirculatory defect in patients with microangiopathy.[35–37] Studies have shown a reduced hyperaemic response to heating of the skin,[38] reduced hyperaemia in response to injury (axon flare reflex), and other microcirculatory deficits.[39–41] However, in spite of these microcirculatory deficits, microangiopathy probably does not play a major role in the pathogenesis of skin ulceration. Otherwise it is difficult to see how removal of mechanical causes of ulceration or treatment of large-vessel disease can lead to healing of ulceration in a great proportion of cases.

Joint and gait abnormalities

The importance of deformity of the foot in the pathogenesis of ulceration has been discussed above. It is also important to mention the contribution to ulceration made by limited joint mobility (LJM).[42] There is a strong association between LJM and abnormal foot pressures in people with diabetes. Rigidity of the first metatarso-phalangeal joint results in abnormal stress on the skin overlying this joint during lifting of the heel on walking, increased by loss of ankle joint movement and eversion at the subtalar joint. Abnormalities of the foot shape due to Charcot's joints or pes cavus and abnormalities of gait due to motor weakness or loss of position sense also increase foot pressure abnormalities.

Trauma

Minor trauma is the initiating factor in almost all cases of the diabetic foot ulceration. Penetrating injuries by stepping on sharp objects such as glass may be a result of walking barefoot. Ill-fitting shoes probably account for the majority of ulcers. These ulcers can be caused by low pressures over a long period of time; for example, ulceration over the PIP joint of a claw toe due to tight shoes. (Fig. 17.4). Such ulcers are more characteristic of ischaemia than neuropathy. Ulcers may also be caused by high pressures sustained for short periods. These may be the result of shoes that are too loose, allowing the foot to move inside the shoe, resulting in shear stresses. This, together with vertical forces, are the cause of the majority of neuropathic ulcers. Thus it is important that people with diabetes wear shoes that

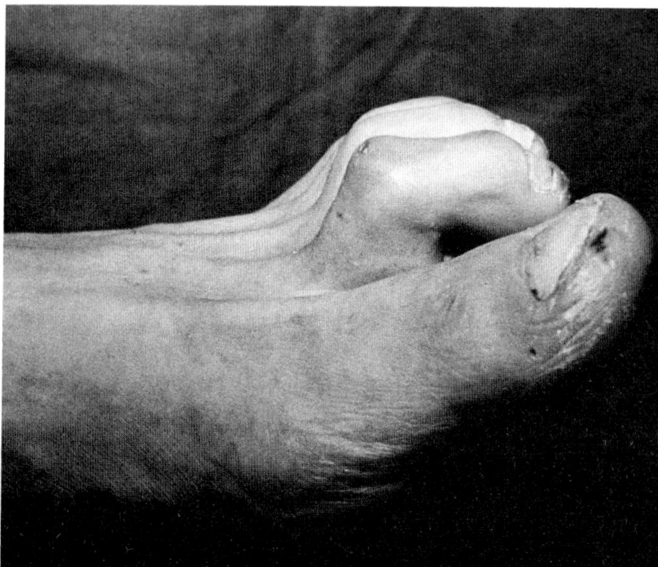

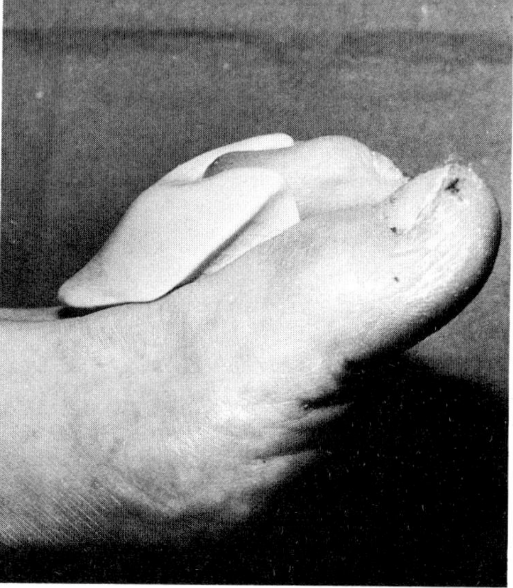

Fig. 17.4 Claw toes with ulcer over PIP joint of second toe. The picture on the right shows a protective silicon prosthesis in place.

accommodate the shape of the foot, are tight enough not to allow excessive movement inside them, and have shaped insoles which allow distribution of the patient's weight over a larger area, so reducing the pressure at any one point.

Ulceration may also occur from thermal injuries. This can be from cold, causing chilblains or frostbite, especially in a limb that is compromised by large-vessel disease. It can also be from heat; for example, from having the foot too close to a heater or using a hot-water bottle that is too hot(Fig. 17.5).

Infections

Infections are rarely a precipitating cause of diabetic ulcers. However, as soon as ulceration occurs, secondary infection follows. The infection is usually of mixed aerobic and anaerobic organisms. This infection may or may not be clinically significant. It may be limited to the surface of the ulcer or may involve deeper tissues such as subcutaneous fat, muscle and bone. The infection may lead to abscess formation in the planter spaces, and may extend upwards along muscles and tendons to involve the lower leg. Infection of the foot without ulceration also occurs. The site of entry may be through minor skin abrasions; for example, from fungal infection between the toes or from dryness and fissuring of the skin due to loss of sweating.

The multidisciplinary approach

A multidisciplinary approach to the prevention and treatment of foot complications results in improved care and a reduction in amputations.[4] It also offers patients a united front and avoids conflicting advice being given. The team should include diabetologist, vascular surgeon, orthopaedic surgeon, chiropodist and general practitioner. Shoe-maker, limb-fitter, dietician, physiotherapist and occupational therapist are also needed in the management of these patients. The role of the main team members will be discussed briefly.

Diabetologist

The diabetologist's role is central. He or she should not be concerned only in the management of the blood sugar and overall well-being of the diabetic patient, but also provide patient education and refer the patient to the vascular surgeon, chiropodist, etc. as appropriate.

Vascular surgeon

The vascular surgeon is responsible for investigating the patient who is either at risk of developing or currently has an ulcer or has symptoms suggestive of large-vessel disease. Doppler pressure can be misleading in diabetes owing to inelasticity of the vessels, and angiography is often necessary to determine if a revascularization procedure is appro-

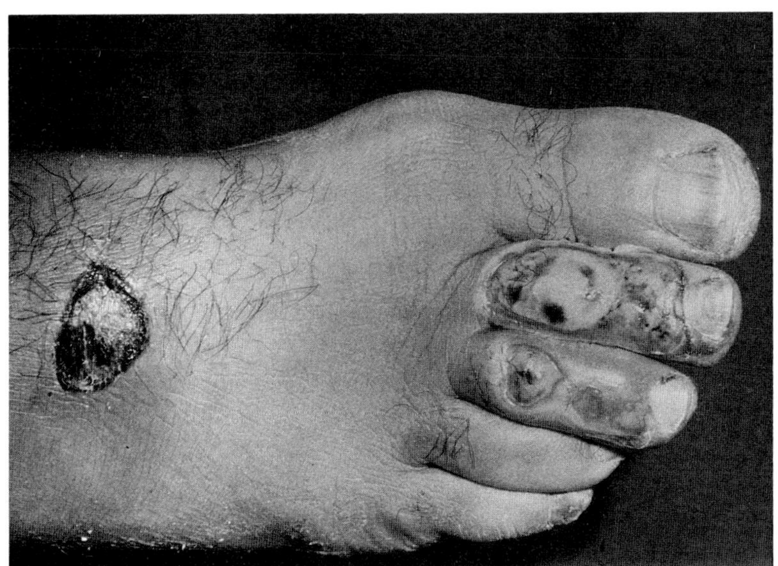

Fig. 17.5 Ulcers caused by a hot-water bottle.

priate. In this respect there is no difference in treatment between the diabetic and non-diabetic patient.

Orthopedic surgeon

The orthopaedic surgeon, in cooperation with the maker of shoe insoles is responsible for redistributing pressure in a deformed foot. If this cannot be done with insoles, operative measures may be needed to prevent or help heal ulceration. Minor procedures such as extensor tenotomies, arthroplasties or reimplantation of flexor tendons on to extensor expansions may be needed for correction of clawing of the toes, or more major procedures for correction of high arches or 'rocker sole' deformities in patients with Charcot's joints (Fig. 17.6).

Chiropodist

The role of the chiropodist is in the provision of routine foot care, debridement of ulcers, callus removal and patient education. Chiropodists are also involved in staffing special clinics where foot pressure studies can be performed, insoles made, and advice given regarding footwear.

General foot care and removal of callus

The chiropodist plays an important role in the prevention of ulceration in the diabetic patient. Cutting, filing down hard nails and general foot care by a professional avoids injury, neglect and ingrown toe nails, which may occur if the patient were to deal with this alone. Removing callus and hard skin reduces pressure on that area of the skin and allows softer skin to be in contact with footwear. This reduces shear forces between hard skin and underlying bone. Removing callus and debridement of dead tissue hastens the healing of ulcers. Chiropodists are also capable of cushioning bunions, claw and hammer toes and bony prominences with a variety of methods, including making silicon prostheses and can thus avoid ulceration from trauma to these areas by footwear (Fig. 17.7).

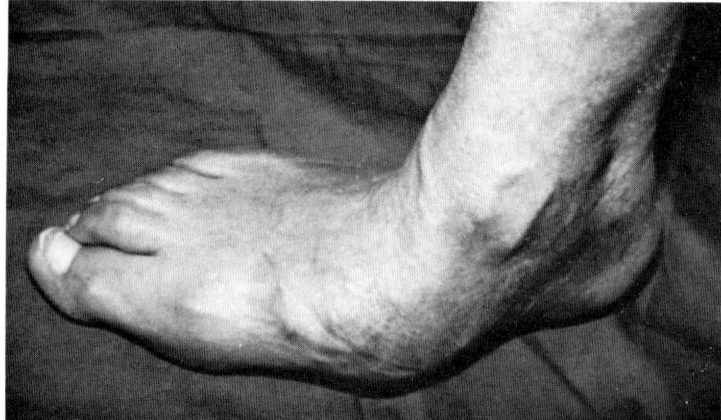

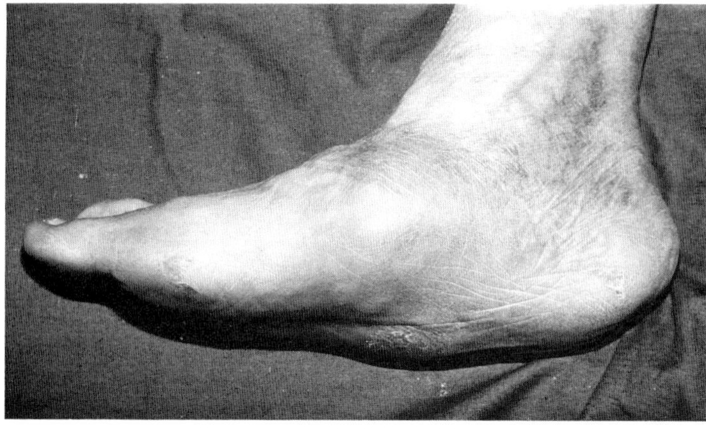

Fig. 17.6 'Rocker sole' deformity of Charcot's joint.

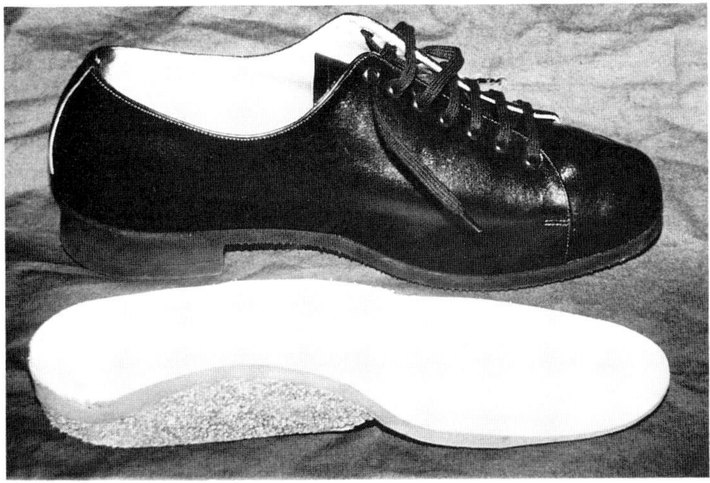

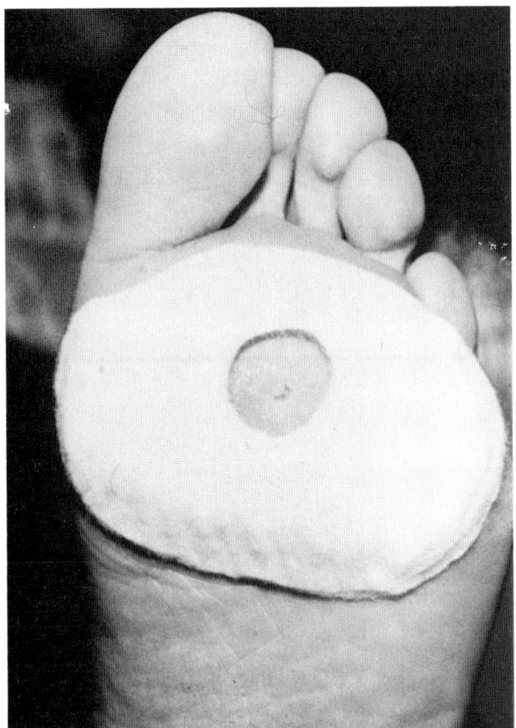

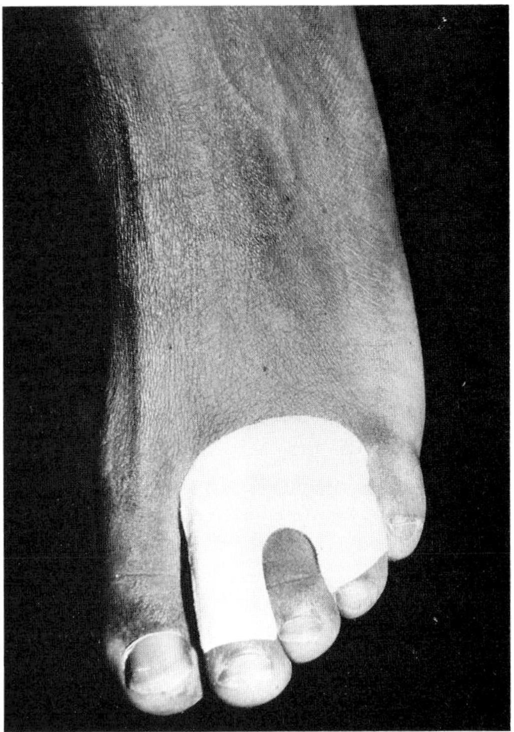

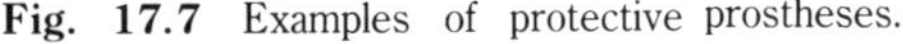

Fig. 17.7 Examples of protective prostheses.

Insoles and footwear

Properly made insoles are very important in the prevention of primary or recurrent ulceration. If a patient walks in his or her normal shoes after healing of an ulcer, recurrence is almost inevitable, and can sometimes occur in a matter of days. The importance of redistribution of stresses in the foot in the prevention of ulceration needs to be emphasized. Insoles specifically designed to reduce the longitudinal horizontal shear forces help to prevent this. These insoles are best made in three layers to a cast of the foot. The upper layer is made of 6 mm standard-density plastazote which moulds with wear to the dynamic forces of the foot, reducing peak loads and shear. The middle layer is made of either Cleron or Poron which are shock-absorbing extensible materials and move with the forefoot to reduce shear. Both of these layers are flattened under the heel and reduced in bulk under the mid-foot which is then filled with Burco cork. This forms a rigid mid-foot cradle to cut down excessive pronation, elongation and forward movement of the foot within the shoe. The insoles need to be housed in surgical shoes with full length lacing to reduce this motion further and thus reduce the shearing stresses. Using this method the majority of healed ulcers will remain healed.

General practitioner

The general practitioner plays a pivotal role in the management of the patient in the community. It is important that the hospital specialists communicate with the GP regarding management decisions.

Patient education

All members of the team should be involved in patient education. This may be in the form of special classes, audiovisual demonstrations in clinics, or through personal communications. Patients should be encouraged to keep their feet clean, free of hard skin and to examine them regularly, especially between the toes. They should also understand the importance of avoiding barefoot walking, having their shoes fitted by an expert, regular visits to the chiropodist, and good control of their blood sugar.

Prevention of ulceration

The prevention of ulceration is dependent on the removal or minimization of factors leading to ulceration and the identification of patients at risk of ulceration. Tables 17.2 and 17.3 list these factors.

Table 17.2 Principles of prevention of the 'diabetic foot'

Good control of blood sugar
Daily cleaning and inspection of feet
Avoiding walking barefoot
Wearing good quality supportive shoes
Moulded insoles and surgical shoes for deformed feet, especially if pressure areas develop
Inspection of shoes for foreign objects, nails, and rough edges before putting them on
Prompt treatment of all developing foot lesions
Regular visits to chiropodists

Table 17.3 Diabetes patients at risk of foot ulceration

Previous foot ulceration
Peripheral arterial disease
No protective sensation
Foot deformity or limited joint mobility
Long history of diabetes
Age

Management of the patient with ulceration

Particular attention must be paid to the vascular and neurological systems when taking a history from and examining a patient with a foot lesion. The musculoskeletal system of the lower limb and gait of the patient must also be carefully assessed.

Assessment and investigations of the arterial system

Assessment of the arterial tree in patients with diabetes does not differ from others and this has been covered in depth in other chapters. There are, however, some points to remember:

1. Diabetic patients are more prone to medial sclerosis of vessels. This results in reduced compressibility of vessels and may give misleadingly normal or high pressure readings in Doppler measurement of the vessels. If Doppler pressures appear normal, the Doppler waveform may be indicative of disease.
2. Diabetic patients are more prone to atherosclerosis in the medium-sized vessels, such as the tibial and peroneal vessels. However, the foot vessels are often spared, making them suitable for distal bypass surgery.

No diabetic patient should undergo major amputation without arteriography.[25] This should include good, preferably magnified, views of foot vessels to determine if there are any that a graft can be anastomosed to. Prediction of ulcer and amputation level healing have been attempted using a number of techniques in both diabetics and non-diabetics.[43] None, however, has gained widespread acceptance and these methods are still regarded as research tools. It is important not to forget the nutritional aspect of the patient. Healing is more likely to take place in a nutritionally sound patient, and indicators of the nutritional status, such as serum albumin, should be monitored.

Assessment and investigation of the peripheral neurological system

An account of a full neurological history and examination is beyond the scope of this chapter and can be obtained from a standard neurological textbook, so only a brief account of the important factors will be given.

In the neurological history it is important to determine if there is evidence of central or peripheral neuropathy. Symptoms of central neuropathy include: fainting spells, postural dizziness, nausea, vomiting of retained foods and, in men, impotence. Symptoms of peripheral neuropathy include: motor weakness, dry feet, numbness or loss of sensation in the feet, hyperaesthesia or pain in the legs.

On examination, a general idea of muscle strength can be obtained by assessing the patient's ability to walk on his toes and heels, rise from a kneeling position, and by testing the intrinsic muscles of the hand. Sensation in the limbs can be assessed using cotton wool and sharp and blunt points.

Quantitative assessment of both myelinated and unmyelinated fibres is desirable, especially to monitor progress. Motor and large sensory fibres can be assessed using traditional electrophysiological nerve conduction studies. However, smaller myelinated and unmyelinated fibres are more difficult to examine quantitatively. These can be assessed using the following techniques.

Myelinated fibres

Threshold to sensation. This can be tested quantitatively using Semmes–Weinstein fibres. These are monofilament fibres of differing diameters that bend at a force proportional to their diameter. The patient is tested with increasing diameter fibres until the threshold to sensation is obtained. Being able to detect a 10 g force (filament no. 5.07) being applied to the skin has been taken as being sufficient sensation to prevent ulceration.[44] This makes the 5.07 filament a good screening test for protective sensation.

Threshold to vibration. The sensation of vibration is conducted to the central nervous system through myelinated A-beta fibres. There are many different methods for testing the threshold to vibration and a number of commercially available instruments are available. The Ohio Bio-Thesiometer (Bio-Medical Instruments Co., Newbury, Ohio, USA) (Fig. 17.8) is one of the simplest to use and produces reproducible results. It can be applied to any point on the skin, usually on the big toe, medial or lateral malleolus. The threshold to vibration is obtained by gradually increasing the intensity of the vibration and asking the patient to indicate when the stimulus is felt.

Threshold to cooling. The sensation of cooling of the skin is transmitted to the central nervous system through small myelinated A-delta fibres. Different devices are available for testing the threshold to cooling of the skin. We use the 'Middlesex Thermal Tester' which consists of a thermode made up of a Peltier junction sandwiched between a copper plate

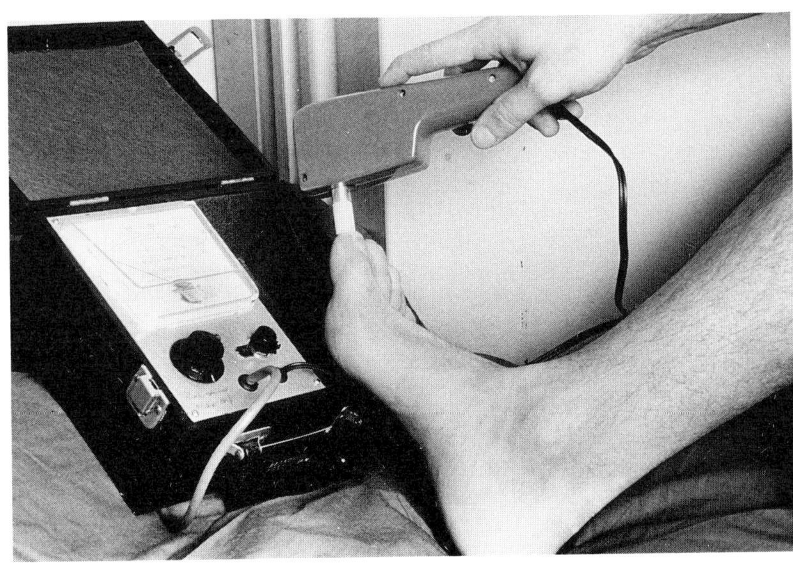

Fig. 17.8 The Ohio Bio-Thesiometer for measuring vibration sense.

and cooling fins. The copper plate incorporates a thermocouple which measures the change in temperature at the plate. When a current is passed to the Peltier junction, cooling on one side of the junction and warming on the other side occurs. This change in temperature is transmitted to the copper plate and the thermocouple detects the amount of change. A current passed in the opposite direction causes reversal of the situation. The duration and voltage of the current passed determines the degree of temperature change. This thermode is connected to a power source controlled by microcomputer with specially written software. A series of temperature changes are given to the patient until the threshold is reached. It is important to give 'sham' signals while testing to check the reliability of the patient's responses.

Unmyelinated fibres

Threshold to warming. The sensation of warming of the skin is conducted to the central nervous system via unmyelinated slowly conducting C fibres. This can be tested with the same equipment and in exactly the same way as the threshold to cooling.

Sympathetic fibres. Preganglionic sympathetic nerves are made up of small myelinated B fibres and are difficult to test clinically. The postganglionic fibres are made up of unmyelinated C fibre type and are more amenable to testing. The two functions of the peripheral sympathetic nerves that can be tested in the skin are the vasoconstrictor response and the sudomotor (sweat) response to sympathetic stimulation.

Assessment of the musculoskeletal system and gait

Abnormalities of gait and foot shape result in abnormal foot skin pressures. These pressures can be studied using a number of static and dynamic methods. The earliest method was to use an inked rubber matt over which a paper was laid; the patient stood on this, thus providing a footprint. This has been susequently developed to show ridges of different depth on the footprint depending on the pressure applied, giving a semi-quantitative method of measuring vertical pressure on the sole of the foot. Later optical and strain gauge systems for measurement of foot pressures were invented.[45,46] More recently, foot plates with special sensors attached to a microcomputer allow footprints to be obtained with different colours denoting different pressures. Fig. 17.9 shows a monochrome reproduction. These prints can be done in a standing static position or dynamically while walking on a special sensor mat. Transducers that measure shear stresses are also being developed and these will provide further information needed to identify patients at risk and help design appropriate footwear.

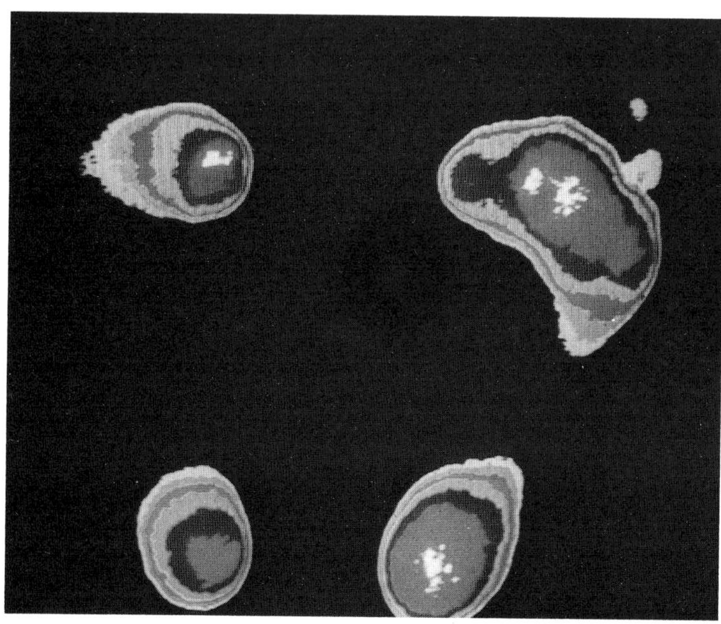

Fig. 17.9 Foot pressure footprints.

Specific treatments

Once a lesion has developed, it is important to classify it into a neuropathic, ischaemic or mixed lesion and determine if it is simple or complicated. Predominantly neuropathic ulcers are easier to heal and have a better prognosis than ischaemic ulcers. Fig. 17.10 shows a flow chart summarizing the management of patients with lesions of the foot.

Complicated lesions

These are initially best managed in hospital. The patient's diabetes is usually out of control due to the presence of infection or frank pus, and glycaemic control may be difficult until the infection is dealt with. This necessitates good cooperation between the medical and surgical teams treating the patient.

Infection

By definition, infection is present in complicated lesions. It is important to obtain swabs for culture from the infected area and start systemic antibiotics, with parenteral administration for at least the first 48 hours. The choice of antibiotics is dependent on personal preferences, but it is important to cover both aerobic and anaerobic organisms as the majority of ulcers will have mixed flora. Antibiotics should be continued until all signs of deep infection disappear. If cellulitis or rigors are present, blood cultures must also be taken. If osteomyelitis is present or suspected, then a deep swab or, preferably, a bone biopsy is necessary to establish the nature of the invading organism. The choice of antibiotics can be reconsidered when culture and sensitivity results become available. Cleaning of the ulcer, bed-rest and elevation of the limb to get rid of oedema (provided this is not contraindicated by vascular disease) will promote healing.

Debridement

It is important to debride all dead tissue and incise and drain any pockets of pus as soon after admission as possible. However, excessive removal of viable tissue should be avoided to minimize skin loss. Debridement can usually be done without anaesthesia owing to the neuropathy. Frequent debridement is often required until infection is under control. An X-ray of the foot is essential in order to exclude osteomyelitis. In general, with diligence and repeated debridement, it is possible to save the majority of limbs. Occasionally minor amputations or removal of infected bone is necessary if osteomyelitis is present (Fig. 17.11). These should be done with removal of a minimal amount of normal tissue.

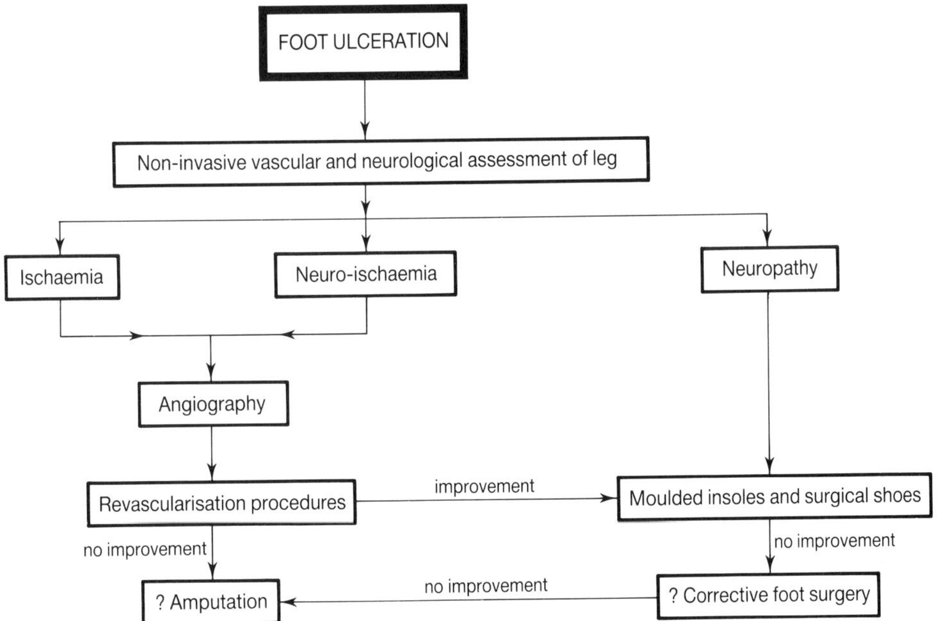

Fig. 17.10 Simplified flow chart showing the management of diabetic foot ulceration.

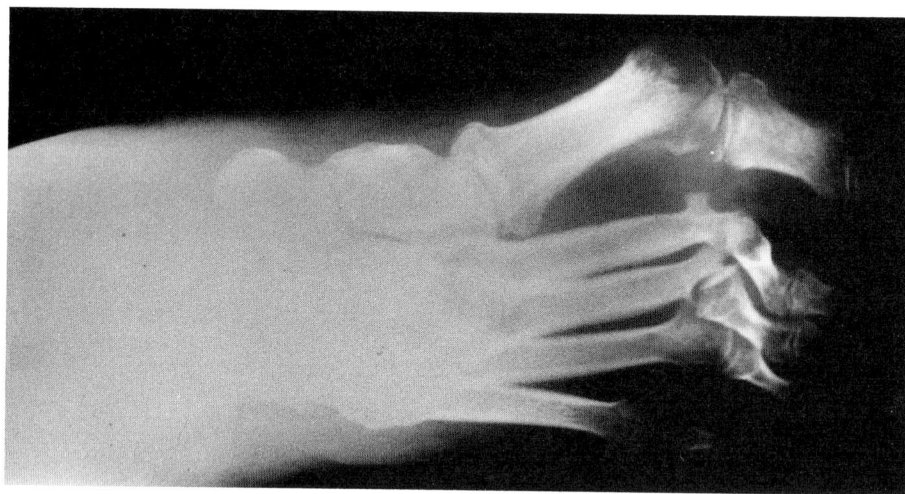

Fig. 17.11 X-ray showing bony destruction due to osteomyelitis.

Vascular assessment

Vascular assessment is mandatory to determine whether revascularization procedures are needed to save the limb. Surgery or angioplasty are sometimes carried out immediately, but often can be delayed for a few days until gross infection has settled and glycaemic control of the patient has been achieved. Sympathectomy does not tend to be a useful option in diabetic patients with foot lesions since the majority of them will have had 'auto-sympathectomy' due to autonomic neuropathy.

Amputation

If the above measures are not successful in controlling the infection, and revascularization is not possible or has failed, amputation may be necessary. Minor foot amputation should be performed, keeping in mind functional rather than cosmetic considerations. It is important to preserve as much as possible of the weight-bearing area of the foot. As mentioned earlier, the nutritional status of the patient should be monitored.

With the foregoing measures, provided amputation has not been needed, the foot will improve within a few days and antibiotics can be administered orally. Once infection has settled down the ulcer can be managed in the same way as for an uncomplicated ulcer (see below). If large skin defects are present after treatment, reconstructive plastic surgery may be needed.

Uncomplicated lesions

These are predominantly neuropathic ulcers and can be healed by diverting the pressure away from the ulcer site. A number of methods of doing this are available.

Bed-rest

This is an effective way of removing pressure from an ulcer but is not cost-effective. A period of bed-rest, however, may be necessary in an ulcer resistant to healing by other pressure-relieving methods.

Removing callus

This aids the healing of ulcers by reducing vertical and shear pressures on the ulcer base and is used in conjunction with other methods to achieve ulcer healing.

Total contact plaster

This is essentially a below-knee plaster applied with minimal padding and a rocker sole on the base. The function of this is to reduce both vertical and shear forces on the area of the ulcer by redistributing them over a wider area. Plasters will need to be changed regularly to allow inspection and removal of callus from around the ulcer.

Moulded insoles and surgical shoes

These have been described earlier. If they are made properly they probably result in a rapid ulcer healing as total contact casts. If a patient does not need special shoes, it is important that the feet are measured correctly and shoes fitted by an experienced salesman. These facilities are available at a number of shoe shops. If special shoes are not needed but there is still stress over a part of the foot such as a bony protuberance, then an appropriate hole can be cut in the shoe. Special padded socks, as worn by athletes, are becoming available for diabetics. It is claimed that these help redistribute pressure on the foot.[47]

Antibiotics

There is much controversy over the use of antibiotics in simple ulcers with no underlying tissue involvement. We restrict their use to complicated ulcers. Much has been written on the topical treatment of ulcers. Topical antibiotics are of no use, and probably encourage the emergence of resistant strains. Many antiseptics have been shown to delay wound healing, possibly by damage to fibroblasts. The clinical significance of this is not established. Provided that the ulcer is laid open and there are no deep pockets of pus, cleaning with sterile saline should suffice.

Other methods

A number of other methods for healing or preventing ulcers have been tried, but there is a lack of controlled clinical trials demonstrating their effectiveness. Topically applied platelet and other growth factors have been used in diabetic ulceration and each manufacturer claims accelerated healing using them. Healing of wounds by the use of hyperbaric oxygen (patient placed in chamber pressured to 3 atmospheres and breathing 100% oxygen) may be useful, but it is costly and the equipment is not generally available. Certainly, if it is to be successful, the whole patient has to be pressurized, and not just the affected limb.

Success with the implantation of silicon to replace the 'fat pads' or to act as cushions on areas of high pressure or on previously ulcerated areas has been reported.[48]

Other complications

Diabetic arthropathy

This is an aseptic arthritis sometimes seen in diabetic patients and is similar to a Charcot's arthropathy. There is usually an abnormality of gait and these patients have to be treated with specially made footwear to stabilize the foot and prevent further deformity. Surgery is sometimes needed to correct severe deformity. Some cases are associated with ulceration, and treatment is then no different from the principles discussed above.

Painful neuropathy

Ulceration in painful neuropathy is rare. Patients complain of burning feet. Other causes of this have to be excluded and treatment is difficult, usually consisting of analgesics, phenothiazines or antidepressants.

Conclusions

The 'diabetic foot' is a distressing but common complication of diabetes mellitus and usually affects the older patient. These lesions are usually caused by neuropathy or vascular disease or a combination of both. Treatment can be difficult and costly. Prevention and treatment are best mediated through patient education and a multidisciplinary approach.

References

1. Williams DRR. Hospital admissions of diabetic patients: information from hospital activity analysis. *Diabet Med* 1985; **2:** 27–32.
2. Most RS, Sinnock P. The epidemiology of lower extremity amputations in diabetic individuals. *Diabet Care* 1983; **6:** 87–91.
3. Bild DE, Selby JV, Sinnock P, Browner WS, Braveman P, Showstack JA. Lower extremity amputation in people with diabetes. *Diabet Care* 1989; **12:** 24–31.
4. Thomson FJ, Veves A, Ashe H, Knowles EA, Gem J, Walker MG, Hirst P, Boulton AJM. A team approach to diabetic foot care: the Manchester experience. *The Foot* 1991; **2:** 75–82.
5. Oakley W, Catterall RCF, Martin MM. Aetiology and management of lesions of the feet in diabetics. *Br Med J* 1956; **2:** 953–7.
6. Wagner FW. The dysvascular foot: a system for diagnosis and treatment. *Foot Ankle* 1981; **2:** 64–7.
7. Gibbons GE, Ellopoulous GM. Infection of the diabetic foot. In: *Manaegment of Diabetic Foot Problems*. Philadelphia: WB Saunders, 1984: 97–102.
8. Coleman W. Footwear in a management program of injury prevention. In: *The Diabetic Foot*, 4th edn. St Louis: CV Mosby, 1988: 293–308.
9. Frykberg RG. Diabetic foot ulceration. In: *The High Risk Foot in Diabetes Mellitus*. Edinburgh: Churchill Livingstone, 1991: 185–6.
10. Boulton AJM, Knight G, Drury J, Ward JD. The prevalence of symptomatic neuropathy in an insulin-treated population. *Diabet Care* 1985; **8:** 125–8.
11. Newrick PG, Boulton AJM, Ward JD. The distribution of diabetic neuropathy in a British clinic population. *Diabet Res Clin Pract* 1986; **2:** 263–8.
12. Lundborg G, Myers R, Powell H. Nerve compression injury and increased endoneurial fluid pres-

sure: a 'miniature compartment syndrome'. *J Neurol Neurosurg Psychiat* 1983; **46:** 1119–24.
13. Rydevik BL, Myers RR, Powell HC. Pressure increase in the dorsal root ganglion following mechanical compression. *Spine* 1989; **14:** 574–6.
14. Myers RR, Kalichman MW, Reisner LS, *et al.* Neurotoxicity of local anesthetics: Altered perineurial permeability, edema, and nerve fiber injury. *Anesthesiology* 1986; **64:** 29–35.
15. Powell HC, Kalichman MW, Garrett RS, *et al.* Selective vulnerability of unmyelinated fiber Schwann cells in nerves exposed to local anesthetics. *Lab Invest* 1968; **59:** 271–80.
16. Myers RR, Mizsin AP, Powell HC, *et al.* Reduced nerve blood flow in hexachlorophene neuropathy. *J Neuropath Exp Neurol* 1982; **41:** 391–9.
17. Myers RR, Powell HC. Galactose neuropathy: impact of chronic endoneurial edema on nerve blood flow. *Ann Neurol* 1984; **16:** 587–94.
18. Myers RR, Murakami H, Powell HC. Reduced nerve blood flow in edematous neuropathies: a biomechanical mechanism. *Microvasc Res* 1986; **32:** 145–51.
19. Flynn MD, Edmonds ME, Tooke JE, Watkins PJ. Direct measurement of the capillary blood flow in the diabetic neuropathic foot. *Diabetologia* 1988; **31:** 652–6.
20. Delbridge L, Ctercteko G, Fowler C, *et al.* The aetiology of diabetic ulceration of the foot. *Br J Surg* 1985; **72:** 1–6.
21. Brand FN, Abbott RD, Kannel WD. Diabetes, intermittent claudication, and risk of cardiovascular events: the Framingham study. *Diabetes* 1989; **38:** 504–9.
22. Jonason T, Ringqvist I. Diabetes mellitus and intermittent claudication: relation between peripheral vascular complications and location of the occlusive atherosclerosis in the legs. *Acta Med Scand* 1985; **218:** 217–21.
23. Strandness DE, Priest RE, Gibbons RE, Seattle MD. Combined clinical and pathological study of diabetic and non-diabetic peripheral artery disease. *Diabetes* 1961; **13:** 366–72.
24. Gibbons GW. Vascular surgery. In: *Proceedings of the First International Symposium on the Diabetic Foot,* Bakker K, Nieuwenhuijzen Kruseman AC (eds). Amsterdam: Excerpta Medica, 1991: 117–24.
25. Dormandy J (ed). *European Consensus Document on Critical Limb Ischaemia.* Berlin: Springer-Verlag, 1989.
26. Gilcrease MZ, Hoover RL. Activated human monocytes exhibit receptor-mediated adhesion to a non-enzymatically glycosylated protein substrate. *Diabetologia* 1990; **33:** 329–33.
27. Setiadi H, Wautier J, Courillon-Mallet A, *et al.* Increased adhesion to fibronectin and MO-1 expression by diabetic monocytes. *J Immunol* 1987; **138:** 3230–4.
28. Brownlee M, Vlassara H, Ceranii A. The pathogenetic role of non-enzymatic glycosylation in diabetic complications. In: *Diabetic Complications: Scientific and Clinical Aspects*, Crabbe MJC (ed). Edinburgh: Churchill Livingstone, 1987: 94–139.
29. McCord JM. Oxygen-derived free radicals in postischaemic tissue injury. *N Engl J Med* 1985; **312:** 159–63.
30. Wolff SP. The potential role of oxidative stress in diabetes and its complications: novel implications for theory and therapy. In: *Diabetic Complications: Scientific and Clinical Aspects*, Crabbe MJC (ed). Edinburgh: Churchill Livingstone, 1987: 167–200.
31. Jennings PE, Jones AF, Florkowski CM, Lunec J, Barnett AH. Increased diene conjugates in diabetic subjects with microangiopathy. *Diabet Med* 1987; **4:** 452–6.
32. Collier A, Wilson R, Bradley H, *et al.* Free radical activity in type 2 diabetes. *Diabet Med* 1900; **7:** 27–30.
33. Jennings PE, Chirico S, Jones AF, Lunec J, Barnett AH. Vitamin C metabolites and microangiopathy in diabetes mellitus. *Diabet Res* 1987; **6:** 151–4.
34. Feher MD, Stevens J, Lant AF, Mayne PD. Importance of routine measurement of HDL with total cholesterol in diabetic patients. *J Roy Soc Med* 1991; **85:** 8–11.
35. Tooke JE. Microcirculation and diabetes. *Br Med Bull* 1989; **45:** 206–23.
36. Flynn MD, Edmonds ME, Tooke JE, *et al.* Direct measurement of the capillary blood flow in the diabetic neuropathic foot. *Diabetologia* 1988; **31:** 652–6.
37. Rayman G, Hassan A, Tooke JE. Blood flow in the skin of the foot related to posture in diabetes mellitus. *Br Med J* 1986; **292:** 87–90.
38. Rayman G, Williams SA, Spencer PD, Smaje LH, Wise PH, Tooke JE. Impaired microvascular hyperaemic responses to minor skin trauma in type 1 diabetes. *Br Med J* 1986; **292:** 1295–8.
39. Parkhouse N, LeQuesne PM. Impaired neurogenic vascular response in patients with diabetes and neuropathic foot lesions. *N Engl J Med* 1988; **318:** 1306–9.
40. Walmsley D, Wales JK, Wiles PG. Reduced hyperaemia following skin trauma: evidence for an impaired microvascular response to injury in the diabetic foot. *Diabetologia* 1989; **32:** 736–9.
41. Aronin N, Leeman SE, Clements RS. Diminished flare response in neuropathic diabetic patients: comparisons of effects of substance P, histamine and caspaicin. *Diabetes* 1987; **36:** 1139–43.
42. Delbridge L, Perry P, Marr S, *et al.* Limited joint mobility in the diabetic foot: relationship to neuropathic ulceration. *Diabet Med* 1988; **5:** 333–7.
43. Sarin S, Shami SK, Shields DA, Scurr JH, Coleridge Smith PD. Selection of amputation levels: a review. *Eur J Vasc Surg* 1991; **5:** 611–20.
44. Kumar S, Fernando DJS, Veves A, Young MJ,

Boulton AJM. Semmes–Weinstein monofilaments: a simple screening device to identify patients at risk of foot ulceration. *Diabet Med* 1990; **7** (Suppl 2): 4A.
45. Elftmann HO. A cinematic study of the distribution of pressure in the human foot. *Anat Rec* 1934; **59:** 481–90.
46. Hutton WC, Drabble GE. An apparatus to give the distribution of vertical load under the foot. *Rheum Phys Med* 1972; **11:** 313–17.
47. Veves A, Masson EA, Fernando DJS, Boulton AJM. Use of experimental hoisery to reduce abnormal foot pressure in diabetic neuropathy. *Diabet Care* 1989; **12:** 653–5.
48. Balkin SW, Kaplan L. Injectable silicon and the diabetic foot: a 25-year report. *The Foot* 1991; **2:** 83–8.

18

Vascular trauma

Aires AB Barros D'Sa

The treatment of vascular trauma before the turn of this century mainly involved control of haemorrhage to save life. Through two world wars and subsequent major conflicts, increasingly sophisticated methods of vascular repair have been employed to save both organ and limb.[1–5] Despite the augmented wounding power of weaponry used in successive wars, limb salvage rate improved as a consequence of more rapid evacuation, definitive repair of arteries and veins, and the increased use of autogenous vein grafts. That experience was applied to the management of vascular injuries sustained in civilian practice[6–10] and in terrorist violence,[11–16] the favourable results in the latter being mainly attributable to innovative approaches in management.[17–27] Iatrogenic vascular trauma following diagnostic and therapeutic catheterization or complicating certain operations presents an episodic burden on the vascular surgeon.[28–30]

Mechanisms of vascular trauma

Penetrating vascular trauma is caused by glass, sharp weapons, bullets and fragments of shrapnel. Stabbing results in minimal soft tissue injury, but the wounding force of a missile depends on its mass, muzzle velocity and distance travelled. The energy dissipated at right-angles to the trajectory of a high-velocity bullet results in temporary cavitation with extensive destruction and contamination of tissue. These effects are also observed when a shotgun is discharged at close range or in injury caused by fragments and secondary missiles from a bomb explosion.

Blunt vascular trauma, observed particularly in road traffic accidents, results directly from a bone fragment or indirectly due to the intense shearing forces generated during the sudden fracture of long bones such as the femur,[31–33] dislocations of the knee[34,35] and severe open tibial fractures[36] in which extensive tissue loss and contamination inevitably account for dismal amputation rates. Crush injury resulting from falling masonry, railroad and mining accidents predictably leads to the 'crush syndrome' and may be compounded by direct injury to major vessels.

The invasive nature of modern diagnostic and therapeutic angiography and cardiac catheterization is responsible for most cases of iatrogenic vascular trauma manifesting as haemorrhage, thromboembolism, dissection, false aneurysm, arteriovenous fistula or catheter retention.[29,30] Atherosclerotic vessels are particularly vulnerable to accident, flawed judgement or poor technique, especially during interventional procedures such as balloon angioplasty, stenting, thrombolysis, atherectomy and insertion of the intra-aortic balloon pump.[37] Orthopaedic operations performed in areas of anatomical proximity to major vessels – namely, lumbar discectomy, total hip replacement and lateral menisectomy – can each result in vascular injury.[29,38]

Irradiation therapy for certain tumours can injure adjacent vessels: for example, the great vessels and carotid arteries in head and neck tumours, the subclavian and axillary arteries in lymphomas and breast cancer,[39] and the iliofemoral arterial system in tumours of the ovary, cervix and testes. In most cases the endothelium, and internal elastic lamina, as well as the outer layers of the vessel are damaged.[40]

Types of vascular trauma

Blunt vascular injury manifests itself variously as an intramural haematoma which obstructs flow, thrombosis in continuity, or an intimal fracture which may form a flap and by dissection inevitably lead to thrombotic occlusion, especially if the fracture is circumferential. A presumptive diagnosis of arterial spasm engenders inactivity and may obscure serious injury. Lacerations, whether clean or ragged, prevent circumferential contraction, leading to persistent bleeding either externally or into a tense enlarging pulsatile haematoma which occludes the artery. Arterial flow through a gap in the wall forces its way into a haematoma to create an endothelium-lined false aneurysm which may thrombose, expand, compress adjacent veins and eventually rupture. A completely divided artery (Fig. 18.1), either simply transected or as a result of avulsive traction, usually retracts and is sealed by a plug of thrombus. Simultaneous penetration of major artery and adjoining vein will result in an arteriovenous fistula (Fig. 18.2) which short-circuits distal flow and is recognized by a continuous thrill, audible bruit, and in some cases a high-output cardiac state.

Pathophysiology of vascular trauma

The compensatory rising afterload and falling stroke volume, following exsanguination from large vessels, further compromise the already reduced tissue perfusion and oxygenation of an organ or extremity resulting from the vascular injury. Unreplaced clotting factors and platelets aggravate bleeding. Tissue hypoxia raises capillary membrane permeability, facilitating fluid exudation into the interstitial space. In vascular injury of a limb, swelling of striated muscle raises the pressure within inelastic fascial compartments, impairing arterial inflow already attenuated by other factors: damage to bone, soft tissue and collateral vessels, haematoma, impaired drainage due to vein injury and progressive microvascular thrombosis.[20] The injurious effect of reperfusion of ischaemic tissue[41] may be the cumulative effect of factors such as tissue pO_2, pH, lactate, calcium ion, prostaglandins, proteases, histamines and leucocytes. The latter are either involved in free radical production or are released in response to free radical interaction with membranes. Prolongation of warm ischaemia time beyond 6–8 hours may result in

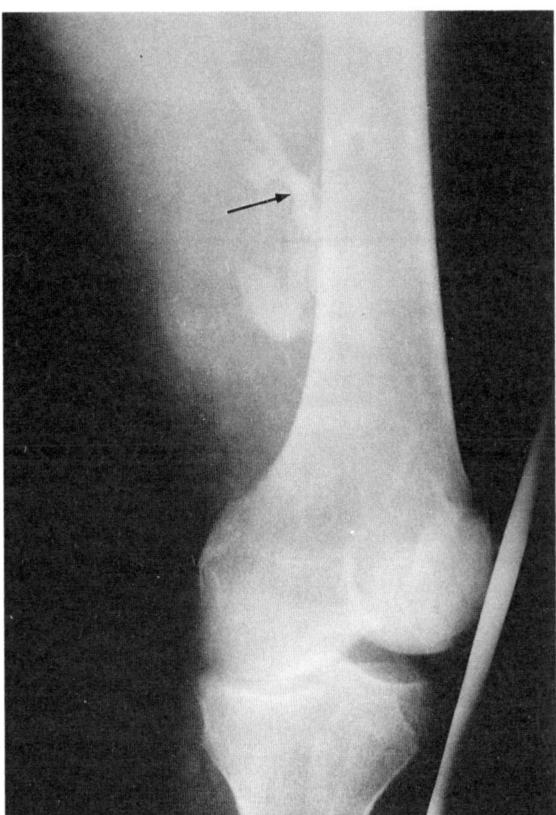

Fig. 18.1 Angiogram showing an irregular atherosclerotic lower femoral artery transected (arrow) in a road accident. Bleeding is occurring both externally and into a haematoma.

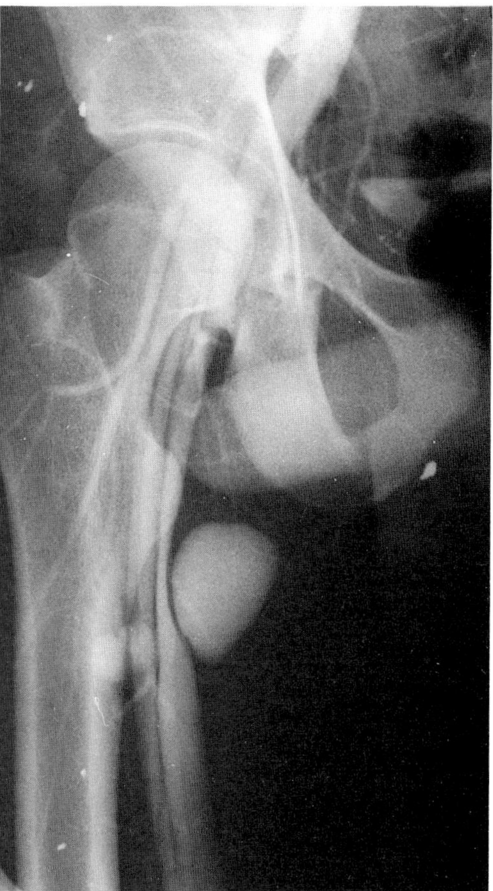

Fig. 18.2 Angiogram showing a superficial femoral arteriovenous fistula with false aneurysms caused by shrapnel injury.

aseptic muscle necrosis, myoglobinuria, acute renal tubular necrosis, Volkmann's ischaemic contracture and limb loss.

Wounds sustained in road accidents, high-velocity bullet injury and bombs are contaminated by Gram-positive cocci, Gram-negative bacilli and Clostridia, some of which can act synergistically to produce cellulitis, fasciitis, gas gangrene or fatal secondary haemorrhage from the site of vascular repair. These complications are more likely when there is delay or if exploration and debridement are incomplete.

Lower limb vascular trauma

Primary clinical care

A firm pad and bandage or digital compression will control external bleeding. Tourniquets should be avoided as they can actually increase bleeding. The blind application of clamps will endanger vessels and nerves. Standard resuscitative measures are adopted in the shocked or multiply injured patient. Information on the wounding agent, muzzle velocity of the gun and distance from which it was fired as well as estimated blood loss are of assistance in management. Tetanus toxoid and prophylactic cefuroxime and metronidazole are given.

Clinical examination should determine if bleeding is arterial or venous, if a haematoma is pulsatile or expanding, if a thrill or bruit is present, if distal pulses are palpable and if signs of ischaemia are present – including pallor, mottling, coolness, hypoaesthesia and lack of movement. Subtle signs such as transient ischaemia, minimal neurological deficit or nonexpanding haematoma[42] may be missed in closed injuries of the femur or knee. An audible Doppler signal does not necessarily mean that the proximal artery is intact, whereas measurement of Doppler pressure, not always practicable, with an ankle–brachial index less than 0.90 should be regarded with suspicion. Duplex scanning is showing promise but angiography remains the most reliable method of imaging an injured artery.

Nearly a third of major military arterial injuries[4] and a tenth of civilian arterial injuries[7] are accompanied by long-bone fracture. X-ray films of bone are essential in assessment.

Angiography

With penetrating wounds, biplane angiography localizes an arterial injury, which usually makes exploration mandatory; and if it excludes vascular injury the surgeon has the confidence not to intervene.[43] Against this, the angiographic yield of arterial injury in wounds in close proximity to the femoral and popliteal vessels is low,[44] but in foregoing this investigation the risk of missing an injury should be borne in mind. In institutions lacking angiography, the clinician relies on meticulous and repeated physical examination and, if there is doubt, early exploration.

Complex limb vascular trauma

High energy injuries of limbs are caused by sudden deceleration, crush trauma, high-velocity gunfire or explosions. They are characterized by damage to both artery and vein, comminuted fractures with periosteal stripping, nerve damage, soft tissue and skin loss, contamination and multiple injury. Salvage of the critically injured lower limb has improved with advances in operative technique; but if the obviously irreparable and mutilated limb is treated too zealously, the patient and surgeon are committed to a protracted series of operations, inevitable morbidity, poor rehabilitation and eventual limb amputation. Objective clinical criteria in the form of scoring systems can predict outcome,[45] but as neither of the two key factors responsible for late amputation (namely, failed vascular repair and sepsis) can be foreseen at admission, those systems are limited in their scope.

The importance of time

The unforgiving effect of warm ischaemia time on striated muscle is a key arbiter of outcome and is the single factor which can be influenced by resuscitation, early diagnosis and definitive treatment. A finite and irreducible period of time, nevertheless, is required for exploration, control of haemorrhage, identification of nerves, wound debridement, bone fixation, preparation of vessels, harvesting of vein and arterial and venous repair. Pressures to expedite vascular repair may introduce lapses of principle and technique. Lateral suture of arteries or end-to-end anastomosis are quicker but may be flawed, and large venous channels may be hurriedly ligated. Robust manipulation of bone fragments may disrupt previously completed vascular repairs. Reduction and fixation of a fracture before vascular repair ensures that grafts used are of optimal length and that they will remain undisturbed. However, high-quality orthopaedic surgery does take time, and if rushed in order to shorten ischaemia time, technical imperfections may occur which can result in delayed or failed union. These concerns are immediately resolved if both artery and vein are bridged temporarily by intraluminal shunts (Fig. 18.3), a policy which fosters a logical multidisciplinary approach to complex vascular trauma.[17–27]

Operative treatment

Standard longitudinal incisions are employed and a muscle-splitting retroperitoneal approach for external iliac artery control is effective in groin vascular trauma. A gentle S-shaped posterior incision in an oblique axis provides good access to the popliteal artery.[11,12] After controlling bleeding, the injured vessel is trimmed back to intact wall. Proximal clot in an artery is flushed out, and distal thrombus removed by balloon catheter. If there has been a delay the leg is milked upwards to express clot, following which heparinized saline is infused into the distal vessels. A suitable indwelling shunt is inserted to restore arterial flow, and after ensuring that the adjoining injured vein is clear of thrombus a similar shunt re-establishes venous flow (Fig. 18.3). In the absence of commercially available shunts, simple silicone elastomer or plastic tubing of suitable consistency (with smoothly trimmed ends to avoid intimal damage) can be used.

The arterial shunt terminates warm ischaemia time, and by holding down intracompartmental pressure significantly reduces the need for fasciotomy. When there is extensive destruction of lengthy segments of vessels and contamination of soft tissue, long outlying shunts may be used to revitalize the distal limb and drain it adequately. Before re-establishing venous drainage, stagnant venous blood (low in pH and rich in potassium and toxic metabolites likely to endanger the myocardium) is flushed out. This can be done most conveniently via the side-arm of a Brener shunt which can be used later for intravenous treatment. If this shunt is placed in an artery, the side-arm can be used for blood sampling, blood gas estimations, injection of anticoagulants or contrast for on-table angiography.

Reperfusion sharpens the distinction between viable and dead muscle. The latter is recognizable by its purplish discoloration and failure to bleed or contract. There is ample time for wound survey, identification of nerves, removal of bone fragments, dirt, debris and foreign bodies, and copious irrigation to reduce bacterial innoculum.

Skeletal integrity is then restored accurately by

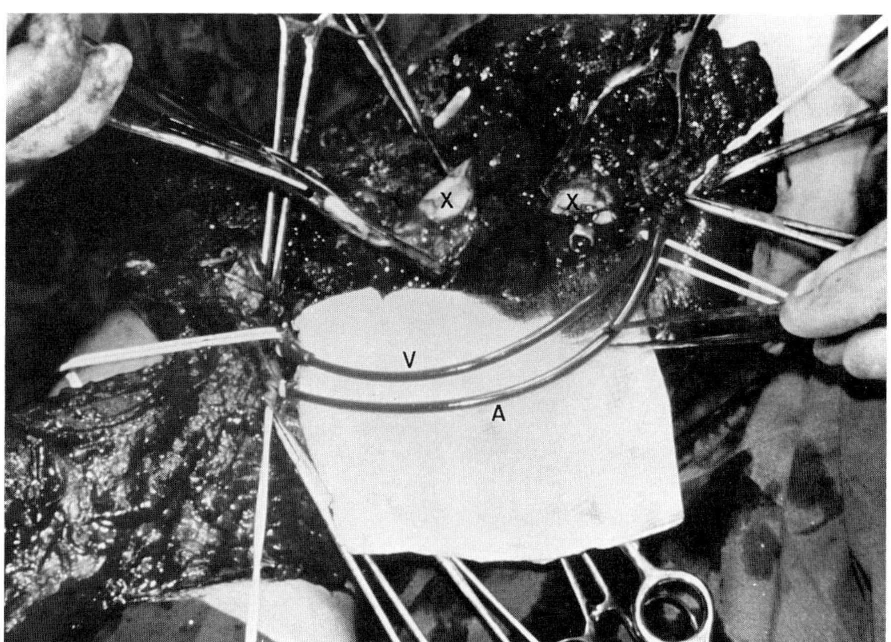

Fig. 18.3 A Javid shunt (A) bridging a lengthy gap in the femoral artery and perfusing the distal limb, and another such shunt (V) bridging a similar gap in the adjoining femoral vein and draining the limb. The picture shows the ends of a fractured femur (XX) being manipulated prior to fixation – see also Fig. 18.4. (Reproduced from reference 22 with permission.)

internal or external fixation in preparation for vascular repair. Although lateral suture is adequate for puncture wounds and small lacerations, vein patch angioplasty is required to repair longitudinal lacerations so as to maintain vessel diameter. Direct end-to-end repair is effective in clean transections, but if loss of a damaged segment introduces anastomotic tension, any length of excised vessel can be replaced easily with reversed autogenous vein (Fig. 18.4).

With shunts in place, time is taken to fashion panel[11,12,46] (Fig. 18.5) or spiral[25] compound vein grafts of a diameter matching that of the host vessel. Neither artery nor vein merits priority of repair if both vessels have been shunted. Precise suture technique is facilitated by a shunt which acts as a stent. In situations of extensive tissue and vessel damage, outlying shunts provide a safety margin of time for the construction of an extra-anatomic graft tunnelled through untraumatized viable tissue, for example, from the proximal femoral to the distal popliteal or anterior tibial artery.[25]

In severe open tibial fractures there appears to be some enthusiasm for repair of either the anterior or posterior tibial artery irrespective of the discouragingly ischaemic appearance of the foot. Despite favourable reports[10] of repair using PTFE grafts, account has to be taken of the inherent risks of sepsis, secondary haemorrhage and limb loss, particularly when such prostheses are used in combat wounds. False aneurysms and arteriovenous fistulae are excised and repaired by lateral suture, patch repair or vein graft replacement. A reconstructed major venous channel enhances the patency of an adjacent arterial repair. Vein repair by lateral suture or patch angioplasty is effective, but when there is greater damage the segment should be replaced by a simple or compound vein graft. Ligation leads to obstructive venous insufficiency, may predispose to deep vein thrombosis and pulmonary embolism and, rarely, precipitates acute venous gangrene and amputation.

The use of indwelling shunts lowers the fasciotomy rate by maintaining compartment pressures within a safe range. Delayed restoration of flow, evidence of marked oedema or limited muscle necrosis, complex injury, fixed plantar flexion at the ankle or compartment pressures exceeding 40 mmHg, are each indications for fasciotomy, the anterior compartment being the most vulnerable of the four. Fasciotomy should be both timely and adequate and all compartments can be decompressed using two incisions.[47] Viable adjacent tissue is used for vessel

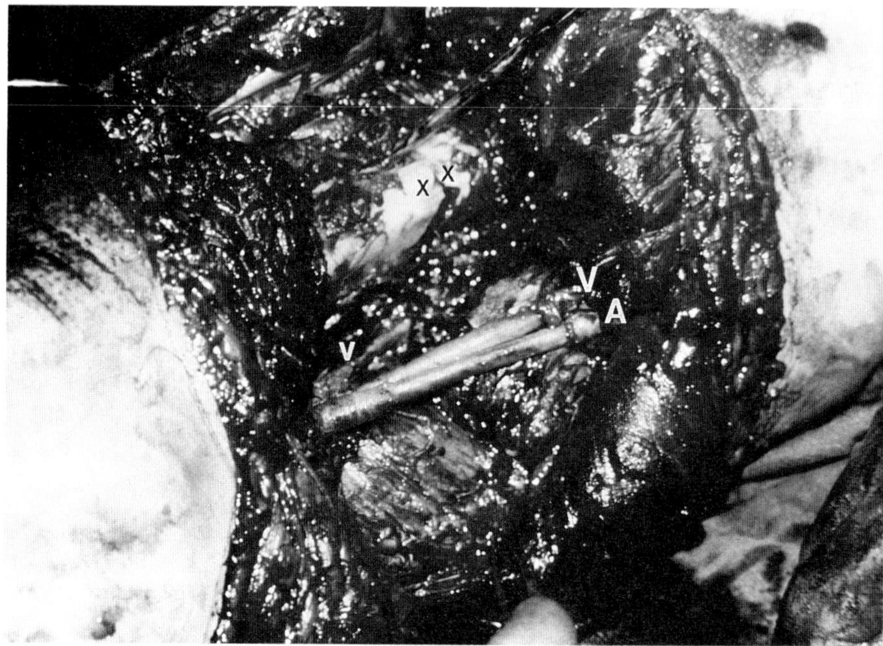

Fig. 18.4 After stabilization of the fracture (XX), interposed vein grafts restore flow through superficial femoral artery (A) and vein (V) and the deep femoral vein (v). Vessel and bony cover followed. (Reproduced from reference 22 with permission.)

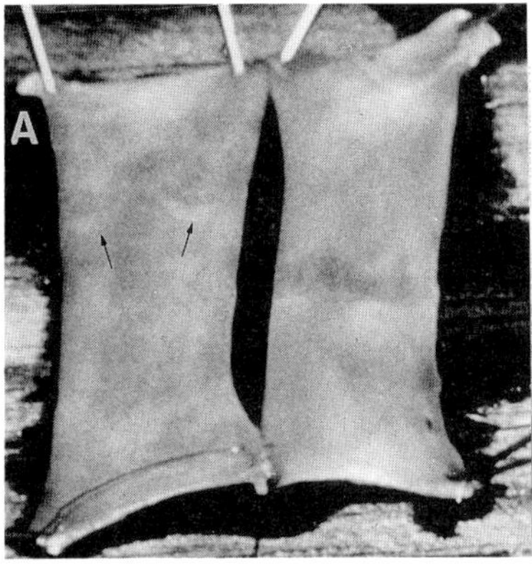

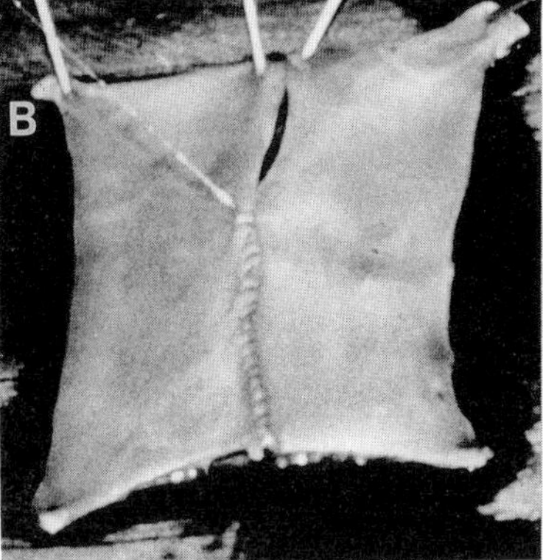

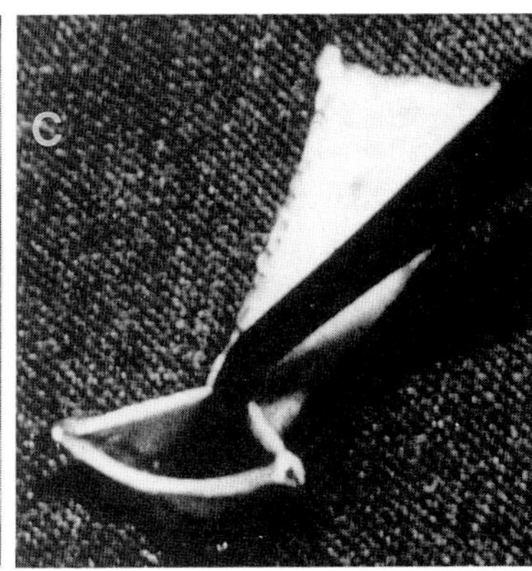

Fig. 18.5 Steps in the construction of a panel compound vein graft. (a) Two segments are opened longitudinally and pinned down, the flow surface resting on heparinized saline irrigant. Attachments of excised valves (arrows) are just visible through the wall. (b) First everting suture line in progress. (c) On completion of the second suture line the result, observed end-on, is a graft of larger calibre. (Reproduced from reference 46 with permission.)

cover, to eliminate dead space and to prevent dessication of a graft; but if tissue loss has been excessive, freed but well-vascularized sartorius or gracilis muscle may be swung over to ensheath the graft. Alternatively, plastic-surgery skills are brought in to construct a vascularized musculocutaneous flap. In a closed injury, primary suture is satisfactory, but in contaminated wounds delayed suture should be the norm, if necessary after inspections and further debridement.

The disciplined sequence of key steps in the operative care of complex limb vascular injury based on the use of shunts is illustrated in a simple alliterative aide mémoire (Fig. 18.6). The validity of this systematic approach is borne out by years of surgical practice,[17–27] the dividends of which have been a low complication rate and early discharge from hospital.

Postoperative care

A mannitol infusion may assist in lowering compartmental hypertension, in part by accelerating the inactivation of oxygen-derived free radicals and thereby limiting reperfusion injury. Adequate fluid replacement and low-dose heparin encourage graft patency, tissue perfusion and good healing. Vigilance is essential in monitoring peripheral flow and, if graft occlusion is suspected, angiography followed by urgent re-exploration may be necesary. The weaknesses of vascular repair techniques which result in graft failure include inadequate excision of damaged vessel, use of vein grafts which are too long or of small calibre, and commonly anastomotic defects such as poor intimal coaptation, constriction and tension.

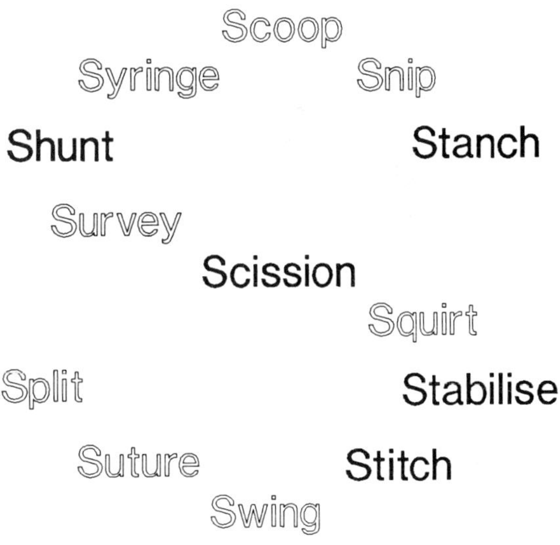

Fig. 18.6 Aide-mémoire for the Sequence of Steps in the operative management of complex limb vascular injury: *stanch* the bleeding, *snip* damaged ends of vessels, *scoop* out clot, *syringe* in heparinized saline, *shunt* both artery and vein, *survey* the wound and identify nerve injury, perform *scission* of non-viable soft tissue, *squirt* saline to irrigate wound, *stabilise* fractured bones, *stitch* vessel grafts, *swing* tissue for cover, *suture* the wound (delayed primary if contaminated) and, if necessary, *split* fascia to decompress muscle. (Reproduced from reference 27 with permission.)

Thoracic vascular trauma

The magnitude of battlefield injuries of the thoracic aorta and great vessels, and the time lag before treatment, contribute to a high fatality rate. In civilian practice firearm injuries,[48] even when associated with pulmonary, oesophageal and cardiac trauma, can be successfully treated by experienced surgical teams.[7,49–51] Success often depends on the first few minutes of care when a brisk but orderly routine is followed in restoring and supporting vital functions; namely, maintenance of airway, ventilation and circulatory support, insertion of chest drains and pericardiocentesis. If vital signs stabilize it is reasonable to proceed to plain X-rays and even aortography. Failure to respond to resuscitation may be due to unrelieved cardiac tamponade, myocardial contusion or intracardiac injury. Continuing haemorrhage or a major air leak demand urgent thoracotomy. As a desperate measure in the moribund patient, and if facilities exist, emergency-room thoracotomy will enable direct relief of cardiac tamponade as well as control and repair of cardiac and even vascular injuries.[52]

Sudden deceleration accidents, particularly on the road but also in air crashes and in falls from a great height,[53,54] are responsible for partial or complete tears of the thoracic aorta at the isthmus just distal to the origin of the left subclavian artery (Fig. 18.7). Fatal exsanguination occurs instantly in 10–20% of cases. Even when the tear is contained within the adventitia and overlying pleura as a haematoma and false aneurysm, 30% of untreated survivors die within 6 hours, 40% within 24 hours, 72% by 8 days, 83% by 3 weeks, 90% by 10 weeks, and a few after many years of complete stability.[53] Other common sites of rupture include the ascending aorta, just distal to the aortic valve, and the great vessels of which the innominate artery is the most vulnerable.

Thoracic aorta

If the direction and depth of a knife wound is not clear, and as the path of a bullet can be capricious, shock or haemothorax cannot be attributed specifically to the heart, lung, thoracic aorta or its branches. Bleeding into the superior mediastinum may be contained retrosternally, a bruit and peripheral pulse deficit possibly being the only clues to this serious situation. Wounds of the ascending aorta, aortic arch or great vessels can be repaired via a median sternotomy in most cases without resorting to cardiopulmonary bypass.[55,56] A left thoracotomy provides adequate access to the descending thoracic aorta.

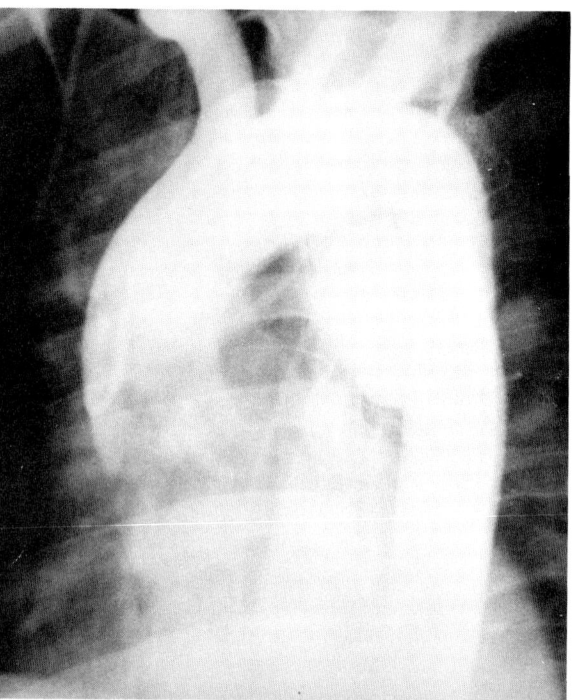

Fig. 18.7 Aortogram showing isthmic rupture of thoracic aorta sustained in a road accident, presenting as a false aneurysm. At operation a haematoma extended proximally to the aortic root and distally to the mid-descending thoracic aorta. Continuity was successfully restored with a Dacron graft. (Reproduced from reference 46 with permission.)

Clinical symptoms of disruption of the thoracic aortic isthmus are pain, cough, hoarseness, dysphagia, haemoptysis and respiratory distress. Associated physical signs may include a steering wheel bruise of the chest wall and a poor pulse and pressure in the left arm. Impending exsanguination should be suspected when high-risk signs such as prominent left haemothorax, pseudocoarctation or superior mediastinal haematoma extending above the clavicle are present. In such cases immediate thoracotomy is required, but patients still die en route to the operating theatre or during induction of anaesthesia. A plain chest X-ray film in a stable patient may reveal widening of the superior mediastinum, distortion of the aortic contour, apical 'capping' of the medial aspect of the left upper lung field by haematoma, depression of the left main bronchus or fractures of the first and second rib. CT diagnosis is quite informative, whereas aortography (Fig. 18.7), which is a more accurate diagnostic device, is potentially dangerous. A standard posterolateral thoracotomy through the fourth space provides access. While debate continues amongst advocates of partial bypass, external shunts or simple aortic clamp-and-repair in reducing the incidence of the most feared outcome of paraplegia,[57] the last of the three, expeditiously accomplished by means of a Dacron tube graft, is gratifyingly successful.

Innominate artery

Injuries of the innominate artery[50] are mainly caused by low-velocity gunshot wounds, occasionally by a sudden deceleration tear at its origin from the arch. Rarely, a tracheo-innominate arterial fistula can result from erosion caused by the tip of an improperly placed tracheostomy tube, a fatal condition unless immediate endotracheal intubation is followed by arterial repair. A median sternotomy offers adequate access for repairs of the innominate artery either by standard methods or alternatively by closing the proximal artery and taking a Dacron graft from the proximal ascending aorta.

Great veins

Penetrating injury to the great veins of the mediastinum and neck by knife or bullet[58] can cause catastrophic exsanguination. Simple lateral suture, direct anastomosis or ligation to save life are each acceptable.

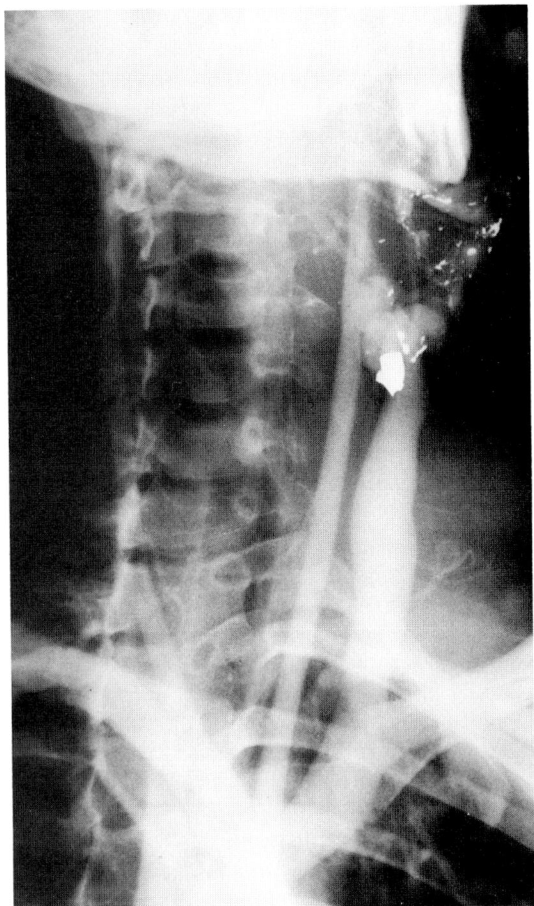

Fig. 18.8 Fragmented missile injury resulting in a carotico-jugular fistula.

Vascular trauma of the neck

Vascular injury to the neck mainly results from penetrating neck trauma by knife or missile (Fig. 18.8). Blunt trauma is rare and may remain unsuspected because external evidence of injury is usually absent. Penetrating vascular trauma may be associated with injury to the trachea, pharynx, oesophagus, superior mediastinum, lungs, spine, cranial nerves or brachial plexus. Immediate endotracheal intubation with the cuff inflated prevents extravasated blood entering the lungs. External bleeding is controlled by direct pressure and a chest drain is sometimes also necessary. Endoscopy or contrast studies to locate injury to the upper respiratory and alimentary tracts tend to be unhelpful. A nasogastric tube may pass through a tear, causing mediastinitis, and should be avoided.

In general, all penetrating wounds in the anterior triangle of the neck piercing the platysma should be explored. Operation is mandatory for severe bleeding, expanding haematoma, bloodstained sputum, escaping air from a wound or subcutaneous emphysema in the absence of pneumothorax. In some cases injury to the carotid and subclavian arteries may demand control of the great vessels through a median sternotomy.

Carotid artery

Blunt trauma to the carotid artery may be caused by a direct blow, by sudden rotation and hyperextension of the head and neck, by base-of-skull fractures, or through the classical injury of a child falling forward on a pencil held in its mouth. Injuries include dissection, pseudoaneurysm or frequently mural thrombosis which may lead eventually to stroke. The neurological sequelae of a penetrating injury proceed from the interruption of arterial flow, hypotension, hypoxic cerebral oedema and, in some patients, an inability to compensate for arrested flow due to an anomaly of the Circle of Willis. An increasing neurological deficit is associated with a progressively unfavourable prognosis and is a critical factor in deciding treatment.

Routine angiography in stable patients yields only a small number of penetrating arterial injuries. Negative angiography is reassuring in the patient who has suffered blunt trauma and who is potentially at risk of developing stroke.

Penetrating carotid injuries can be considered in three zones; below the clavicle (I), between the clavicle and angle of the mandible (II), and above the angle of the mandible (III).[59] Preliminary angiography is helpful in defining the type of injury in zones I and III. For zone II, stable patients may proceed to operation with or without angiography, but those with a neurological deficit should be operated on immediately. A CT scan is not particularly helpful in deciding whether a carotid artery repair should be deferred or not.

Fears of haemorrhagic infarction following restoration of flow to ischaemic areas of the brain have generally proved to be unfounded. The consensus of opinion favours prompt carotid thrombectomy and repair as long as prograde flow is seen to be present, regardless of neurological deficit or shock.[60] If the internal jugular vein is torn, sometimes in association with a carotico-jugular fistula (Fig. 18.8), swift head-down tilt is necessary to prevent air embolism. It is advisable to use an indwelling carotid shunt particularly if systemic pressure is low.[12–14]

Standard methods of vascular repair are employed, with the additional option of replacing a damaged and possibly diseased proximal internal carotid by a distally detached external carotid artery.

Subclavian artery

Subclavian vessels, protected skeletally by sternum and clavicle, are usually injured by severe blunt trauma,[8,9,12,51] which also injures the adjacent brachial plexus.[61] A penetrating injury may present with torrential haemorrhage externally or into the chest, abnormal arm pulses, nerve injury and fractures. Angiography should be reserved for the stable patient.

The first part of the right subclavian artery can be exposed by excising the medial third of the clavicle. The first part of the left subclavian is relatively inaccessible and is best approached by the 'open book' or 'trapdoor' approach which combines a median sternotomy, a left supraclavicular incision, a third-space left anterior thoracotomy and division of the mid-clavicle.[62] The second and third parts of either subclavian are exposed through a supraclavicular incision and, given a rich collateral circulation, will tolerate ligation.

Tissue cover for vascular repair is scanty and, although replacement with PTFE grafts has been successful,[51] caution is required in potentially contaminated wounds.

Vertebral artery

The position of the vertebral artery renders it less vulnerable to penetrating trauma. In closed head and neck injuries it may be damaged in its course up to the sixth cervical vertebra, above which it lies beyond the scope of the vascular surgeon. Bleeding is unusual and injuries often progress to thrombosis, aneurysm or arteriovenous fistula formation. Aplasia of the contralateral vertebral artery must first be excluded by angiography before the injured artery is either ligated or subjected to percutaneous transluminal embolisation.

Upper limb vascular trauma

Penetrating upper-limb vascular trauma occurs six times more commonly in military than in civilian practice[7–9] and blunt trauma is much less commonly observed.[63]

Axillary artery

In general, the rich network around the shoulder girdle allows the upper limb to tolerate axillary artery injury. Concomitant injury to elements of the brachial plexus remain an obstacle in rehabilitation. Dislocations of the shoulder, fractures of the humeral neck and even clavicle can injure the axillary artery (Fig. 18.9). Angiography is an essential prelude to operative treatment.

In penetrating injuries of the first part of the axillary artery, from which bleeding may be profuse, it is wise to control the subclavian artery above the clavicle. A classical infraclavicular and deltopectoral groove incision, dividing the tendons of the pectoralis major and minor in exsanguinating situations, gives good access. Care should be taken to protect surrounding nerves during vascular repair.

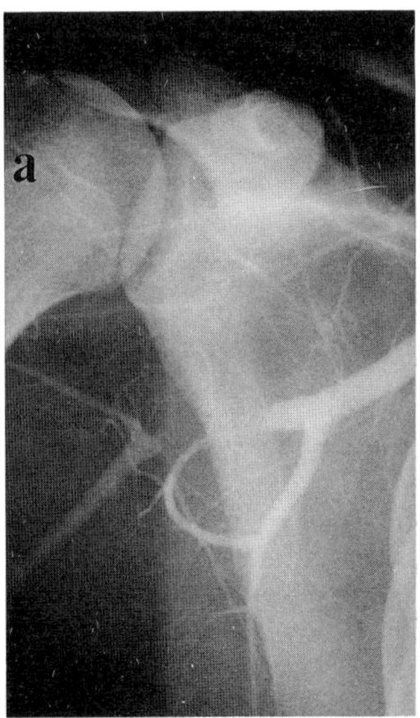

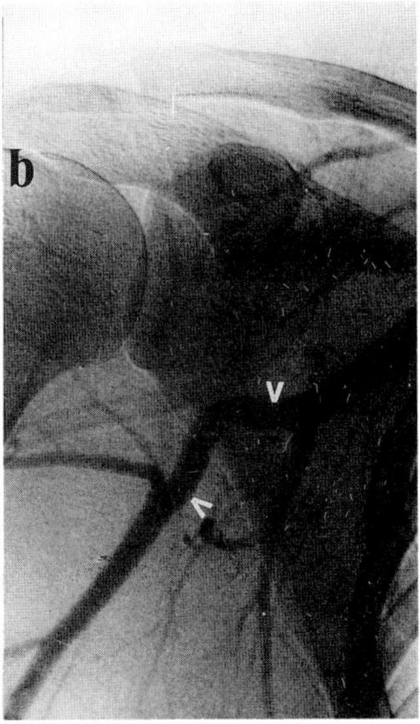

Fig. 18.9 (a) Angiogram of a forestry worker struck on his right shoulder by a falling tree, injuring his axillary artery, brachial plexus and humerus. The angiogram shows the transected artery. (b) This postoperative angiogram shows the interposed graft (between the arrows) with enough laxity to permit safe abduction of the arm. (Reproduced from reference 46 with permission.)

Brachial artery

The brachial artery is vulnerable to injuries of violence, in association with supracondylar humeral fractures in the young, and also during catheterization procedures. Despite a fair collateral circulation, the complacent diagnosis of 'spasm' of the brachial artery may have long-term sequelae such as Volkmann's ischaemic contracture and suboptimal limb growth. Thrombectomy and meticulous repair are necessary and the chances of success diminish with each additional attempt. While the use of intraluminal shunts can be advantageous,[25,26] open flexor and extensor fasciotomy extended into the hand may be necessary to save the limb. Injuries to the radial and ulnar arteries, typically self-inflicted or caused by a pressure monitoring catheter, are unimportant as long as patency of one of the two can be assured by Allen's test.

Vascular trauma of the abdomen

The numbers of patients admitted with penetrating abdominal vascular injury on the battlefield are much smaller than in civilian practice, reflecting both the wounding power of the weapons responsible and the speed of evacuation. Even after admission, mortality rates for aortic and caval injury range from 30 to 70%.[18,64] The incidence of blunt injury to the abdominal aorta, ranging from contusion to transverse rupture, may conceivably rise with the increasing use of car seat-belts.[65]

A 'scoop and run' approach, attending to airway, ventilation and volume replacement en route to hospital for early operation, should be the objective. The MAST or G-suit applied slowly or unskillfully wastes vital time when a hospital is in close proximity. Intrathoracic injuries are also frequently present in gunshot wounds of the abdomen,[14] and so the chest, back and perineum must be examined. In closed injuries, the presence of abrasions and bruises, abdominal distension and shock suggest injury of an underlying solid organ or major vessel trunk. Immediate laparotomy is necessary before the situation becomes irretrievable. In a few well-equipped trauma centres, emergency-room thoracotomy to clamp the aorta, when the patient is obviously moribund or developing hypovolaemic cardiac arrest, has been successful in improving myocardial and cerebral perfusion and in reducing abdominal losses.[66,67]

The sequence following midline laparotomy should be rapid subdiaphragmatic aortic compression to stop torrential bleeding, delivery of the bowel outside the abdominal cavity, and rapid evacuation of blood and clot using packs. This will allow identification of the main sites of injury such as the liver, spleen, mesentery, hollow viscera and the main vasculature. A contained retroperitoneal haematoma should not be disturbed until control of the vessel trunks is complete.

Abdominal aorta

The aorta may have bled into the abdominal cavity or the losses may be contained in a tense expanding retroperitoneal haematoma. Access to the infrarenal aortic injury is quite straightforward. An injury in the vicinity of the right renal artery is best approached by reflecting the right colon and duodenum to the left; damage close to the left renal artery or suprarenally is exposed by displacing the left colon, spleen and pancreas to the right.[68,69] Puncture wounds and lacerations are easily closed, and in through-and-through wounds the anterior opening is extended for access to the posterior wall. If the aortic segment is grossly disrupted a Dacron tube graft is interposed. However, this is an option which is precluded in the presence of faecal contamination; in such a case the aortic ends should be oversewn and obliterated and a temporary extra-anatomic axillofemoral bypass constructed.

Iliac artery

Penetrating iliac artery injuries carry a mortality of 30–40%, particularly when other abdominal vascular injuries are present.[68,70,71] Unlike with aortic trauma, which may be held in check retroperitoneally, iliac artery injuries bleed freely and often fatally into the abdomen. Access through a midline incision and standard methods of repair are used, making sure that at least one internal iliac artery is preserved. If there is evidence of faecal contamination, the ends of the severed iliac artery are ligated and an extra-anatomic femorofemoral crossover bypass constructed.

Renal artery

The impression that penetrating trauma was responsible for most renal artery injuries has altered with the increasing recognition of tears, thrombosis and even complete avulsion of the renal artery, particularly on the left side, as a consequence of deceleration injury (Fig. 18.10). A history of trauma associated with flank pain and haematuria or an unidentifiable kidney on intravenous urography makes angiography mandatory, partly to establish if there is a functioning opposite kidney.

The dissection forces of a haematoma under pressure facilitate access to the renal artery. The viability of the kidney may be preserved by minimal flow through collaterals, and if the renal vein is still intact, arterial repair is worthwhile. Nephrectomy is preferable and may indeed be inevitable in the multiply injured and shocked patient, but if it is the only kidney at least part of it should be autotransplanted into the ipsilateral iliac fossa.

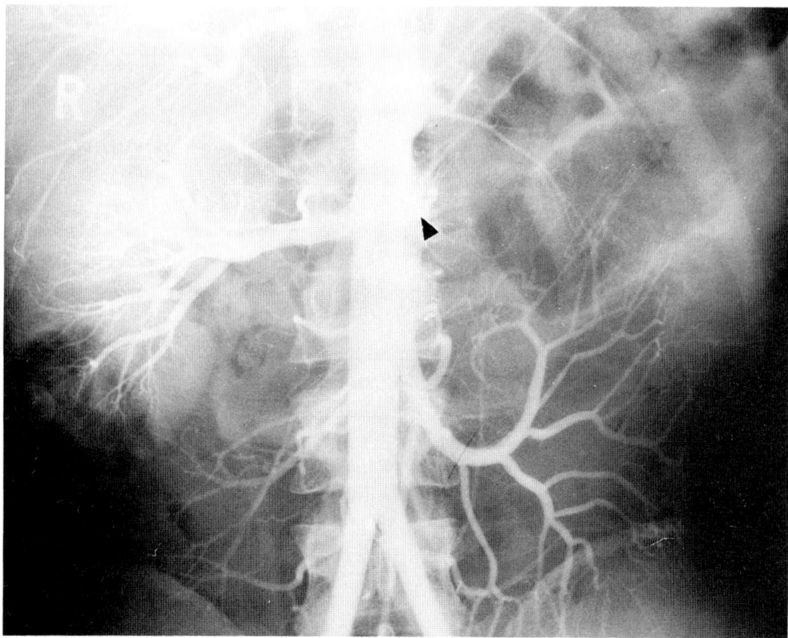

Fig. 18.10 A road accident victim with injuries involving spleen, pancreas and left kidney. The angiogram shows a stump of left renal artery (arrow) caused by near-avulsion of the kidney. (Reproduced from reference 46 with permission.)

Mesenteric arteries

Injuries to the coeliac and mesenteric arteries, well documented in military[4] and in civilian practice,[7,8,68,72,73] pose unique problems of exposure, control of bleeding, prevention of irreversible gut ischaemia and the management of concurrent damage to the pancreas and other organs. After clamping the aorta below the diaphragm the coeliac artery is exposed through the gastrohepatic omentum. The hepatic artery, once considered indispensible for liver viability, can be ligated as long as portal blood supply is intact. Fullen's anatomical classification of superior mesenteric artery injuries into three zones, taking into consideration concurrent pancreatic injury, offers an operative approach suitable to each zone.[74]

Access, either through the transverse mesocolon, or alternatively by reflecting the spleen, pancreas and left colon medially, facilitates repair and, if necessary, splenectomy and distal pancreatectomy can be carried out. Routine methods of repair are applied, but additional options include implantation of the artery into the infrarenal aorta or, preferably, the construction of an aortomesenteric bypass. If bowel survival is in doubt, a 'second-look' operation within 24 hours is advisable.

Great veins

The inferior vena cava, formed from iliac veins, receives renal and hepatic veins and is a conduit for flow not only from the entire systemic circulation below the diaphragm but also from the splanchnic bed and liver. The losses from this system can be alarming and may be reduced temporarily by clamping the aorta.

Retrohepatic caval injuries are fraught with difficulties of exposure, torrential bleeding, a risk of air embolism and a danger of cardiac arrest from clamping. A modified Schrock shunt, in the form of a chest drain passed down the right atrial appendage via a median sternotomy into the inferior vena cava down to the level of the renal veins, allows blood to ascend past the snugged and isolated section of injured cava back to the heart. The clamp tube also serves as an excellent route for direct infusion. The suprarenal cava below this level must be reconstructed either by means of a free graft of suitable length taken from the infrarenal cava, or preferably by means of a spiral compound vein graft.[25] Renal vein injuries carry a high mortality and ligation is acceptable. The infrarenal cava is exposed easily except at the confluence of the common iliac veins where bleeding cannot be easily controlled. A method which permits access to this area involves dividing the right common iliac artery temporarily and mobilizing the aortic bifurcation to the left. Severe bleeding from iliac vein injuries may respond to packing and later repair; if necessary the vessels may have to be ligated, later resulting in limb oedema.

Massive blood loss from an injured valveless mesenterico-portal system, which carries up to 60% of the cardiac output, accounts for very high mortality rates.[66,72,73,75] Bleeding may be stemmed by Pringle's manoeuvre, buying time for exposure which is achieved by reflecting the right colon and duodenum to the left. Ligation of the portal vein is generally considered unacceptable if portal hypertension is to be averted, and a host of repair techniques can be employed to restore continuity.[72] Repair of the superior mesenteric vein may prevent venous pooling, hyperaemia and possibly thrombosis and bowel infarction.

References

1. Ogilvie WH. War surgery in Africa. *Br J Surg* 1944; **31:** 313.
2. De Bakey ME, Simeone FA. Battle injuries of the arteries in World War II. *Ann Surg* 1946; **123:** 534–79.
3. Hughes CW. Arterial repair during the Korean War. *Ann Surg* 1958; **147:** 555–61.
4. Rich NM, Hughes CW. Vietnam vascular registry: preliminary report. *Surgery* 1969; **65:** 218–26.
5. Rich NM, Baugh JH, Hughes CW. Acute arterial injuries in Viet Nam: 1000 cases. *J Trauma* 1970; **10:** 359–69.
6. Morris GC, Beall AC, Roof WR, *et al.* Surgical experience with 220 acute vascular injuries in civilian practice. *Am J Surg* 1960; **99:** 775–81.
7. Drapanas T, Hewitt RL, Weichert RC, *et al.* Civilian vascular injuries: a critical appraisal of three decades of management. *Ann Surg* 1970; **172:** 351–60.
8. Perry MO, Thal ER, Shires GT. Management of arterial injuries. *Ann Surg* 1971; **173:** 403–8.
9. Smith RF, Elliot JP, Hageman JH, *et al.* Acute penetrating arterial injuries of the neck and limbs. *Arch Surg* 1974; **109:** 198–205.
10. Feliciano D, Mattox KL, Graham J, Bitondo C. Five year experience with PTFE grafts in vascular wounds. *J Trauma* 1985; **25:** 71–82.
11. Livingston RH, Wilson RI. Gunshot wounds of the limbs. *Br Med J* 1975; **1:** 667–9.
12. Barros D'Sa AAB, Hassard TH, Livingston RH, *et al.* Missile-induced vascular trauma. *Injury* 1980; **12:** 13–30.

13. Barros D'Sa AAB. Management of vascular injuries of civil strife. *Injury* 1982; **14:** 51–7.
14. Johnston GW, Barros D'Sa AAB. Injuries of civil hostilities. In: *International Medical Reviews: Surgery, Vol. 1, Trauma,* Carter DC, Polk HC (eds). London: Butterworths, 1981.
15. Archbold JAA, Barros D'Sa AAB, Morrison E. Genito-urinary tract injuries of civil hostilities. *Br J Surg* 1981; **68:** 625–31.
16. Graham ANJ, Barros D'Sa AAB. Missed arteriovenous fistulae and false aneurysms in penetrating lower limb trauma: relearning old lessons. *Injury* 1991; **22:** 179–82.
17. Barros D'Sa AAB. Missile injuries of popliteal vessels. In: *Proceedings of the XVth Congress of the Latin American Chapter of the International Cardiovascular Society,* Acapulco, 1980.
18. Barros D'Sa AAB. A decade of missile-induced vascular trauma. *Ann Roy Coll Surg Eng* 1981; **64:** 37–44.
19. Barros D'Sa AAB. Vascular injuries. In: *Lecture Notes on Trauma: 107,* Templeton J, Wilson RI (eds). Oxford: Blackwell Scientific, 1983.
20. Barros D'Sa AAB. How do we manage acute limb ischaemia due to trauma? In: *Limb Salvage and Amputation for Vascular Disease,* Greenhalgh RM, Jamieson CW, Nicolaides AN (eds). London: WB Saunders, 1988: 135–50.
21. Barros D'Sa AAB. Leading article: The rationale for arterial and venous shunting in the management of limb vascular injuries. *Eur J Vasc Surg* 1989; **3:** 471–4.
22. Barros D'Sa AAB, Moorehead RJ. Combined arterial and venous intraluminal shunting in major trauma of the lower limb. *Eur J Vasc Surg* 1989; **3:** 577–81.
23. Best B, Barros D'Sa AAB. Popliteal vessel injury caused by plastic bullets. *Injury* 1987; **18:** 428–9.
24. Elliott J, Templeton J, Barros D'Sa AAB. Combined bony and vascular limb trauma: a new approach to treatment. *J Bone Joint Surg (Br)* 1984; **66:** 281.
25. Barros D'Sa AAB. Upper and lower limb vascular trauma. In: *Vascular Surgical Techniques,* Greenhalgh RM (ed). London: Ballière Tindall, 1989: 47–65.
26. Barros D'Sa AAB. Shunting in complex lower limb trauma. In: *Emergency Vascular Surgery,* Greenhalgh RM, Hollier L (eds). London: WB Saunders, 1992: 331–44.
27. Barros D'Sa AAB. Editorial: Complex vascular and orthopaedic limb injuries. *J Bone Joint Surg (Br)* 1992; **74:** 176–8.
28. Natali J, Benhamou AC. Iatrogenic vascular injuries: a review of 125 cases excluding angiographic injuries. *J Cardiovasc Surg* 1979; **20:** 169–76.
29. Mills JL, Wiedeman IE, Robison JG, *et al.* Minimizing mortality from iatrogenic arterial injuries: the need for early recognition and prompt repair. *J Vasc Surg* 1986; **4:** 22–7.
30. Graham ANJ, Barros D'Sa AAB. Missed arteriovenous fistulae and false aneurysms in penetrating lower limb trauma: relearning old lessons. *Injury* 1991; **22:** 179–82.
31. Doty DB, Treiman RL, Rothschild PD, *et al.* Prevention of gangrene due to fractures. *Surg Gynecol Obst* 1967; **125:** 284–5.
32. Smith RF, Szilagyi DE, Elliott JP. Fracture of the long bones with arterial injury due to blunt trauma. *Arch Surg* 1969; **99:** 315–24.
33. Connolly J. Management of fractures associated with arterial injuries. *Am J Surg* 1971; **120:** 331–5.
34. Alberty RE, Goodfried G, Boyden AM. Popliteal artery injury with fracture dislocation of the knee. *Am J Surg* 1981; **142:** 36–40.
35. Sher MH. Principles in the management of arterial injuries associated with fracture/dislocation. *Ann Surg* 1975; **182:** 630–4.
36. Gustilo RB, Mendoza RM, Williams DN. Problems in the management of type III (severe) open fractures: a new classification of type III open fractures. *J Trauma* 1984; **24:** 742–6.
37. Pace PD, Tilney NL, Lesch M, *et al.* Peripheral arterial complications of intra-aortic balloon counterpulsation. *Surgery* 1977; **82:** 685–8.
38. De Saussure RL. Vascular injury coincident to disc surgery. *J Neurosurg* 1959; **16:** 222–8.
39. McCallion WA, Barros D'Sa AAB. Management of critical upper limb ischaemia long after irradiation injury of the subclavian and axillary arteries. *Br J Surg* 1991; **78:** 1136–8.
40. Benson EP. Radiation injury to large arteries. *Radiology* 1973; **106:** 195–7.
41. Granger DM, Hollwarth ME, Parks DA. Ischaemia–reperfusion injury: role of oxygen derived free radicals. *Acta Physiol Scand* 1986; Suppl 548: 47–63.
42. Snyder WH, Thal ER, Bridges RA, *et al.* The validity of normal arteriography in penetrating trauma. *Arch Surg* 1978; **113:** 424–6.
43. Sirinek KR, Gaskill HV, Dittman WI, *et al.* Exclusion angiography for patients with possible vascular injuries of the extremities: a better use of trauma centre resources. *Surgery* 1983; **94:** 599–603.
44. McCormick TM, Burch BH. Routine angiographic evaluation of neck and extremity trauma. *J Trauma* 1979; **19:** 384–7.
45. Gregory RT, Gould RJ, Peclet M, *et al.* The mangled extremity syndrome (MES): a severity grading system for multisystem injury of the extremity. *J Trauma* 1985; **25:** 1147–50.
46. Barros D'Sa AAB. Arterial injuries. In: *Arterial Surgery,* 3rd edn, Eatcott HHG (ed). London: Churchill Livingstone, 1992: 355.
47. Mubarak SJ, Owen CA. Double-incision fasciotomy of the leg for decompression in compartment syndromes. *J Bone Joint Surg (Am)* 1977; **59:** 184–7.
48. Rapaport AR, Feliciano DV, Mattox KL. An epi-

demiological profile of urban trauma in America – Houston style. *Texas Med* 1982; **78:** 44–50.
49. Hardy JD, Raju S, Neely W, *et al.* Aortic and other arterial injuries. *Ann Surg* 1975; **181:** 640–53.
50. Graham JM, Feliciano DV, Mattox KL, *et al.* Innominate vascular injury. *J Trauma* 1982; **22:** 647–55.
51. Graham JM, Feliciano DV, Mattox KL, *et al.* Management of subclavian vascular injuries. *J Trauma* 1980; **20:** 537–44.
52. Beall AC, Patrick TA, Okies JE, *et al.* Penetrating wounds of the heart: changing patterns of surgical management. *J Trauma* 1972; **12:** 468–73.
53. Parmley LF, Mattingly TW, Manion WC, *et al.* Nonpenetrating traumatic injury of the aorta. *Circulation* 1958; 1086–101.
54. Sevitt S. The mechanisms of traumatic rupture of the thoracic aorta. *Br J Surg* 1977; **64:** 166–73.
55. Billy LJ, Amato JJ, Rich NM. Aortic injuries in Vietnam. *Surgery* 1971; **70:** 385–91.
56. Symbas PN, Sehdeva JS. Penetrating wounds of the thoracic aorta. *Ann Surg* 1970; **171:** 441–50.
57. Mattox KL. Editorial: The debate goes on. *J Trauma* 1989; **29:** 1298–9.
58. Reul GJ, Beall AL, Jordan GL. Injuries of the great vessels. *Surgery* 1973; **74:** 862–74.
59. Monson DO, Saletta JD, Freeark RJ. Carotid–vertebral trauma. *J Trauma* 1969; **9:** 987–99.
60. DiVicenti FC, Weber BB. Traumatic carotid artery injuries in civilian practice. *Am Surg* 1974; **40:** 277–80.
61. Brawley RK, Murray GF, Crisler C. Management of wounds of the innominate, subclavian and axillary vessels. *Surg Gynecol Obst* 1970; **131:** 1130–40.
62. Imamoglu K, Read RC, Huebl HC. Cervicomediastinal vascular injury. *Surgery* 1967; **61:** 271–80.
63. Borman KR, Snyder WH, Weigelt JA. Civilian arterial trauma of the upper extremity: an 11-year experience in 267 patients. *Am J Surg* 1984; **148:** 796–9.
64. Halpern NB, Aldrete JS. Factors influencing mortality and morbidity from injuries to the abdominal aorta and inferior vena cava. *Am J Surg* 1979; **137:** 384–5.
65. Dajee H, Richardson ITN, Iype MO. Seat-belt aorta: acute dissection and thrombosis of the abdominal aorta. *Surgery* 1979; **85:** 263–7.
66. Sankaran S, Lucas C, Walt AJ. Thoracic aortic clamping for prophylaxis against sudden cardiac arrest during laparotomy for acute massive haemoperitoneum. *J Trauma* 1975; **15:** 290–6.
67. Baker CC, Thomas AN, Trunkey DD. The role of emergency room thoracotomy in trauma. *J Trauma* 1980; **20:** 848–55.
68. Buscaglia LC, Blaisdell FW, Lim RC. Penetrating abdominal vascular injuries. *Arch Surg* 1969; **99:** 764–9.
69. Mattox KL, McCollum WB, Jordan GL, *et al.* Management of upper abdominal vascular trauma. *Am J Surg* 1974; **128:** 823–7.
70. Mattox KL, Rea J, Ennix CL, *et al.* Penetrating injuries to the iliac arteries. *Am J Surg* 1978; **136:** 663–7.
71. Ryan W, Snyder W, Bell T. Penetrating injuries of the iliac vessels. *Am J Surg* 1982; **144:** 642–5.
72. Graham JM, Mattox KL, Beall AC. Portal venous system injuries. *J Trauma* 1978; **18:** 419–22.
73. Courcy PA, Brotman S, Oster-Granite ML, *et al.* Superior mesenteric artery and vein injuries from blunt abdominal trauma. *J Trauma* 1984; **24:** 843–5.
74. Fullen WD, Hunt J, Altemeier WA. The clinical spectrum of penetrating injury to the superior mesenteric arterial circulation. *J Trauma* 1972; **12:** 656–64.
75. Bussutil RW, Kitahama A, Cerise E, *et al.* Management of blunt and penetrating injuries to the porta hepatis. *Ann Surg* 1980; **191:** 641–8.

19

Carotid artery disease

Peter R F Bell

The importance of lesions of the internal carotid artery in the neck as a cause of strokes has been recognized for a long time.[1] The carotid artery can be affected by a variety of pathological processes, by far the commonest being stenosis of the origin of the internal carotid artery. Rarely the vessel can also become aneurysmal[2] and can kink or coil,[3] producing similar symptoms requiring the attention of the vascular surgeon.

Carotid artery stenosis

For some years there has been considerable controversy about the correct treatment of patients with carotid artery stenosis, and particularly the place of operation.[4] The escalation in the number of operations for this problem, particularly in the USA, and the suspicion that surgery was actually causing strokes, led to the construction of multicentre trials, two examples being the European trial[5] and the NASCET study.[6] The European trial has now conclusively shown that operation is the treatment of choice under certain circumstances and the American study has produced similar results.

If patients are symptomatic then the likelihood of an ipsilateral stroke in the subsequent three years is much higher if they are treated by medical means such as aspirin than by operation, provided the stenosis is greater than 70%. If the stenosis is less than 30% operation is not indicated unless there are special reasons such as continuing TIAs. Management when the stenosis is between 30% and 70% remains uncertain until further results are available. If, however, the lesion progresses or remains symptomatic then it should probably be operated on. For asymptomatic lesions the problem remains unresolved and the risk of a patient developing a stroke with an asymptomatic lesion is of the order of 2% per annum,[7] which means that unless the stroke rate for interventional surgery is much less than this an advantage cannot be claimed. There may be some patients with an asymptomatic lesion where operation is indicated. One group, for example, may be those where progression of the stenosis towards 80% occurs,[8] and another when a coronary artery bypass graft is proposed.[9]

With these points in mind, when should we operate on patients with carotid artery stenosis, and what should we do in the way of investigations prior to treatment?

Pathophysiology

Although the eventual effect of a stenosis is occlusion, and occlusion is often accompanied by a stroke, it is also the case that this event can be silent. Most of the available evidence suggests that symptoms from carotid artery stenosis are embolic[10] and caused by loose material from the plaque in the internal carotid artery. The evidence for this includes the relative inability to find a cohort of symptomatic patients with cerebral hypoperfusion, the presence of infarcts in the brain on CT scanning in the absence of occlusion, and the correlation between patients with symptoms and plaque morphology on duplex scanning.[11] Other evidence includes the relative lack of symptoms in patients who have a re-stenosis after operation,[12] which is often smooth and does not usually contain atheromatous debris in the lumen of the artery, and the appearance of the lesion at the time of operation (Fig. 19.1). The fact that the majority of symptoms are caused by emboli does influence the investigation, treatment and surgical management of these patients (see later). The fact that aspirin does not prevent progression to stroke is hardly surprising in view of the material which is seen within the carotid artery.

Asymptomatic presentation

Patients are often sent for an opinion because a bruit has been heard in the neck in the course of a clinical examination and symptoms are not present. It is

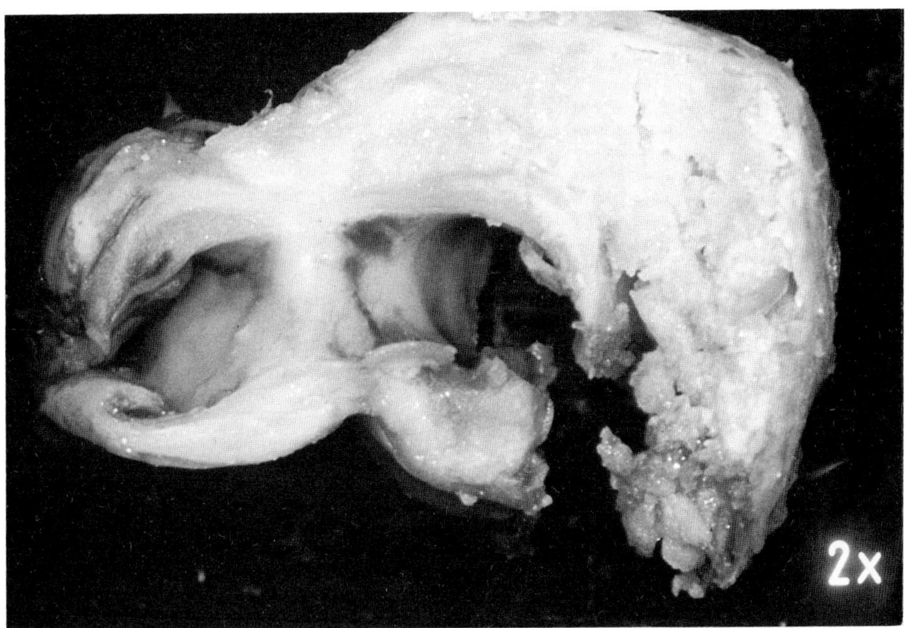

Fig. 19.1 Cross-section of the carotid artery showing stenosis, ulceration and loose material within the lumen of the vessel.

important to point out at this stage that the intensity of the bruit does not necessarily equate with the severity of the stenosis.

Symptomatic lesions

Patients will, in the classical situation, present with transient ischaemic attacks (TIAs) which result in focal symptoms. It is important that they are focal and that the patient's complaints of weakness, loss of function or sensation are on the opposite side and are transient, lasting for a few minutes or hours. These can include loss of speech, 7th nerve palsies, and changes in muscular activity or sensation. If the attack lasts for longer than this, it is referred to as a repetitive intermittent neurological deficit (RIND) and is again reversible. A third symptomatic presentation is loss of vision in the ipsilateral eye (amaurosis fugax), which will classically be described by the patient as though a curtain has been pulled across the eye. Other symptoms such as blurring of vision, deterioration of the eyesight etc. are not typical and should usually be ignored. The patient can also experience a stroke which recovers completely or partially after several weeks, and may also present with an evolving stroke where signs of focal ischaemia are present and rapidly worsen over a period of hours. Lastly, the patient can present with nonfocal symptoms which are vague and commonplace, such as dizziness, loss of memory, attacks of vagueness etc. These symptoms, however, are rarely caused by carotid stenosis unless it is severe and bilateral.

Which patients should be considered for operative treatment?

Asymptomatic bruits

At present there is no good evidence that patients with asymptomatic bruits should be operated upon routinely.[13] However, the still unreported North American trial on asymptomatic bruits has not been concluded, which suggests that there are no significant disadvantages from surgical intervention at present. It is likely, and preliminary evidence suggests, that patients with severe asymptomatic carotid lesions will probably also be candidates for surgical treatment. At present, however, these patients should usually not be operated on as the risk of stroke is less than 2% and the risk of operation is of the same order if not more in a number of surgical centres.[14]

What does one do in a situation where a patient has asymptomatic bruits and is due to have another operation such as an aortic aneurysm repair, coronary artery bypass grafting or general surgical procedures? At present there are no controlled data to suggest that these patients are more prone to intraoperative stroke than patients without severe stenosis.[15] Most reports are anecdotal, and my own practice is not to operate on such patients except when they are having a coronary artery bypass graft done. The reason for this is the undoubtedly high risk of stroke during CABG procedures in such patients, being as high as 20% in those with bilateral disease.[9] Again, however, a controlled study has not been done and should be before a definitive statement can be made. As the danger of death from coronary thrombosis is high in these patients, my practice is to undertake carotid endarterectomy synchronously with the CABG graft. The advantage of this approach is that, should the patient get into trouble, bypass can be started immediately. This policy has been safe in our hands with a permanent stroke rate of <3% in over 50 cases. Others, however, prefer to stage the operations and deal with the coronary arteries first and the carotids second, or vice versa. If a patient is to have a CABG graft and presents with carotid stenosis, if the stenosis is over 70% and is unilateral it should be dealt with. Any stenosis less than this should be left alone, and in patients with bilateral stenoses of over 75% I tend to operate on the dominant side. Again these is no evidence to support these views and trials are needed.

Another group of patients with asymptomatic bruits who may require operation are those who on repeated investigation show progression of the stenosis towards 80%. In these patients the literature suggests that there is a higher stroke rate,[8] but again the studies were not controlled.

Symptomatic presentation

Patients who present with definite focal symptoms such as a TIA, RIND, amaurosis fugax or a completed stroke should have a carotid endarterectomy provided that the stenosis is greater than 70%. If the stenosis is less than this then conservative treatment (aspirin 75 or 150 mg daily) should be offered in the first instance unless the attacks are repeated. In the case of a stroke, where the vessel is totally occluded no further treatment is possible or required but the other side should be examined carefully. If, however, the vessel is not occluded, then at least 3 months should be allowed to pass before operation, as early revascularization may cause bleeding into the infarct which can make matters worse.

For evolving strokes the mortality and morbidity are high, but recent evidence suggests that these should be operated on as aggressive treatment gives better results than conservative treatment.[16] Timing the operation for these patients is difficult, but if the stroke appears to be progressing and if the duplex scan shows thrombus to be present, urgent intervention is indicated.

For those patients with vague nonfocal symptoms such as dizzy attacks, loss of memory etc., the question of surgery is controversial. If, however, the patient has bilateral carotid disease along with vertebral stenoses, it may be acceptable to deal with the carotid stenosis on one or other side to alleviate the symptoms, although this is rarely needed, and there are few data to support this approach.

Investigation

Having decided which patients should be operated upon (a clinical decision) the next stage is to decide which investigations should be done. At present a duplex scan is undoubtedly the best way of assessing carotid stenosis, because the scan not only provides an accurate measurement of the degree of stenosis but will also demonstrate the morphology of the lesion. As mentioned previously, smooth concentric calcified lesions are probably fairly benign (Fig. 19.2), whereas lesions with soft material in them and ulceration are certainly more dangerous (Fig. 19.3).[11] A colour duplex scan does not provide much greater information but is more useful for defining complete occlusion which can sometimes be missed or falsely diagnosed with the black and white machine. Colour duplex scanning can also demonstrate lesions such as a carotid stump syndrome,[17] where thrombus from an occluded carotid artery embolises retrogradely through external carotid collaterals into the brain. Duplex techniques have now reached the state of sophistication where it is also possible to

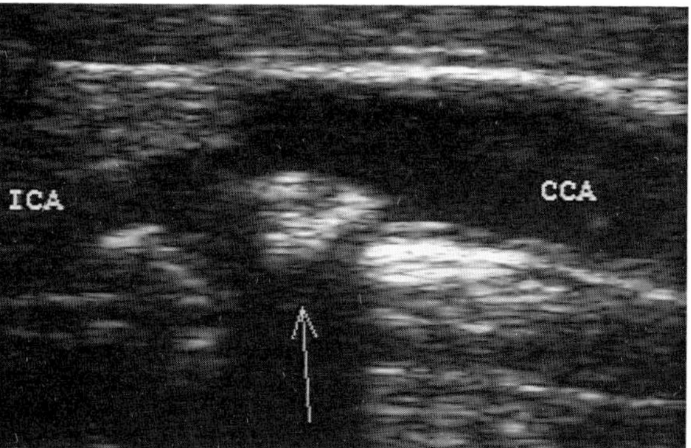

Fig. 19.2 Duplex scan showing echo-dense calcified plaque, with sonic shadow under it.

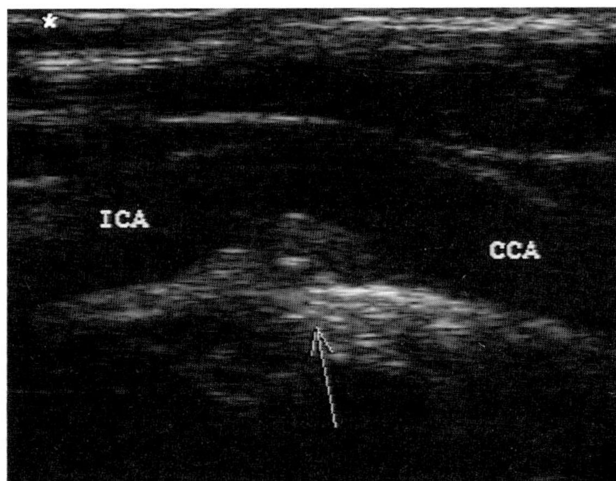

Fig. 19.3 Duplex scan showing echo-lucent stenosis.

diagnose proximal damped flow and disease in the common carotid artery along with more distal internal carotid disease.

Having obtained a good duplex view of the carotid vessels and the morphology of the plaque, is it necessary to proceed to an angiogram? An angiogram is known to be dangerous,[18] but the risks are getting smaller with arch arteriography, DSA and MRI being more commonly used. There are a number of publications which suggest that a duplex scan alone is all that is needed prior to operation;[19,20] but there are undoubtedly cases where the duplex scan does not show the extent of the disease, particularly in the common carotid artery, where occasionally the disease can extend into the aortic arch making the problem almost inoperable. The question, therefore, of angiography being necessary or not remains unresolved. Most surgeons plough a middle course and use duplex alone in most cases, adding angiography if there is any suspicion of proximal or distal disease. If a patient is to have an operation and has had symptoms, then a CT scan of the brain should also be done to exclude other causes of focal symptoms. If this is not done an occasional cerebral tumour will be missed.

After the diagnosis has been made and a decision to operate taken, my own practice is to give the patient aspirin up to the time of the operation, but others feel this leads to peroperative bleeding and prefer not give it.

The operation for carotid artery stenosis

Carotid artery stenosis is a good marker for coronary artery disease and death from myocardial infarction.[21] It is therefore reasonable that these patients should have an ECG and possibly an exercise ECG before operation. In any case where there is doubt they should have a cardiac opinion and even angiography to decide whether they should have a synchronous CABG graft performed. Blood should be cross-matched although transfusion is rarely necessary in these patients.

Before the operation patients must be carefully told about the risks involved. They must be given details of the likelihood of stroke without an operation, and also clearly made to understand that surgery involves a risk of causing a stroke (although the risk is much less). It is particularly important that the surgeon makes it his business to ensure that the relatives are also aware of these risks.

There are a number of controversies surrounding the procedure itself. One of these is whether general or local anaesthesia should be used. Advocates of local anaesthesia[22] claim that it allows selection for shunting and is safer, but there are no data to support this. Proponents of general anaesthesia point out that this allows better brain blood flow and that if isoflurane is used cerebral blood flow is improved.[23] For these reasons I prefer to use general anaesthesia. Antibiotics are not usually necessary unless one is using a synthetic patch, when a single dose of a cephalosporin should be given. The usefulness of other types of pharmacotherapy is uncertain, but steroids may reduce cerebral oedema in the event of ischaemia. Other agents which protect against ischaemia will undoubtedly be available in the future.

The other area of controversy is whether to shunt the patient during the operation. My own view is that, because none of the techniques available for intraoperative monitoring of cerebral function is foolproof, a shunt should be inserted in all cases. A variety of shunts are available and my own preference is the Pruitt (Fig. 19.4), because it is easier to retain in place and allows proximal and distal extension of the carotid incision if necessary. If the surgeon is to use selective shunting then some form of monitoring must be used, and this can either be EEG,[24] stump pressure measurement[25] or the use of sensory evoked potential.[26] More recently, transcranial Doppler[27] has been used for this purpose and is particularly useful to follow shunt flow (Fig. 19.5). It ensures that the surgeon is aware if the shunt stops working for any reason.

Technical aspects

The patient is placed on his or her back with a

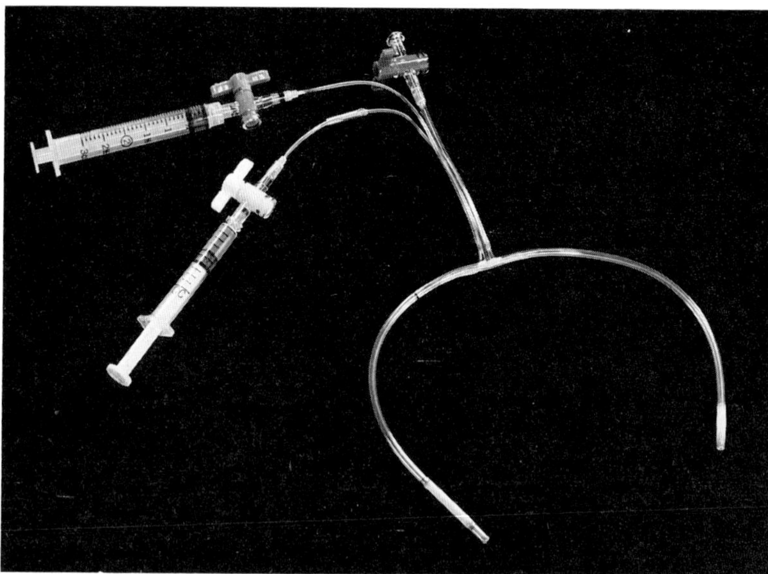

Fig. 19.4 A Pruitt shunt which is kept in place by inflating the balloons at each end.

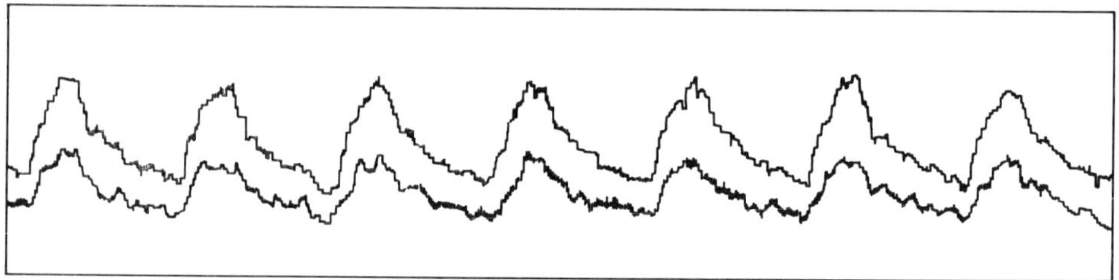

Fig. 19.5 Velocity curve from middle cerebral artery obtained by transcranial Doppler showing a good velocity prior to clamping.

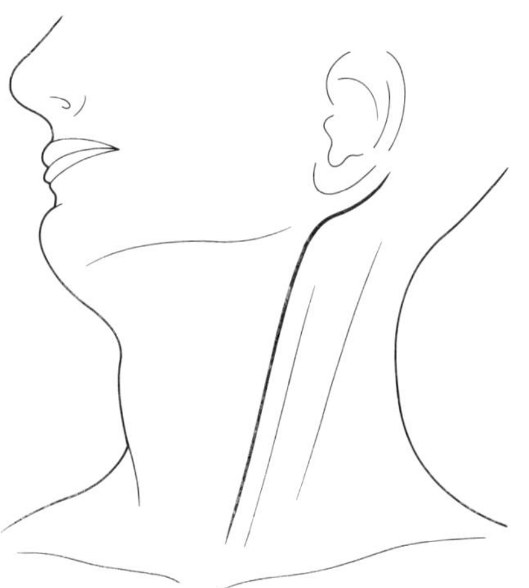

Fig. 19.6 The incision used for carotid endarterectomy.

sandbag under the shoulders and a ring under the head which is turned slightly away from the side of the operation. An incision is made along the anterior border of the sternomastoid, curving slightly posteriorly at the upper end (Fig. 19.6) and the artery exposed after dividing the fascia to reveal the internal jugular vein. At this point the anterior facial vein is doubly ligated and divided and the carotid artery should then be visible. The surgeon should be careful not to disturb the bifurcation area, and the dissection should be well away from this point or loose material can be disturbed and embolise.

The external carotid artery is encircled carefully with a sling and the internal carotid similarly encircled after careful dissection. When this has been done and a little traction placed on the sling, the 12th nerve will be seen crossing the carotid vessels (Fig. 19.7); this must be carefully preserved. The patient

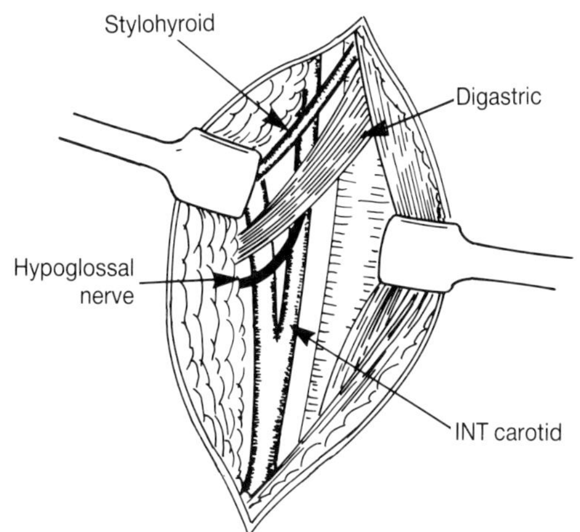

Fig. 19.7 Exposure of the carotid artery.

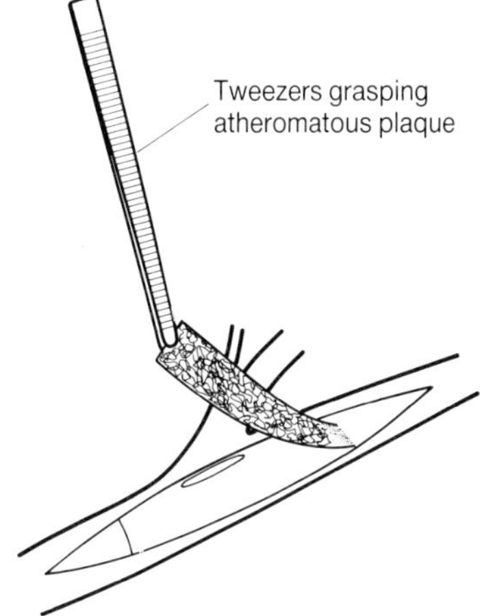

Fig. 19.8 The plaque has been divided proximally and stripped distally to the point where it becomes very thin.

is then given 5000 units of heparin and clamps used to occlude the common carotid artery first and the internal carotid second, well beyond the stenosis. The best clamps for this are the atraumatic Dardik type. The vessel should be opened longitudinally, care being taken not to damage the posterior wall of the artery. The incision is extended to normal carotid artery above and below and any debris washed out with heparinized saline.

A Pruitt shunt is now inserted, placing the proximal balloon first and inflating it. All air is carefully flushed out and the distal end inserted into the internal carotid artery. The distal balloon should not be inflated too much otherwise flow will be reduced. A transcranial Doppler will allow the sequence of events to be followed easily and ensure that the shunt is working.

The endarterectomy is then performed, being careful to get into the right layer. If difficulty is experienced, a stay suture inserted into the adventitia will be helpful. The intima at the proximal end is divided obliquely with a scalpel to leave a bevelled edge of intima in the external carotid artery. When the upward extent of the lesion has been reached the intima usually becomes very thin and should be divided with fine scissors transversely and peeled off in a circular fashion (Fig. 19.8). The atheroma in the external carotid artery is then grasped with a pair of artery forceps and the atheroma pulled out, everting the artery and allowing the thickened area to be divided distally. When this has all been done attention should be paid to the distal area of intima in the internal carotid; if there is any doubt at all that this is not adherent to the muscular wall, sutures should be inserted (Fig. 19.9), with the knot tied on the outside to secure the distal edge so avoiding problems when the circulation is restored. The same applies to the proximal edge, and any area which may form a nidus for thrombus formation should be stitched down. It is helpful to use a loupe for this part of the procedure; a 3.5 magnification loupe, which allows a clear view of the entire segment and ensures that the operator can see and remove every last vestige of atheromatous material, is appropriate. Again, strips of retained material are best removed by stripping in a radial fashion. When this has been done it is wise to inject saline forcibly along the endarterectomized segment of artery to see if there is any other loose tissue present which needs to be removed.

Next a decision must be made about closing the artery. Recent evidence has shown that by using a patch to close the vessel the incidence of re-stenosis in the long term is much lower.[28] At present, either long saphenous vein or a piece of synthetic material can be used to patch the artery, but no controlled

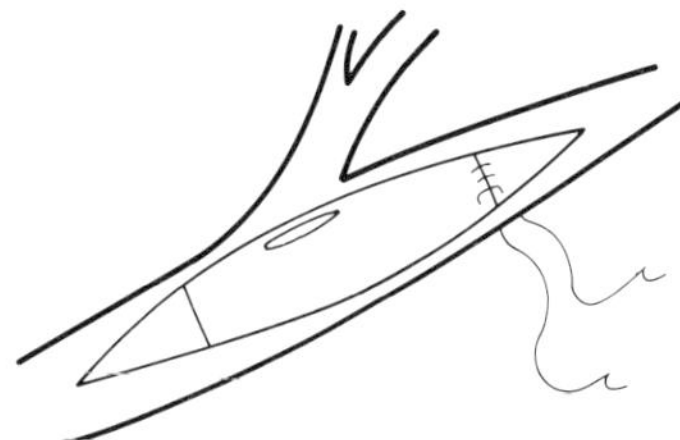

Fig. 19.9 The distal layer of intima being stitched down with interrupted sutures.

studies are available to suggest which of these should be used. It has been suggested that if the saphenous vein is used it should be taken from the upper end of the saphenous vein and not from the ankle, as the latter has been known to rupture and is weaker than the proximal vein.[29] If the vessel is large or if a patch is being used, the arteriotomy should be closed with continuous 6/0 Prolene. The sutures should go around each end of the patch and finish in the middle of one side (Fig. 19.10).

The shunt is then removed after deflating the balloons and the clamps reapplied, care being taken to ensure that all air is removed from the artery by allowing back-bleeding to fill the vessel. When suturing has been completed the internal carotid artery should be clamped at the bifurcation, the proximal clamp released and blood allowed to flow first of all into the external carotid artery in case emboli are present. Haemostasis can usually be secured by pressing some haemostatic foam over the suture line.

Most surgeons do nothing further at this stage, but others suggest that assessment of the operation using intraoperative arteriography,[30] duplex scanning or Doppler waveform analysis should be used to look for technical faults. If any are found the arteriotomy should be opened and these should be dealt with. Unfortunately there is no evidence to prove that this is necessary, or indeed to suggest which patients should be reopened. Because these patients tend to bleed, a drain should be inserted and the wound closed in layers.

Postoperative problems

The most obvious one is a stroke. If this occurs it will either be apparent when the patient wakes from the anaesthetic or will appear in the first 48 hours postoperatively. If it occurs immediately on waking or during the first few minutes or hours, the patient should be returned to the operating theatre and the carotid artery explored and an embolectomy performed to remove any clot that may be present and any defects corrected. If no problem is found then the patient should be given steroids for 24 hours to reduce cerebral oedema. If the problem occurs later, a duplex scan should be used to ensure that the carotid is still patent (which it usually will be) and a CT scan done to look for an infarct. If the vessel is for some reason thrombosed it should be re-explored. Some patients bleed from the neck wound, but this is rare and if it does occur the bleeding should be stopped by re-exploration. The 10th and 12th cranial nerves can sometimes be damaged and injury to the 9th nerve can occur in a small percentage of cases; however, these usually recover spontaneously.[31] Care should be taken to avoid serious fluctuations in blood pressure in the early postoperative period. Inadvertent damage to cutaneous nerves around the neck can lead to irritating areas of numbness postoperatively.

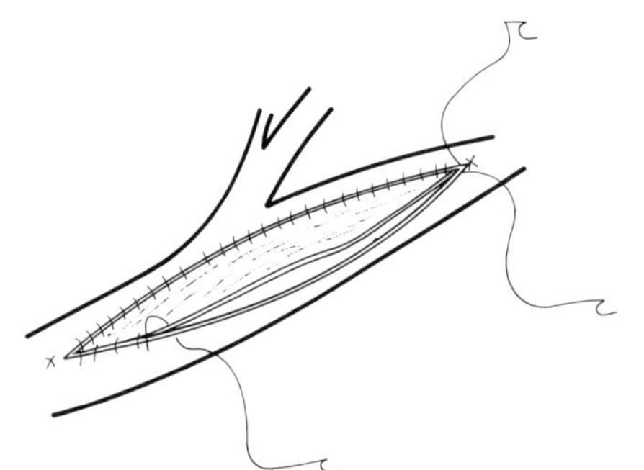

Fig. 19.10 The arteriotomy is closed with a patch of saphenous vein, Dacron or PTFE.

Follow-up

Patients should be followed-up regularly in the first year and duplex scans performed at these times to look for a re-stenosis. There is no real reason for long-term follow-up unless symptoms recur.

The results of carotid endarterectomy are now excellent, with a stroke rate in most large series of less than 2%.[32] There is controversy about who should do these operations and it is generally the view that an endarterectomy should not be done by surgeons doing the occasional procedure. Exactly how many operations a surgeon should do to remain proficient remains a matter for discussion, but there is evidence to show that the results are surgeon dependent. The two carotid trials have shown that the results are durable and the operation does reduce ipsilateral strokes.[5,6]

Angioplasty

Angioplasty is being used by some centres to treat carotid stenosis.[33] However, there is no evidence to suggest that this is the right thing to do. The fact that these lesions are mostly embolic would in fact suggest that angioplasty is dangerous, and it would seem to be difficult to improve on existing surgical results. However, angioplasty will no doubt continue to be used in some of these patients and its place may well be in those who have a smooth stenosis with hypoperfusion.

Carotid aneurysms

These are rare and are usually discovered because of a swelling in the neck (Fig. 19.11) or because of TIAs. They are dangerous lesions and should be resected before they embolise. The best treatment is to remove them, insert a shunt and place a graft of vein or artificial material such as Dacron or PTFE[34] to bridge the gap.

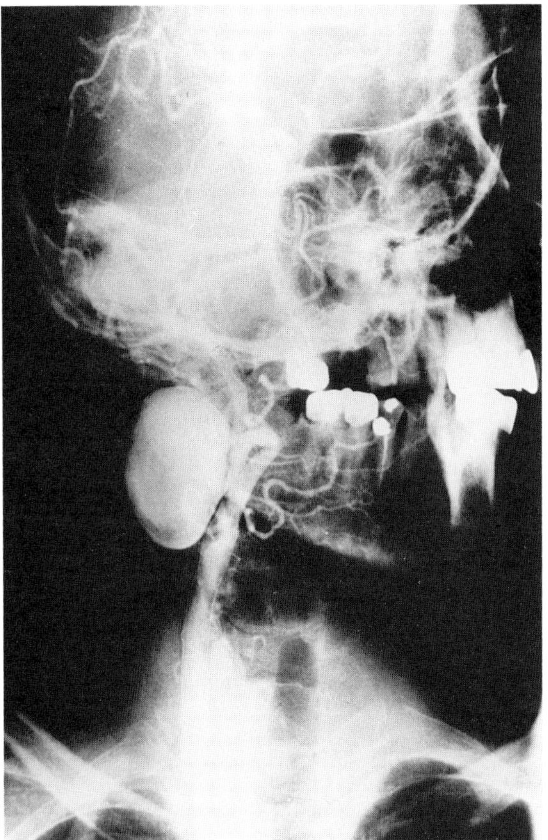

Fig. 19.11 Angiogram showing a large carotid artery aneurysm.

Kinking and coiling

Kinking and coiling of the arteries is commonly seen incidentally (Fig. 19.12) and should not be assumed to be the cause of vague symptoms unless these can be reproduced by a kink occurring during angiography.[35] If they are found, and if they are proved to be causing symptoms, they can be dealt with by shortening the artery in a variety of ways or by removing the excess artery causing the coil and reanastomosing it. However, there is no controlled evidence available and I doubt whether these lesions really cause many problems. They should be left alone in most cases.

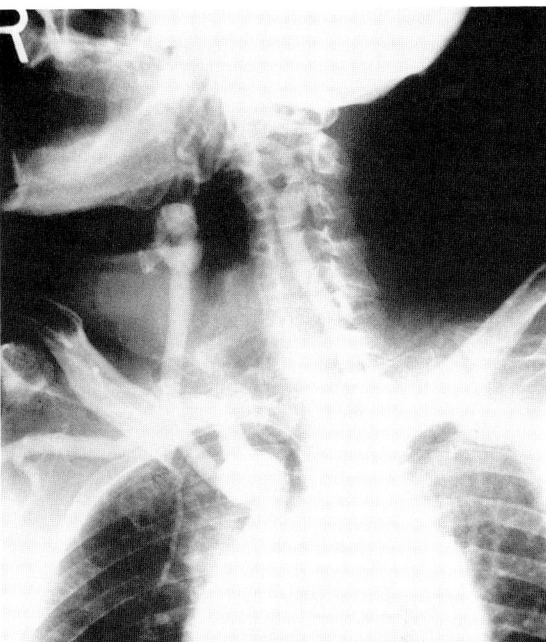

Fig. 19.12 A coiled carotid artery.

Carotid body tumours

Tumours of the carotid body are rare but should be remembered as a cause of a painless lump in the neck over the carotid artery.[36] They are very vascular and should be investigated by duplex scanning, angiography and isotope scanning. Most of them can be removed by close dissection of the carotid vessels, but a minority will need excision and carotid artery grafting. They are of low malignancy and grow slowly to a large size. A swelling over the carotid artery must not be biopsied or excised by a junior surgeon unaware of the possibility of a carotid body tumour, otherwise tragedies will occur.

Conclusions

Carotid artery stenosis is a very common and serious problem. It should be operated on, by experienced surgeons, in patients who are symptomatic and have a stenosis of greater than 70%. If this is done it should be possible to achieve excellent results with very low stroke rates of less than 2%. Management of asymptomatic lesions remains unresolved.

References

1. Hass WK, Fields WS, North R, *et al.* Joint study of extra-cranial arterial occlusion. II: arteriography techniques, sites and complications. *JAMA* 1968; **203:** 961.
2. Welling RE, Taha A, Goel T, *et al.* Extra-cranial carotid artery aneurysms. *Surgery* 1983; **93:** 319.
3. Wiechowski W, Mierzecki AM. Surgical treatment of cerebrovascular insufficiency in patients with pathological elongation of the internal carotid artery. *Eur J Vasc Surg* 1988; **2:** 105.
4. Warlow C. Carotid endarterectomy – does it work? *Stroke* 1984; **15:** 1068.
5. European Carotid Surgery Trialists collaborative group. MRC European Carotid Surgery Trial: interim results for sympatomatic patients with severe [70–99%] or with mild [0–29%] carotid stenosis. *Lancet* 1991; **337:** 1235–41.
6. North American Symptomatic Carotid Endarterectomy Trial collaborators. Beneficial effect of carotid endarterectomy in symptomatic patients with high graft stenosis. *N Engl J Med* 1991; **5:** 33–9.
7. Chambers B, Norris JW. Outcome in patients with asymptomatic neck bruits. *N Engl J Med* 1986; **315:** 860.
8. Roederer GD, Langluis YE, Luslani L, *et al.* Natural history of carotid artery disease on the side contralateral to the endarterectomy. *J Vasc Surg* 1984; **1:** 62–8.
9. Barnes LW, Leibman PR, Marszalak PB, *et al.* The natural history of asymptomatic carotid disease in patients undergoing cardiovascular surgery. *Surgery* 1981; **90:** 1075.
10. Harrison MJG. In: *Pathogenesis in Transient Ischaemic Attacks*, Warlow C, Morris PJ (eds). New York: Marcel Decker, 1982: 162–73.
11. Aldoori MI, Baird RN, Al-Sam SZ, *et al.* Duplex scanning and plaque histology in cerebral ischaemia. *Eur J Vasc Surg* 1987; **1:** 159.
12. Hunter GC, Palmaz JC, Hay Ashi HH, *et al.* The etiology of symptoms in patients with recurrent carotid stenosis. *Arch Surg* 1987; **122:** 311.
13. Barnett HJM, Plum F, Walton JN. Carotid endarterectomy: an expression of concern. *Stroke* 1984; **15:** 941.
14. Fode N, Sundt TM, Robertson JT, *et al.* Multicentre retrospective review of results and complications of carotid endarterectomy. *Stroke* 1986; **17:** 370.
15. Roper AH, Wechsler LR, Wilson LS. Carotid bruit and the risk of stroke in elective surgery. *N Engl J Med* 1982; **307:** 388.
16. Greenhalgh RM, McCollum CN, Bourke BM, *et al.* Emergency carotid endarterectomy. In: *Vascular Surgical Emergencies*, Bergan J, Yao JT (eds). New York: Grune & Stratton, 1987: 139.
17. Quill DS, Wiseman SA, Carter G, *et al.* Carotid stump syndrome: a colour coded Doppler flow study. *Eur J Vasc Surg* 1989; **3:** 79–85.
18. Hankey GJ, Warlow CP, Sellar RJ. Cerebral angiographic risk in mild cerebrovascular disease. *Stroke* 1990; **21:** 209–22.
19. Goodson SF, Flanigan DP, Bishara RA, *et al.* Can carotid duplex scanning supplant arteriography in patients with focal carotid territory symptoms. *J Vasc Surg* 1987; **5:** 551.
20. Gender JW, Camparello PJ, Riles TS, *et al.* Is duplex scanning sufficient evaluation before carotid endarterectomy. *J Vasc Surg* 1989; **9:** 193.
21. Riles TS, Kopelman I, Imparato AM. Myocardial infarction follows carotid endarterectomy: A review of 683 operations. *Surgery* 1979; **85:** 249.
22. Haffner CD, Evans WE. Carotid endarterectomy with local anaesthesia: results and advantages. *J Vasc Surg* 1988; **7:** 232–9.
23. Murkin JM, Farrar JK, Tweed WA, *et al.* Cerebral blood flow, oxygen consumption and EEG during isoflurane anaesthesia. *Anaes Analg* 1986; **65:** 107.
24. Ward J, Flynn R, Kelley JT, *et al.* Electroencephalogram monitoring during carotid endarterectomy. *J Cardiovasc Surg* 1981; **22:** 127–34.
25. Beebe MW, Starr C, Slack D. Carotid artery stump pressure: its variability when measured serially. *J Cardiovasc Surg* 1989; **30:** 419–23.
26. Gentill F, Lougheed WM, Ghato H, Shichijd F. The role of intra-operative monitoring of sensory evoked potentials during cerebro-vascular surgery. In: *Advances in Surgery for Stroke*, Suzuki J (ed). Tokyo: Springer Verlag, 1988; 675–8.
27. Naylor AR, Wildsmith JAW, McClure J, *et al.* Transcranial Doppler monitoring during carotid endarterectomy. *Br J Surg* 1991; **78:** 1264–8.
28. Eikelboom BC, Ackerstaff FGA, Hoeneveld H, *et al.* Benefits of carotid patching: a randomised study. *J Vasc Surg* 1988; **7:** 240.
29. de Vries AC, Riles TS, Lamparello PJ, *et al.* Should proximal saphenous vein be used for carotid patch angioplasty: a critical study of the need for vein in subsequent operations. *Eur J Vasc Surg* 1990; **4:** 301–4.
30. Larson SR, Gaspar MR, Morius HJ, *et al.* Intraoperative arteriography in cerebrovascular surgery. In: *Cerebrovascular Insufficiency*, Bergen J, Yao JT (eds). New York: Grune & Stratton, 1983: 353.
31. Rosenbloom M, Friedman SG, Lamparello PJ, *et al.* Glossopharyngeal nerve injury complicating carotid endarterectomy. *J Vasc Surg* 1987; **5:** 469.
32. Browse NL, Ross-Russel AO. Carotid endarterectomy and the Javid shunt: the early results of 215 consecutive operations for transient ischaemic attacks. *Br J Surg* 1984; **71:** 53.

33. Bookenheimer S-AM, Mathias K. Percutaneous transluminal angioplasty in arteriosclerotic internal carotid artery stenosis. *AJNR* 1983; **4:** 791.
34. Welling RE, Taha A, Goel T, *et al.* Extra-cranial carotid artery aneurysms. *Surgery* 1983; **93:** 319.
35. Vannix RS, Joergenson FJ, Carter R. Kinking of the internal carotid artery: clinical significance and surgical management. *Am J Surg* 1977; **134:** 82.
36. Barros D'Sa AB. Chemodectoma. In: *Surgical Management of Vascular Disease,* Bell PRF, Jamieson CW, Ruckley RV (eds). London: WB Saunders, 1992: 721–37.

20

Venous thrombosis and pulmonary embolism

C Vaughan Ruckley

The distribution of thromboembolism among all specialties ensures that few clinicians acquire sufficient specialist experience to be confident that they are providing optimal care. It is an elusive disorder, often being clinically silent, especially in its most dangerous phase. When symptoms are present it is frequently misdiagnosed. Even when it is correctly diagnosed, the spectrum of severity, signs, symptoms and sequelae are so protean as to create problems for the formulation of a coherent management policy. Nevertheless the formulation of such a policy is both possible and necessary in today's clinical practice.

In this chapter the term 'thromboembolism' will be employed to refer to the combined disease of venous thrombosis (DVT) and pulmonary embolism (PE). The 'oneness' of DVT and PE is an important starting point which deserves special emphasis since many medical texts are apt to discuss the two in isolation, reflecting a tendency amongst clinicians to focus in blinkered fashion on one or other depending on specialty and presentation.

There is no standard or universal treatment of thromboembolism. Therapy depends on the severity, site, duration and extent of DVT and whether it is actively embolising. Fundamental is the view that anticoagulants, being dangerous drugs, should not be prescribed unless thrombosis has been unequivocally confirmed.

First the broad principles of management will be outlined, providing practical strategies which can be applied at unit or hospital level. This is followed by short sections specifically addressing some of the common types of presentation and questions which may give rise to clinical difficulty or uncertainty.

Epidemiology

Pulmonary embolism remains one of the commonest causes of death in hospital patients.[1,2] It is a particular threat in major trauma, orthopaedics, malignant disease, abdominal surgery, gynaecology and neurosurgery. It is the commonest cause of maternal perinatal mortality in the UK. It frequently provides the *coup de grâce* in ill patients in medical wards, especially those with cardiorespiratory disease. The major risk factors for thromboembolism are summarized in Table 20.1.

There is some evidence that, over the last decade, the incidence of fatal pulmonary embolism in surgical patients has been falling.[3–6] It seems reasonable to attribute at least a proportion of this improvement to the use of prophylactic measures, but other changes in patient care have no doubt played a part. This trend does not appear to apply to medical patients.

Patient-related risk factors have been defined. The incidence of thromboembolism rises with age. Other risk factors include previous episodes of thromboembolism, a family history of thromboembolism, malignant disease, varicose veins, obesity, blood diseases and oestrogen-containing contraceptives. In both acute medical and postoperative patients the incidence of DVT is significantly higher

Table 20.1 Major risk factors for thromboembolism

Previous thromboembolism
Malignant disease
Age
Varicose veins
Obesity
Immobility
Oestrogen-containing contraceptive
Various blood disorders

in non-smokers than in smokers.[7] Haematological causes of increased risk of thromboembolism, or 'thrombophilia', include deficiencies of protein C, protein S and antithrombin III, polycythaemia, thrombocytosis and hyperfibrinogenaemia.[8]

Pathology

The great advances in the understanding and management of venous thromboembolism in the 1960s and 70s were founded on two avenues of research: autopsy studies and the radiofibrinogen test. The first shed light on the end-results of the disease, the other enabled study of the starting point and evolution of the thrombus. Neither are widely employed now. The universal decrease in autopsy rates is to be deplored, for it has seriously blunted clinical awareness of the frequency and lethal role of thromboembolism.

What have we learnt from autopsy studies? Pulmonary embolism has been shown to be the commonest acute lung disorder in hospital patients.[9,10] Morrel, using careful serial section techniques, found it to be present in more than 50% of lungs of patients dying in hospital.[11] The usual origin of DVT is the veins of the calf, but big emboli usually arise in the iliofemoral segment. Iliofemoral DVT commonly begins in the calf but sometimes arises *ab initio* in the pelvic veins, particularly in obstetric and orthopaedic patients. Pulmonary embolism may arise from other sites of thrombus in the body, notably veins of the head, neck and upper limb (especially in these days of central lines), and from the right heart chambers.[12] Less than a quarter of the patients dying of pulmonary embolism have any prior symptoms or signs detected in the lower limbs.[13] The majority of patients who die of pulmonary embolism do not suffer from a single massive event but have multiple emboli, commonly spread over a period of time.[9,13,14]

The radiofibrinogen test facilitated development of the prophylactic armamentarium now available to surgeons, and it remains a valuable research tool. It showed us that postoperative DVT often begins on the operating table or may even be present before operation. In hip surgery, in obstetric and gynaecological surgery and in major pelvic operations, DVT frequently starts in the pelvic veins. Otherwise the small veins of the calf are a common starting point. Thrombus propagates both distally and proximally. It is generally limited to the calf, but alternatively may extend into the popliteal, femoral and iliac veins and cava within days or even hours. At the time of this early thrombogenesis and propagation the patient is entirely asymptomatic. The classical features of DVT (pain, tenderness and swelling) do not arise until the inflammatory response to the thrombus in the vein wall has had time to develop or the propagation of thrombus has become so extensive as to occlude flow not only in main stem veins but also in collaterals.

The gross features of phlegmasia caerulea dolens only occur when there is widespread coagulation in the microvascular collaterals in addition to the main venous channels. It thus reflects a morbid coagulopathy such as may occur in advanced malignant disease.

Very often, then, the first clue to the presence of DVT is the onset of symptoms of pulmonary embolism. However, it is worth bearing in mind that only about one in eight emboli cause infarction; so, unless they are so large as to obstruct cardiac output or precipitate respiratory insufficiency, they may remain undiagnosed. The serious pathological significance of the small pulmonary embolism has been emphasized earlier.

All these facts have clear implications for management:

1. In the light of the occult nature of early DVT and of the diagnostic difficulties, prophylaxis is crucial.
2. There is a need for heightened clinical awareness of the risk of thromboembolism.
3. The 'at-risk' patient should be identified and prophylaxis started before operation.
4. In the patient with pre-existing cardiorespiratory disease, even a small pulmonary embolism may be fatal.
5. A small pulmonary embolism must be assumed to be a herald of a bigger one until that risk has been excluded.
6. DVT should be assumed to be giving rise to emboli or likely to do so until proven otherwise.
7. Failure to demonstrate DVT in the legs does not exclude thromboembolism.

Prophylaxis

A full discussion of thromboembolism prophylaxis is beyond the scope of this chapter. The following is a broad outline of guiding principles. For an authoritative review the reader is referred to the review by Bergqvist.[15]

The first question for the surgeon is: 'Is prophy-

Table 20.2 Typical frequencies of postoperative thromboembolism

Type of surgery	Method of diagnosis	Frequency
General	I^{125} fibrinogen	29%
Gynaecological	I^{125} fibrinogen	19%
Neurosurgery	I^{125} fibrinogen	29%
Hip fracture	Phlebography	40%
Elective hip surgery	Phlebography	52%

laxis needed in my population of patients?'. Rates of thromboembolism in broad categories of patients and types of surgery are well documented (Table 20.2).[16] Linked to this is the question: 'Is a routine regimen of prophylaxis economically justified?' Next comes the question, since pharmacological methods are the best documented prophylactic agents: 'What are the relative risks of thromboembolism versus bleeding?'

Prophylactic methods are divided into pharmacological and physical (Table 20.3). While low-dose subcutaneous heparin and dextran have both been demonstrated to protect against pulmonary embolism, the mechanical methods have not been studied in large enough clinical trials to demonstrate efficacy against embolism. However, it seems entirely logical to suppose that the latter can be inferred from a demonstrable effect against DVT. The search for an agent with protective effect equivalent to unfractionated heparin but with less bleeding risk has led to the marketing of low-molecular-weight heparins (LMWHs) at several times the cost. It is by no means clear that the benefits of LMWHs are sufficient to justify their use in all areas of surgery. In general surgery, for example, the evidence to date is conflicting. However, in certain categories of patients such as those undergoing major orthopaedic surgery, spinal surgery and pelvic operations for malignancy, the use of LMWH, would appear to be justified.

Table 20.3 Prophylactic methods

Physical methods
Graduated elastic compression
Motorized foot mover
Electrical calf stimulation
Intermittent pneumatic compression

Pharmacological methods
Oral anticoagulants
Antiplatelet agents
Dextran
Low-dose heparin
Low-dose heparin plus dihydoergotamine
Low-molecular-weight heparin
Heparin analogues

Dextran is effective against pulmonary embolism to a degree comparable with low-dose heparin but does not have the same popularity, except possibly in Sweden. Because intravenous infusion is required, it may aggravate renal failure and, rarely, allergic reactions have been reported. The latter can be preempted by the administration of a hapten (i.e. a small infusion of 50 ml of dextran 1 (mean molecular weight 1000)) prior to the main dextran infusion.

Antiembolism stockings (TED Kendall) have been shown in several trials to protect against DVT, as has intermittent pneumatic compression. The latter is less popular, being somewhat unwieldy.

Except where there are serious bleeding risks, low-dose heparin, unfractionated or LMWH, is the prophylactic agent of choice. Graduated compression TED stockings offer an alternative, and where the patient is recognized to be at particular risk pharmacological and physical methods should be combined, the commonest combination being antiembolism stockings plus subcutaneous heparin.

Deep vein thrombosis

Clinical features

A number of conditions can masquerade as DVT, some of the commoner ones being shown in Table 20.4. Distension of superficial veins when the patient is horizontal may be a useful sign. Localized calf tenderness is a fairly consistent, but late, sign. Some DVTs have a strong inflammatory component, particularly iliofemoral DVT in young women. Swelling is also a late sign.

Table 20.4 Differential diagnosis of deep vein thrombosis

Primary and secondary lymphoedema
Dependant oedema
Post-reconstruction oedema
Factitial oedema
Mechanical venous compression
Cellulitis
Arterial occlusion
Synovial leak
Muscle injury
Myositis
Intramuscular haemorrhage

It is important to understand the significance of swelling in relation to the underlying pathology. Any degree of swelling indicates that the thrombus is not trivial. Swelling at ankle level means occlusive thrombus at least up to popliteal vein. Swelling extending up towards the knee means extensive femoral vein thrombus, while thigh swelling means occlusive iliofemoral DVT. Phlegmasia caerulea dolens means that not only are main stem veins occluded but so also are collaterals down to venular size. As noted above, this grave condition, which sometimes leads to venous gangrene, is usually associated with advanced malignant disease. Unless the DVT is exceptionally extensive, swelling can be regarded as a late sign; that is, the thrombus is likely to have been present for a number of days.

Homan's sign is not recommended, being nonspecific and possibly dangerous. Warmth of the overlying skin is said to be an early sign. As soon as there is oedema present the skin will be cooler than normal.

Investigations

Diagnostic tests may be divided into those useful for screening the 'at-risk' population, those employed simply to confirm or exclude a clinical diagnosis, and those capable of defining the extent and characteristics of the thrombus as a basis for treatment.

The best screen remains the radiofibrinogen test, but this is largely reserved for research purposes. For confirmation of a clinical diagnosis, impedence or strain-gauge plethysmography or thermography may be helpful if there is an experienced technician available to provide a service. This is seldom the case in the UK. Duplex scanning will reliably detect thrombus in the popliteal or common femoral veins but not in the calf or pelvis.

Thus these noninvasive tests may be useful in reducing the number of phlebograms requested but do not provide the quality of information necessary for the effective management of thromboembolism, especially if one believes that treatment should be adapted to the characteristics of the thrombus – notably its site, size, extent, adherence, duration and whether it is embolising or not.

The implication of the latter statement is that in the patient presenting with DVT, perfusion lung scanning should be an early investigation (i.e. within the first 24 hours of presentation), not only to show whether there is evidence of embolism but also to provide a baseline image against which to match later scans. The accuracy of lung scanning is discussed later, but in the present context suffice it to say that a single lung scan, performed later in the patient's course in response to some new symptom or event, may be very difficult to interpret. The existence of an earlier baseline scan will resolve this difficulty.

Phlebography is the most important investigation and this is normally done bilaterally by the ascending route. It is discussed later in the chapter.

The management of DVT and of minor pulmonary embolism are now described together.

Pulmonary embolism

Classification

The presenting features of pulmonary emboli are listed in Table 20.5. They are divided into minor or non-life-threatening, and major or life-threatening. This is an important distinction since the management pathways are entirely different.

Table 20.5 Presenting features of pulmonary embolism

Minor embolism	Major embolism
Mild or progressive breathlessness	Collapse
Haemoptysis	Cardiac arrest
Pleuritic pain	Central chest pain
Radiological changes	Severe breathlessness
Asthmatic episodes	Shock
Syncope	
Confusion	

Management of minor embolism

In this category are included any emboli that do not immediately threaten life. The majority of small emboli do not cause infarction and are therefore asymptomatic. Infarction is more likely to occur in pulmonary segments which are already poorly aerated; hence the basal distribution of most infarcts. They present with late symptoms and signs such as haemoptysis or pleuritic pain, or with vague and nonspecific symptoms such as confusion, syncope, general deterioration, mild breathlessness, cardiac failure, episodes of bronchospasm, radiological changes etc. Thus a high index of clinical suspicion in 'at-risk' situations is essential.

Lung perfusion scanning is the principal diagnostic test. It is valuable but clinicians must be aware of its limitations. Studies correlating the findings of lung scanning with pulmonary angiography, which is taken as the reference standard, show that scanning fails to detect approaching 50% of emboli.[17–19] However, as emphasized earlier, a baseline scan performed early in management can be very valuable if the patient subsequently develops new symptoms or signs such as pyrexia, haemoptysis, breathlessness, new radiological changes etc. Hence our policy is to obtain a lung scan within 24 hours of DVT or PE being suspected. Should any new signs or symptoms appear or the patient fail to improve as rapidly as expected, a second scan can be obtained before the heparin treatment is converted to that with warfarin.

Chest X-ray changes, especially early, are non-specific. They include segmental opacities, usually basal, linear atelectasis, pleural effusions and diaphragmatic elevation.

Management of DVT and non-life-threatening PE

The management policy is summarized in Figs 20.1 and 20.2. The patient is started on intravenous heparin 5–10 000 units immediately on clinical suspicion of thromboembolism. He or she is continued on heparin pump infusion at around 2000 units/hour, depending on laboratory monitoring aimed at keeping the APPT or thrombin clotting time at around two to three times control. Within 24 hours a bilateral ascending phlebogram and a perfusion lung scan are obtained. These two crucial diagnostic techniques are discussed below. A ventilation scan usually does not add much unless the patient suffers from chronic obstructive airways disease.

All patients are continued on heparin. I do not use thrombolytic therapy for lower-limb DVT owing to its relatively poor success rates and substantial haemorrhagic complications. This does not apply to upper-limb DVT: subclavian and superior caval thrombosis generally respond well to lytic therapy.[18] By what route should the heparin be given? It is our policy to continue with the intravenous route, unless or until the patient is ready to be mobilized in which case the subcutaneous route is equally effective.[21–22]

How long should heparin be continued? There is no standard course. Common sense suggests that it should be continued until the patient is clearly improving and is not likely to need any other invasive procedures. It may be preferable to repeat the lung scan and compare it with the baseline scan for evidence of recurrent embolism before starting warfarin. A standard course of heparin in my practice would be 7–10 days. The overlap with warfarin

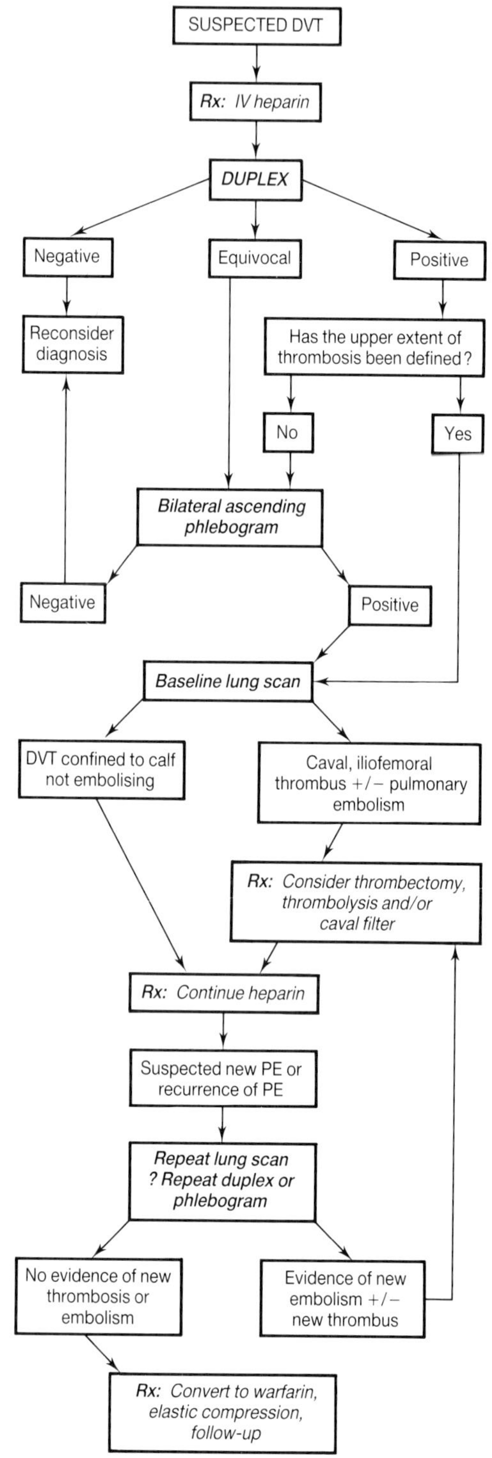

Fig. 20.1 Flow chart for the management of the patient presenting with suspected DVT.

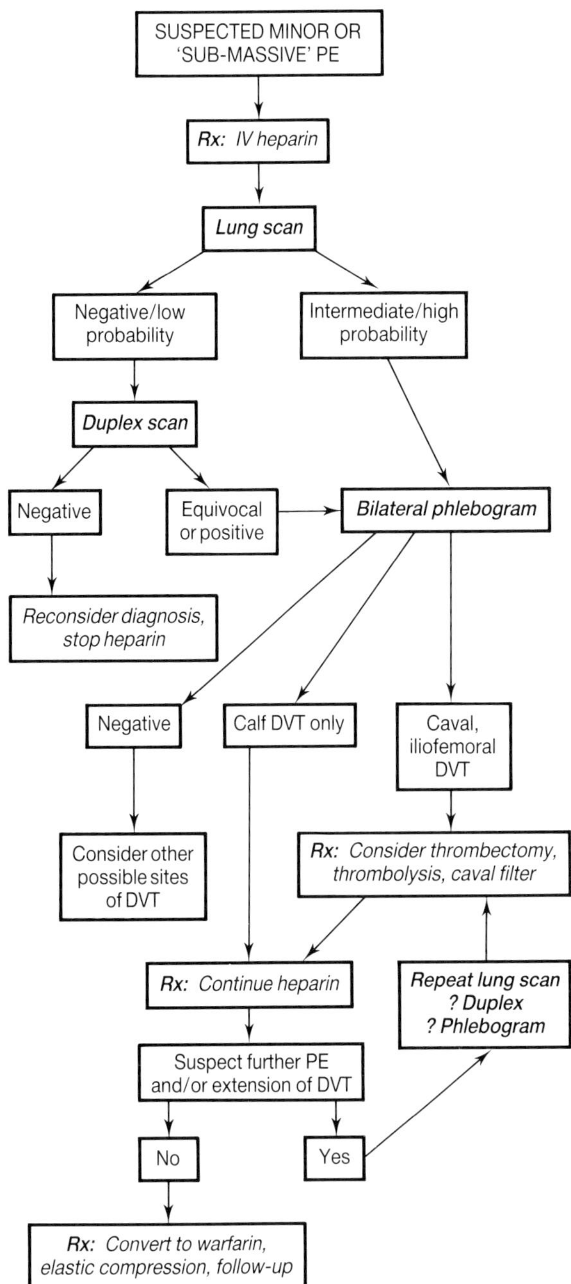

Fig. 20.2 Flow chart for the patient presenting with non-life-threatening pulmonary embolism.

should cover at least 3 days. The duration of the warfarin treatment depends on the severity of the symptoms and whether there is a history of recurrent thromboembolism. With rapid resolution of leg symptoms our practice is to prescribe a 3-month course. For patients with persisting post-thrombotic sequelae a 6–12 month course is preferred; and if the patient has a history of recurrent thromboembolism, life time oral anticoagulant therapy may be advised.

Additional treatment depends mainly on the probability or actual occurrence of further embolism. Thrombus which is recent and free-floating is dangerous particularly if located in femoral, iliac veins or cava.[23,24] Thus, the appearance of the proximal thrombus may suggest the need for insertion of a caval filter, as would the demonstration of recurrent embolism (despite anticoagulation) on follow-up lung scan when compared with the baseline scan. Indications for filter insertion are listed in Table 20.6. Filters such as the LMG or the Greenfield can be placed by the percutaneous transvenous route and have a low complication rate.[25]

Thrombectomy. Is there still a place for venous thrombectomy? This operation has been abandoned in many centres. It is still recommended to avoid venous gangrene and in patients with phlegmasia caerulea dolens in the rare event of there being no evidence of advanced malignancy. In the author's practice, caval or isolated right-sided iliac thrombi are still occasionally removed surgically. But for more extensive or peripheral DVT the benefits of thrombectomy are unproven.

General measures. There is no evidence that the patient needs to be kept on bed-rest. However, severe oedema must first be controlled by high elevation of the limb combined with active exercises.

Table 20.6 Indications for insertion of caval filter

Recurrent embolism not controlled by anticoagulation
Recurrent embolism, or a grave risk of embolism, in a patient in whom for any reason effective anticoagulation is not possible
Caval, iliac or femoral thrombus, especially if:
(a) it is free-floating
(b) the patient has limited cardiopulmonary reserve
(c) the patient is to undergo major operation, orthopaedic manipulation etc.
Thromboembolic pulmonary hypertension
Following pulmonary embolectomy

Once the oedema is controlled the patient is mobilized, with graduated elastic compression. This can be by a shaped tubular support in the first instance, followed rapidly by correctly fitted graduated compression hosiery. If the patient has residual swelling, follow-up by a specialist in venous disease may be advisable.

Management of major embolism

Patients present with collapse, central chest pain, severe breathlessness or cardiac arrest (Fig. 20.3). The diagnosis may be helped by the clinical context in which the event occurs (e.g. following injury, childbirth or operation). The patient is shocked, restless, anxious, breathless and cyanosed. The jugular venous pressure is elevated. A chest X-ray is usually unhelpful and ECG changes are nonspecific. In any case, action is required before any investigation can be performed. A commonly observed mistake is to waste time and further jeopardize the patient's prospects by requesting a lung scan.

Cardiac massage if necessary, oxygen therapy and a large dose of intravenous heparin (e.g. 15 000 units) are given immediately. If the event occurs in a hospital with a cardiothoracic unit the surgeon is notified. If pulmonary angiography is readily available it is immediately performed and, the diagnosis having been confirmed, thrombolytic therapy is commenced via the pulmonary catheter. If a pulmonary angiogram cannot be performed it has to be assumed that the potential benefits of thrombolytic therapy outweigh the hazards consequent upon incorrect diagnosis. The main differential diagnosis is myocardial infarction for which thrombolytic therapy could also be beneficial. If a pulmonary angiogram has not been performed, thrombolytic therapy is started intravenously: 500 000 units streptokinase followed by 100 000 hourly. Monitoring of pulmonary artery pressure and central venous pressure are helpful but systemic arterial pressure is the best criterion of response to therapy. Tissue plasminogen activator or urokinase are effective alternatives to streptokinase but are more expensive and not available in all centres. Pulmonary angiography is repeated at 12–24 hours.

Failure to respond within 15–30 minutes of instituting thrombolytic therapy should suggest the need to consider pulmonary embolectomy. Patients sustaining massive embolism in the near proximity of a cardiothoracic unit may have an additional opportunity for survival, but the fact is that the majority of patients suffering lethal embolism die within an hour.

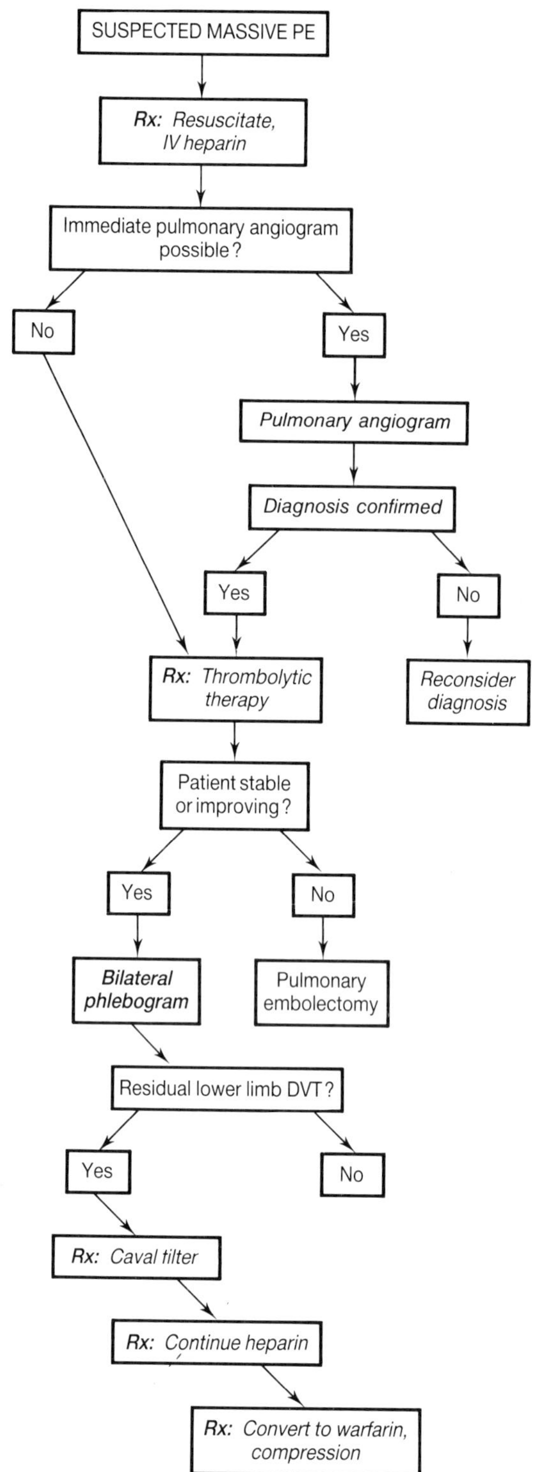

Fig. 20.3 Flow chart for the patient presenting with massive pulmonary embolism.

A patient surviving for an hour after the onset of embolism is likely to survive with prompt and vigorous medical therapy. Thrombolytic therapy is continued for up to 12–24 hours depending on speed of improvement, and is followed by intravenous heparin.

The biggest threat to survival is further embolism. Therefore, as soon as the patient's condition has stabilized, bilateral ascending phlebography is performed. The demonstration of residual thrombus in the cava, iliac or femoral veins is an indication for the percutaneous, transfemoral insertion of a filter such as the LMG or the Greenfield. Thereafter, the patient is managed as for any major thromboembolism with eventual conversion to warfarin and mobilization with properly fitted graduated elastic compression hose.

Caval filter

Caval filter insertion has become easier and safer in the last decade. The early problems of filter migration and caval thrombosis have largely been overcome, and filters such as the LMG and the Greenfield can now be positioned percutaneously, usually via the femoral route.

In my view, filter insertion is an important and at times life-saving measure. It has to be conceded, however, that randomized controlled trials of caval interruption versus conventional thrombolytic or anticoagulant therapy have never been performed. The indications (Table 20.6) should be carefully considered and remain a matter of individual judgement.

Some specific clinical problems and issues in thromboembolism

The patient with a history of 'thromboembolism'

Patients are sometimes labelled as having had previous episodes of thromboembolism. Such a label can radically influence that patient's subsequent management. In my experience it is commonly ill-founded. The first step is to check how well-supported were the diagnoses. Unless DVT was demonstrated by a phlebogram and pulmonary embolism by unequivocal lung scan or pulmonary angiogram, the diagnosis should be regarded with scepticism. The performance and interpretation of phlebograms and lung scans are discussed below.

A well-validated history of recurrent thromboembolism should raise the possibility of underlying predisposing disease such as those listed in Table 20.1. Recurrent thromboembolism in a relatively young person may be due to thrombophilia in the form of protein C, protein S or antithrombin III deficiency.[8] Such a patient may require long-term therapy with an oral anticoagulant.

Phlebography

Despite the benefits of duplex scanning, phlebography remains the most important diagnostic technique, and the reference standard, in the management of venous thromboembolism. Before the advent of non-ionic contrast materials it was not a popular investigation owing to the discomfort and thrombogenicity of the earlier media. When the indication is a suspected DVT, phlebography should always be bilateral for two main reasons. First it may often reveal thrombus in the asymptomatic limb; and second, it ensures a sufficient concentration of contrast at caval level. This is vital since the most important information that the examination can provide is the nature and extent of the proximal end of the thrombus.

The importance of optimal radiological technique and interpretation are well illustrated in Fig. 20.4, which shows phlebograms of a patient recently under my care. The patient presented three weeks after Caesarian section with a 24-hour history of slight thigh and calf swelling plus a tendency for the limb to become cyanosed in the erect position; it appeared normal when horizontal. The bilateral ascending phlebogram was reported as normal, despite the fact that there was greater concentration of contrast on the left and an indistinct filling defect in the left common femoral vein, which was interpreted as overlying bowel gas shadow. No active treatment was instituted. The patient was referred to the vascular unit on the following day where a transfemoral phlebogram was requested. This showed that by this time the thrombus had extended retrogradely to occlude the left common femoral vein. Injection of contrast on the right showed thrombus in the left common iliac vein but, importantly, no significant propagation into the cava. On the strength of this and a negative lung scan it was decided that heparin therapy would suffice.

Phlebography by the ascending route is appropriate for the great majority of patients with suspected DVT, but it should not be attempted when the limb is grossly swollen, since the chances of effectively delineating the proximal thrombus are vir-

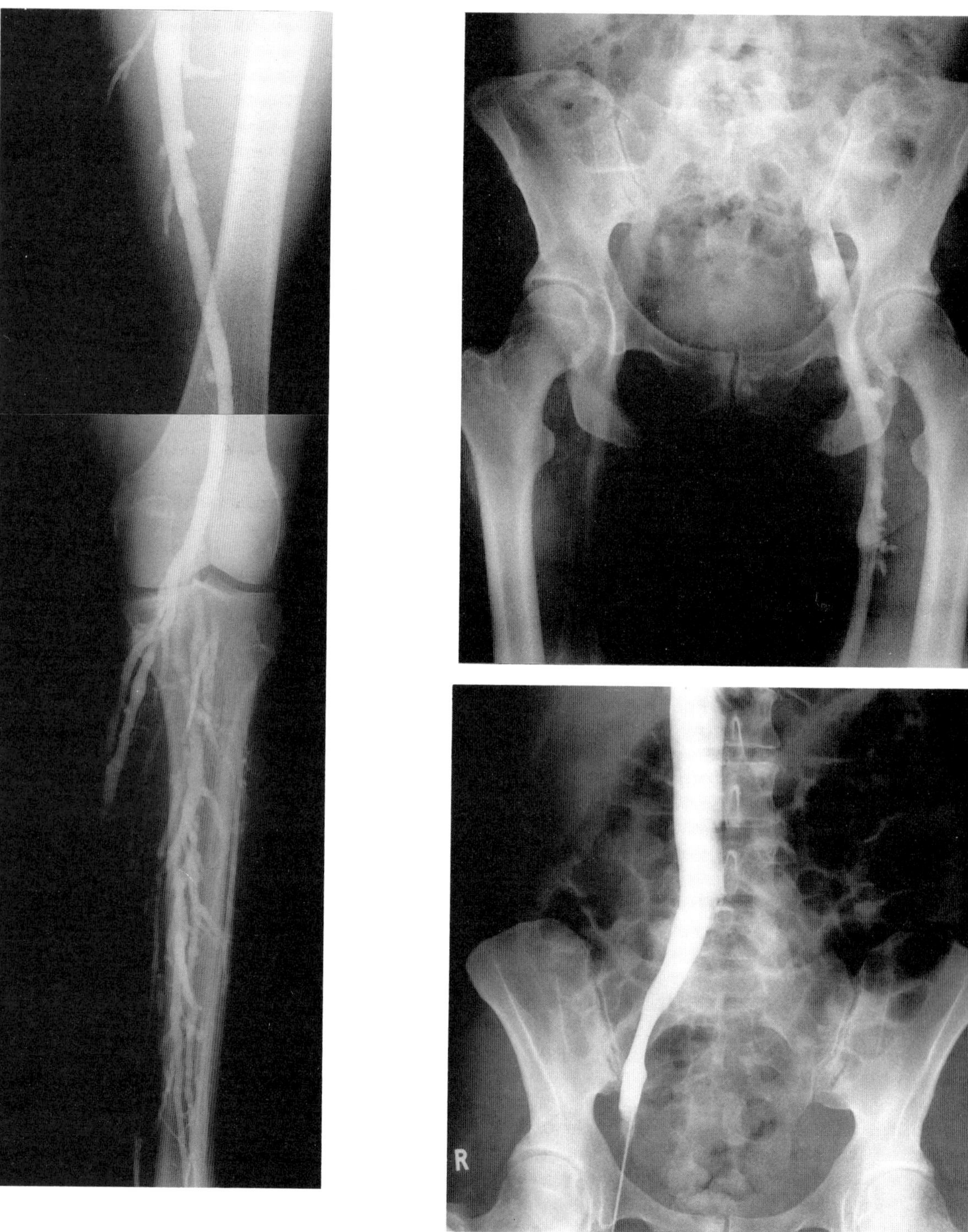

Fig. 20.4 (Left and top right) Bilateral ascending phlebograms in a patient presenting with swelling and cyanosis, coming on only in the erect posture, three weeks after a Caesarian section. (Bottom right) Transfemoral phlebogram in the same patient.

tually nil, and certainly not in the presence of phlegmasia caerulea dolens when it may cause considerable damage. In such cases transfemoral phlebography should be first choice, and often the only feasible access is from the contralateral groin.

Lung scanning

Lung scanning has its limitations. There are interpretation problems, irrespective of the addition of ventilation scanning, which have been much debated in the literature. The correlation with pulmonary angiography, which is regarded as the reference standard, is poor.[20] However, lung scanning remains by far the most valuable diagnostic test for 'submassive' pumonary embolism. It cannot be overemphasized that lung scanning should not be requested in the patient who is critically ill with suspected massive pulmonary embolism since life-endangering delays may ensue.

A clearly negative lung scan is of clinical value, as is a clearly positive scan. The difficulty lies with those of low or intermediate probability since these provide a poor basis for clinical decisions. This is why the concept of obtaining a 'baseline' lung scan at the start of clinical management of a patient with suspected DVT or PE is so useful.

Calf pain and tenderness

Table 20.4 lists the differential diagnosis of DVT. The question is: 'Does this patient, who has a tender calf, have a DVT?' With the patient horizontal, bend the knee to about 45° so that the calf muscles hang relaxed. If on deep palpation the muscle has a 'doughy' feel to it plus localized deep tenderness, there may be DVT present. Tenderness without oedema is unlikely to be associated with clinically significant DVT (i.e. occlusive thrombus of the popliteal vein is unlikely to be present); but to be sure the popliteal vein should be examined with duplex ultrasound. If in doubt bilateral ascending phlebography should be requested.

The swollen leg

Swelling is a commoner presentation of DVT than pain or tenderness. It is a frequent and nonspecific symptom and many of the common causes such as pregnancy, trauma, venous insufficiency, arterial reconstruction, dependent immobility etc. are also risk factors for DVT. The differential diagnosis is enumerated in Table 20.4.

In relation to the evolution of the pathological process, the thrombus and its interaction with vessel wall and peri-venous tissues, swelling is a late symptom, unless the thrombosis is so extensive as to occlude not only the stem veins but also the collaterals, in which case the swelling is likely to be gross.

The main period of risk of pulmonary embolism is before any swelling or other symptoms of any sort have arisen.[13] Duplex ultrasound is a useful initial diagnostic test in the patient with leg swelling. It is an inaccurate diagnostic method in the calf and above the groin, but if a swollen limb is due to DVT there will almost always be thrombus in the popliteal or common femoral veins or both, and duplex will detect it. Phlebography will be required to define the proximal extent and characteristics.

Recurrent thromboembolism

A particularly difficult clinical situation is when a patient with a known history of thromboembolism presents with new symptoms or an exacerbation of symptoms. Increases in swelling or leg discomfort may be induced purely by changes in physical activity, such as the resumption of walking, prolonged dependency, trauma or travel. Likewise new chest symptoms such as pain or breathlessness may be provoked by a variety of causes. Patients who have been labelled as such are often anxious and may readily report symptoms. Furthermore, there is a particular group of patients, usually relatively young women, who manufacture symptoms and may even create swelling by applying tourniquets to the extremities.

Recurrent thromboembolism, when it does occur, may be serious and lead to irreversible pulmonary hypertension. Diagnostic tests are often difficult to interpret. Post-phlebitic damage can be indistinguishable from new occlusions. Likewise the significance of lung scan perfusion defects may be obscure. Once again the existence of prior 'baseline' investigations may be very helpful. This situation is a test of clinical judgement.

Thromboembolism in pregnancy

Pulmonary embolism is the commonest cause of maternal mortality in the UK. Management is complicated by the limitations on anticoagulant therapy and diagnostic irradiation, especially during the first trimester. Hitherto the therapeutic management has therefore been largely based on clinical diagnosis, phlebography only being freely applied in the postpartum period. Lung scanning is not contraindicated in the pregnant patient. The advent of duplex ultrasound has been a definite advance for the care of pregnant patients and makes it possible for the clinician to follow logical sequential patterns of management approximating to those outlined in Figs 20.1–20.3. Both heparin and thrombolytic therapy can be used in pregnancy and during the puerperium, although the latter would be reserved for life-threatening embolism. A prolonged course of heparin during pregnancy can cause osteoporosis.

Compression therapy

The place of compression stockings in DVT prophylaxis is well established (see also Chapter 21). However, in acute DVT the role of compression has never been tested by clinical trial. Often one sees an elastic stocking applied to a swollen leg in a patient who is on bed-rest. In my view there is no good case for this, and stockings may distract from the real need, which is to promote venous return and the reduction of oedema by physical measures. Furthermore it is common to see tourniquet effects above the knee caused by stocking slippage, and compression can be very damaging in patients with diabetes or impaired arterial circulation.[26]

My policy is to rely on elevation and active physiotherapy to reduce oedema while the patient is on bed-rest. Once the oedema has been reduced stockings are fitted, which the patient wears as soon as the erect posture is adopted and walking started.

What type of stocking is required? For the patient whose swelling is confined to the lower leg, below-knee stockings are prescribed. For the patient with iliofemoral thrombosis, with swelling in the thigh, a full-length stocking with a waist-band is preferred. For the average patient the class-3 grade is appropriate, while class-2 is chosen if the patient is frail.

How long should the patient with DVT be kept in bed?

It has long been the policy to keep patients with DVT on prolonged bed-rest. There is no valid reason why this should be so. It is only necessary to keep a patient on bed-rest for as long as it takes to get rid of gross oedema. As noted above, this is achieved by high elevation and active exercises. As soon as possible stockings are fitted and the patient mobilized.

References

1. Hauch O, Jorgensen LN, Khattar SC, *et al.* Fatal pulmonary embolism associated with surgery: an autopsy study. *Acta Chir Scand* 1990; **156:** 747–9.
2. Rubenstein I, Murray D, Hoffstein V. Fatal pulmonary emboli in hospitalised patients: an autopsy study. *Arch Intern Med* 1988; **148:** 1425–6.
3. Knight B, Zaini MRS. Pulmonary embolism and venous thrombosis: a pattern of incidence and predisposing factors over 70 years. *Am J For Med Path* 1980; **1:** 227–33.
4. Ruckley CV, Thurston C. Pulmonary embolism in surgical patients. *Br Med J* 1982; **284:** 1100–4.
5. Dismuke SE, Wagner EH. Pulmonary embolism as a cause of death. *JAMA* 1986; **255:** 2039–45.
6. Bergqvist D, Linblad B. A thirty year survey of pulmonary embolism verified at autopsy: an analysis of 1274 surgical patients. *Br J Surg* 1985; **72:** 105–10.
7. Prescott RJ, Jones DRB, Vasilescieu C, Henderson JT, Ruckley CV. Smoking and risk factors in deep venous thrombosis. *Thromb Haemost* 1978; **40:** 128–35.
8. Lowe GDO, Forbes CD. Predisposing and aggravating factors in arterial and venous thrombosis. In: *Surgical Management of Vascular Disease,* Bell PB, Jamieson C, Ruckley CV (eds). London: Baillière Tindall, 1992: 47–62.
9. Coon WW, Coller FA. Clinico-pathologic correlation in thromboembolism. *Surg Gynae Obst* 1959; **109:** 259–69.
10. Morrell MT, Truelove SC, Barr A. Pulmonary embolism. *Br Med J* 1963; **2:** 830–5.
11. Morrell T, Dunnill MS. Postmortem incidence of pulmonary embolism in a hospital population. *Br J Surg* 1968; **55:** 347–52.
12. Hume M, Sevitt S, Thomas DP. Pathology of pulmonary embolism. In: *Venous Thrombosis and Pulmonary Embolism.* Harvard: Harvard University Press, 1970: 194–229.
13. MacIntyre IMC, Ruckley CV. A clinical and autopsy study of pulmonary embolism. *Scot Med J* 1974; **19:** 20–6.
14. Smith GT, Dexter L, Dammin GJ. Postmortem quantitative studies in pulmonary embolism. In: *Pulmonary Embolic Disease,* Eds Sasahara AA, Stein M (eds). New York: Grune & Stratton, 1965: 120–37.
15. Bergqvist D. The prevention of venous thrombosis and embolism. In: *Surgical Management of Vascular Disease,* Bell PR, Jamieson CW, Ruckley CV (eds). London: WB Saunders, 1992: 1137–50.
16. Bergqvist D. *Postoperative Thromboembolism: Frequency, Aetiology, Prophylaxis.* New York: Springer Verlag, 1983: 6–34.
17. Hull RD, Hirsh J, Carter CJ. Pulmonary angiography, ventilation lung scanning and venography for clinically suspect pulmonary embolism with abnormal perfusion lung scan. *Ann Int Med* 1983; **98:** 891–9.

18. Hull RD, Raskob GE, Coates GE, Panju AA. Clinical validity of a normal perfusion lung scan in patients with suspected pulmonary embolism. *Chest* 1990; **97:** 23–6.
19. Gray HW, McKillop JH, Bessent PG, *et al.* Lung scanning for pulmonary embolism: clinical and pulmonary angiographic correlations. *Quart J Med* 1990; **77:** 1135–50.
20. Ruckley CV, Boulton FE, Redhead D. The treatment of venous thrombosis of the upper and lower limbs with 'APSAC' (P-anisoylated plasminogen-streptokinase complex). *Eur J Vasc Surg* 1987; **1:** 107–12.
21. Walker MG, Shaw JW, Thomson GJL, *et al.* Subcutaneous calcium heparin versus intravenous sodium heparin in treatment of established acute deep vein thrombosis of the legs: a multicentre prospective randomised trial. *Br Med J* 1987; **294:** 1189–92.
22. Pini M, Pattachini C, Quintavalla R, *et al.* Subcutaneous versus intravenous heparin in the treatment of deep venous thrombosis: a randomised clinical trial. *Thromb Haemost* 1990; **64:** 222–6.
23. Norris CS, Greenfield LJ, Herrman JB. Free-floating iliofemoral thrombus. *Arch Surg* 1985; **120:** 806–8.
24. Berry RE, George WE, Shaver WA. Free-floating deep venous thrombosis: a retrospective analysis. *Ann Surg* 1990; **211:** 719–22.
25. Redhead DN, Adam R, Allan PL, Ruckley CV. Radiological evaluation of caval patency and filter migration in patients with caval interruption/plication. *J Interven Radiol* 1989; **4:** 42–5.
26. Callam MJ, Ruckley CV, Dale JJ, Harper DR. Hazards of compression treatment of the leg: an estimate from Scottish surgeons. *Br J Med* 1987; **295:** 1382.

21

Management of the swollen limb

Kevin G Burnand

Limbs may be 'swollen' in whole or in part. The swelling may be associated with swellings elsewhere (e.g. other limbs), and may have been present since birth or have developed either acutely or chronically later in life. It may be caused by a tumour, by overgrowth of tissue (hypertrophy or gigantism) or by fluid (oedema). Tumours are usually relatively easy to diagnose because they typically cause a localized swelling in some part of the limb, although a rapidly growing sarcoma in the thigh or calf may occasionally be initially misdiagnosed as a deep vein thrombosis. Plexiform neurofibromas are also sometimes a source of diagnostic difficulty (Fig. 21.1) Any suspicion of a soft tissue or bony tumour is an indication for plain radiographs of the limb and some form of biopsy – fine needle, trucut, punch or even open. CT scanning of the limb may also be helpful, especially if performed with contrast enhancement when a haemangioma is suspected (Fig. 21.2).

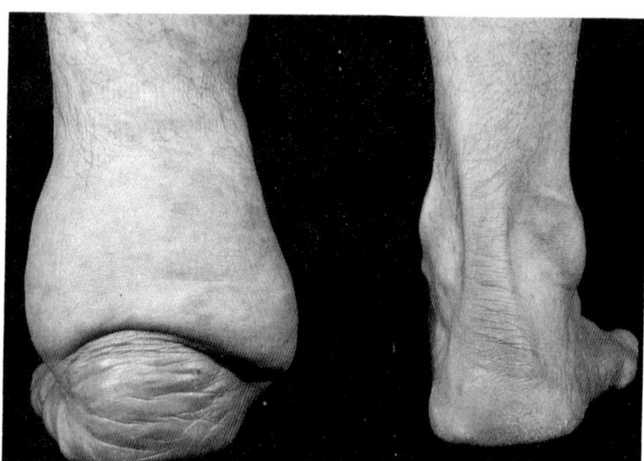

Fig. 21.1 Plexiform neurofibroma.

Gigantism and AV fistulae

Most swollen limbs are as a result of oedema, although this must always be differentiated from local gigantism. The latter may be congenital (Robertson's giant limb) or secondary to increased blood flow (e.g. multiple arteriovenous fistulae or Parkes–Weber syndrome). Limbs with tissue overgrowth do not 'pit' on pressure. Gigantism is suspected when limb length as well as girth is increased (Fig. 2.3). The shoe sizes often differ and the distance from the anterior superior iliac spine to the medial malleolus is increased when compared with the opposite side. The width of the bones may also be increased, which may be detectable clinically, or if less obvious radiologically. Other indications of upper-limb gigantism are asymmetric pectoral muscle bulk or breast size. A Parkes–Weber limb, not to be mistaken for Klippel Trenaunay syndrome, is usually warmer than its pair and machinery murmurs may be audible over the sites of major fistulae. If a tourniquet is applied at the root of a limb affected by the Parkes–Weber syndrome and rapidly inflated, immediate slowing of the pulse (Branham's sign) indicates a sizable left to right shunt. The diagnosis is confirmed by plethysmographic flow measurements and the location of the fistulae may be displayed by arteriography (Fig. 21.4).

There is no treatment for local gigantism other than reassurance, but arteriovenous fistulae may be therapeutically embolised with steel coils, muscle, gelfoam clots, acrylic glues and a number of other materials. This type of treatment may be repeated on many occasions over many years as there is a tendency for new fistulae to keep appearing. Other techniques for obliterating fistulae include skeletonizing (exposing the major limb vessels and ligating all the tributaries) or by excision if they are localized to one part of the limb. Amputation of the limb may be required if the fistulae cannot be effectively blocked despite repeated attempts at embolisation and the patient's life is under threat from high-output cardiac failure. Amputation can be complicated by the continued presence of fistulae within the stump. This may lead to persistant swelling, haemorrhages, blisters and ulceration. Even when fistulae have been successfully obliterated the limb swelling usually does not disappear.

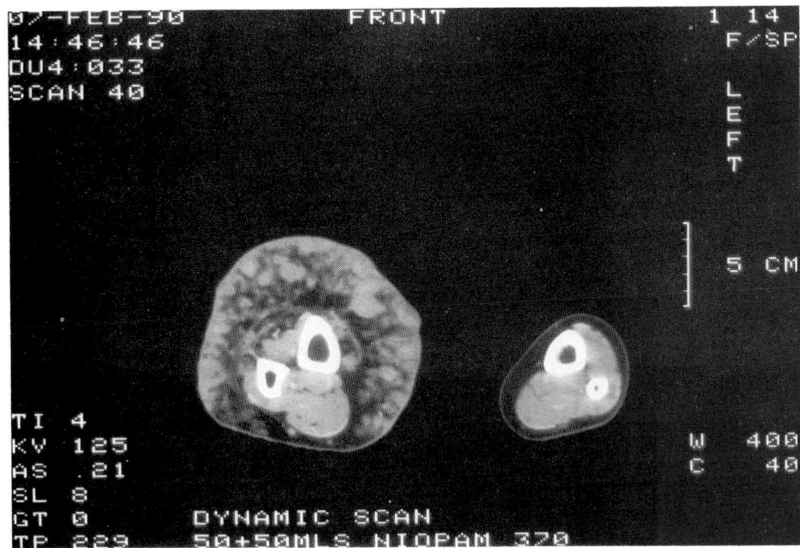

Fig. 21.2 Contrast enhancement showing haemangioma.

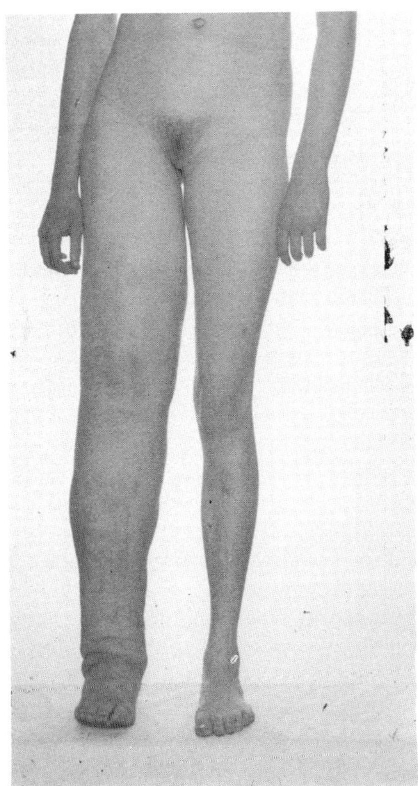

Fig. 21.3 Gigantism of left lower limb and arm.

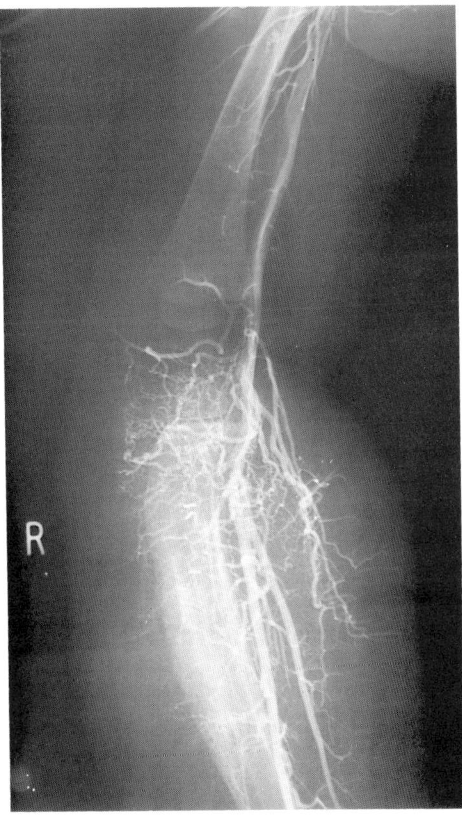

Fig. 21.4 Arteriography showing location of the fistulae.

Oedema

As stated earlier, the major cause of limb swelling is oedema and this can be the result of a systemic or a local cause. The main local causes are venous or lymphatic disorders which can cause unilateral or bilateral oedema. General causes of limb oedema include cardiac failure, renal failure and hypoproteinaemia; these must be excluded by a careful clinical examination supplemented by laboratory investigations such as the serum urea and electrolytes and the plasma protein levels. A chest radiograph and an electrocardiogram may also be helpful. Once a systemic cause of leg oedema (almost always bilateral) has been excluded, attention can be focused on excluding a venous or lymphatic cause.

Venous causes of oedema

Deep vein thrombosis (DVT)

Sudden onset of pain and swelling suggests the possibility of an acute DVT (see Chapter 20). There are few reliable clinical signs of a DVT and any patient with this type of presentation must be considered to have a probable thrombosis until proved otherwise, especially if there is an obvious predisposing cause such as a recent operation or a period of bed-rest. Pyrexia, associated chest pain, or shortness of breath and local calf or thigh tenderness over the course of the axial veins are all supportive evidence, but Homan's sign is no longer considered to be of much diagnostic value. Dilated cutaneous veins, stiff calf muscles, increased skin temperature and mild ankle oedema (Fig. 21.5) are all subtle signs of DVT. There may also be evidence of pulmonary embolism or pulmonary hypertension, with raised neck veins, and a fixed split second heart sound. A pleural rub is occasionally heard.

Some patients presenting with acute leg pain and swelling have no discernible cause, but other conditions which need to be differentiated from deep vein thrombosis include ruptured plantaris or gastrocnemius tendons, achilles tendonitis, a ruptured Bakers' cyst, cellulitis in a lymphoedematous leg, myositis ossificans, a stress fracture of the tibia or fibula, acute arthritis of the knee, hip or ankle, haemarthrosis of the knee, a calf haematoma and a rapidly growing sarcoma. In order to avoid treating up to a third of all patients unnecessarily with anticoagulants, the diagnosis of DVT must be confirmed by special investigations.

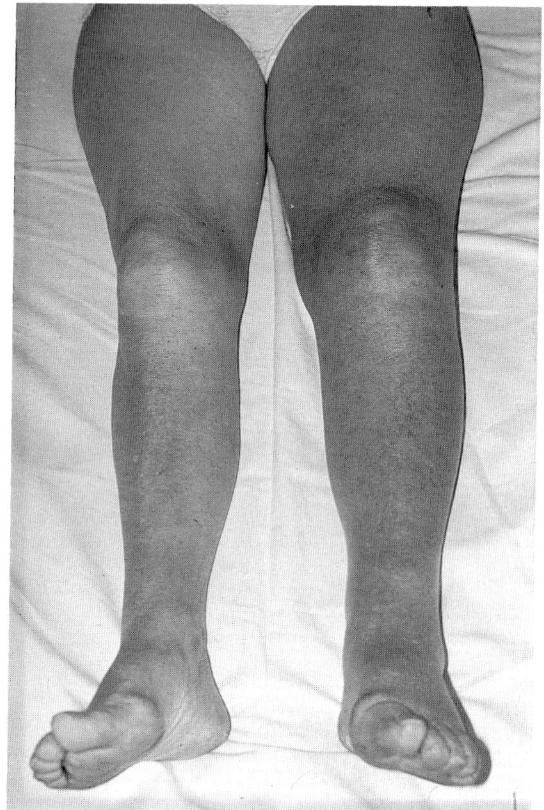

Fig. 21.5 Dilated cutaneous veins and mild ankle oedema demonstrating deep vein thrombosis.

A number of different techniques measure venous outflow obstruction. These include various types of plethysmography and venous Doppler, which are crude and of dubious worth. Thermography is in the same category, as is the measurement of fibrin degradation products which rise after any thrombosis occurring anywhere in the body.

Isotope-labelled fibrinogen used to be given to high-risk patients to image the onset of thrombosis after it had been shown experimentally to enter forming thrombus in animal models. It became a very useful test for scanning high-risk individuals, and for assessing different methods of prophylaxis. Radioactive fibrinogen is now being withdrawn, and other blood constituents which have been labelled with a view to 'thrombus-imaging' include platelets, genetically engineered fibrin fragments and plasminogen activators. It remains open to speculation as to which of these will emerge as the favoured technique.

The thrombus can now be imaged directly by either venography or duplex Doppler. Venography has been available for many years since it was first introduced by Dos Santos in the 1930s. The development of the newer non-ionic iso-osmolar contrast materials has made venography safer and less painful, but the poor quality examinations produced by many radiological departments have discredited this reference investigation. It is impossible to give a precise accuracy for venography in the detection of thrombosis, as there is nothing to compare it with; but if it is properly performed and interpreted, between 95% and 100% accuracy has been claimed (Fig. 21.6). Few patients die of pulmonary embolism derived from the leg veins after a 'normal' venogram, and few patients with unmatched ventilation perfusion defects on lung scans have 'normal' venograms.

Duplex scanning offers an alternative technique for visualizing thrombus in the leg veins. It has been compared with venography in a number of studies and has been shown to be very accurate in detecting thrombus in the main axial veins proximal to the calf (95% plus) (Fig. 21.7). It is, however, only about 70–75% accurate in detecting thrombus in the calf veins. If undetected thrombus in these veins is left untreated, it may well propagate into the stem veins, when it is more liable to fragment and cause a sizeable pulmonary embolism. This must be borne in mind if a policy decision is taken to use duplex Doppler as the first means of investigation.

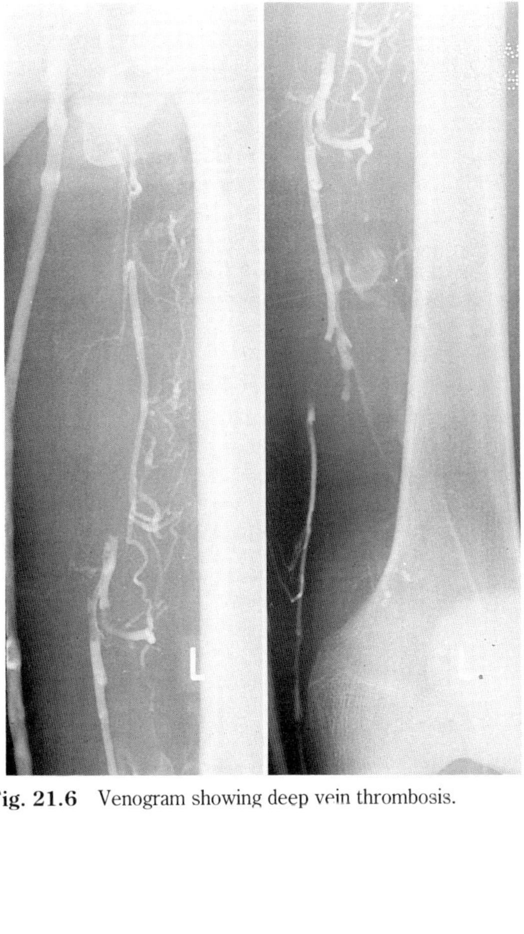

Fig. 21.6 Venogram showing deep vein thrombosis.

Once a thrombus has been diagnosed, a decision has to be taken on the best means of treatment. Most physicians and surgeons would argue that isolated calf thrombus without chest or lung scan evidence of pulmonary embolism is best treated by anticoagulants, although there are some who would simply manage this type of DVT expectantly with stockings and mobilization. This appears to be a foolhardy policy and one liable to lead to malpractice suits should a fatal pulmonary embolism ensue.

When the thrombus is old (more than a week) and occlusive, even if it extends up the limb into the iliac vessels, it is again best treated by anticoagulants (an intravenous continuous infusion of heparin 30–40 000 units/day controlled by the KCCT followed by warfarin for 3–6 weeks to prevent propagation, and pulmonary embolism). Fibrinolytic treatment is not effective at re-establishing flow in occluded veins and is unlikely to be effective once nonocclusive thrombus is more than 48 hours old.

In patients with fresh loose propagated proximal thrombus in the femoral or iliac veins, especially if this extends into the inferior vena cava, there is a

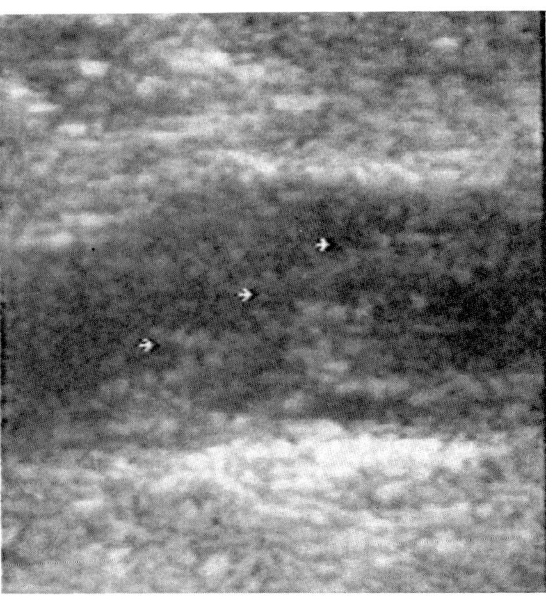

Fig. 21.7 Duplex scan showing thrombus in the main axial veins proximal to the calf.

dilemma over the best method of treatment. Many would again simply use anticoagulants, although this policy has been shown to result in deaths from pulmonary embolism especially where a small 'herald' embolism has already occurred. The policy of using anticoagulants on all-comers means that no attempt is being made to prevent the future development of the post-thrombotic limb. Sadly there is little evidence that active thrombus removal, be it by operation or fibrinolytic treatment, is any more effective in preventing long-term complications of lipodermatosclerosis, ulceration, leg swelling and discomfort which may subsequently develop. Despite this, many young patients with a recently developed non-occlusive proximal thrombus deserve active treatment in an attempt to overcome these potential problems and avoid fatal pulmonary embolism. For this reason thrombectomy may be undertaken, using Fogarty catheters and external limb compression or lysis with streptokinase, urokinase or tissue plasminogen activator. If these measures are not considered appropriate (and many feel that they are not justified), it may be a better option to lock the loose thrombus in the leg and prevent it escaping into the lungs. This is usually accomplished by placement of a vena cava filter. This is best inserted through the right internal jugular vein and passed through the right atrium using an image intensifier before being positioned in the inferior vena cava just below the renal veins. The Greenfield–Kimray filter has stood the test of time and can now be inserted percutaneously if desired. There are a number of different intracaval filters now available such as the helical, bird's-nest and Gunther filters.

The major indication to insert a filter is a patient who continues to have repeated pulmonary emboli despite apparently adequate anticoagulation treatment. Patients with the problem of repeated embolism despite adequate anticoagulation usually have either a hidden malignancy or some type of thrombophilia (antithrombin III deficiency, protein C deficiency, the lupus anticoagulant etc.). Insertion of a caval filter may well preserve life but continued embolisation or *in situ* thrombosis of the filter may lead to further leg swelling.

Post-thrombotic leg

The majority of limbs return to a normal size a month or two after a deep vein thrombosis, although those with a major proximal occlusive iliac thrombosis may not do so. By 6 months there will be a clear indication as to whether the patient has recovered or whether the limb will remain permanently swollen. Persistant leg swelling after a DVT is called the 'post-thrombotic syndrome' and usually indicates a severe proximal extension into the femoral or iliac veins, although total obstruction of the popliteal vein with poor collateral formation can cause marked calf swelling. The risk of post-thrombotic syndrome, which is often accompanied by the development of lipodermatosclerosis and venous ulceration in subsequent years, cannot be accurately predicted during the acute phase of DVT (in the first couple of months after its development) and there is some evidence that its course is unpredictable. Some limbs with apparently severe thrombotic damage develop few, if any, symptoms, while others with minimal changes develop severe pain and swelling. Patients may go for many years (10 or even 20) with few or no symptoms before gradually developing increasing pain, swelling, lipodermatosclerosis and eventually ulceration.

There is little evidence to suggest that the condition can be effectively prevented once the thrombosis has occurred, although successful prophylaxis of venous thrombosis in the postoperative period obviously abolishes the condition. Attempts at lysing or surgically removing fully developed thrombus have not been successful in significantly reducing the risk of future swelling. It is not known how long a thrombus takes to damage valve function irreparably.

Patients presenting with leg swelling are suspected of having the 'post-thrombotic leg or syndrome' if there is a clear history of deep vein thrombosis or pulmonary embolism, if collateral veins are present on either the limbs or abdomen (Fig. 21.8.), or if lipodermatosclerosis, venous flare or ulceration are present in the gaiter region (Fig. 21.9.).

The diagnosis must be confirmed and, at present, bipedal ascending phlebography is still the investigation of choice. Duplex scanning can also be used to image the deep veins and determine valvular reflux, but there are certain segments of the venous system of the lower limb which are difficult to image. Furthermore, abnormal reflux may be the result of congenital valvular aplasia rather than post-thrombotic damage. The iliac veins are also poorly demonstrated by duplex, but duplex assessment of venous reflux may compliment ascending venography which shows the anatomical sites of post-thrombotic damage, and replace descending venography which is often poorly accepted by patients. In addition an estimate of calf pump function

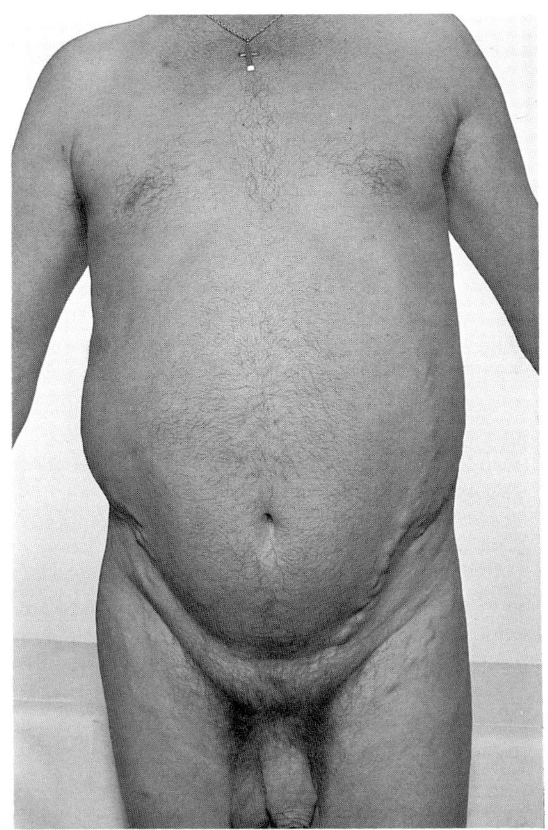

Fig. 21.8 Collateral veins present on abdomen of patient with inferior vena caval obstruction.

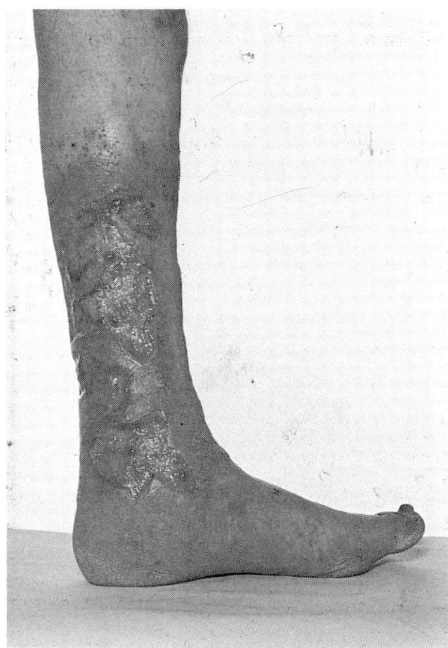

Fig. 21.9 A large irregularly shaped ulcer situated over the gaiter region of the leg. There is marked lipodermatosclerosis in the skin around the ulcer, and an 'ankle flare' is just visible beneath it.

should be made. This can be by venous pressure measurement during exercise, by photoplethysmography or by foot volumetry.

There is little that can be done surgically to improve symptoms if severe post-thrombotic damage is present in the calf and popliteal veins (Fig. 21.10.). Attempts have been made to use the long saphenous vein as a conduit to bypass distal obstruction by anastomising it to the popliteal vein. There is little evidence that this procedure produces a worthwhile improvement in venous claudication or leg swelling, and it is usually no better than the pathophysiological adaption that occurs when incompetent perforating veins 'join' the posterior tibial veins to the long saphenous system to produce a 'natural' bypass. This procedure has therefore largely been abandoned, as has ligation of the perforating veins as this operation may even make the post-thrombotic symptoms worse. Patients should be treated by the prescription of good, graduated-compression below-knee elastic support stockings which must be worn every day for the rest of the patient's life. It is important to prescribe two stockings which must be worn and washed on alternate days, and to prescribe at least four stockings per year (two every six months).

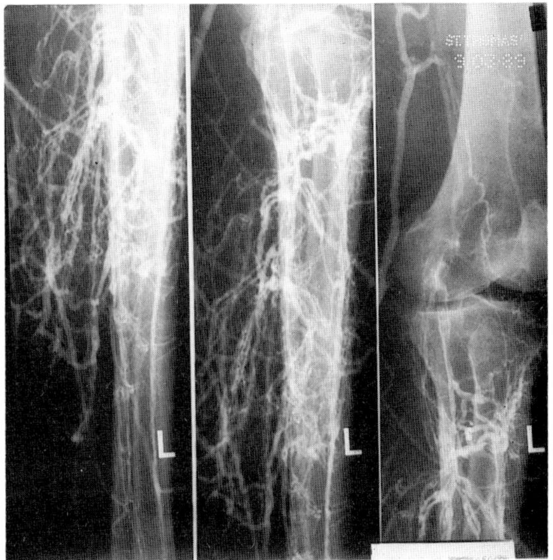

Fig. 21.10 Post-thrombotic damage in the calf and popliteal veins.

Fibrinolytic enhancement with stanozolol may improve painful lipodermatosclerosis.

When there is a proximal obliteration of one iliac vein, a Palma bypass is often very effective in alleviating claudication and improving leg swelling and skin complications. In this operation the long saphenous vein from the 'normal' contralateral limb is mobilized down to the knee without detaching or damaging the saphenofemoral function. The femoral and profunda veins are then mobilized on the affected side and the most normal segment of vein is selected for the saphenofemoral anastomosis. The opposite long saphenous vein is divided at knee level to ensure sufficient length and swung across in a suprapubic subcutaneous tunnel. The end of the long saphenous vein is then anastomosed to the side of the femoral vein with a continuous everting 6/0 Prolene suture. An arterio-venous fistula is then formed between the femoral artery or one of its tributaries and the femoral or profunda femoris veins below the anastomosis, in order to ensure high flows through the bypass during the postoperative period (Fig 21.11). The fistula is closed after 6 weeks. A nonabsorbable nylon ligature may be left around the fistula to enable it to be located more easily at the second operation, although the value of this is debatable as the ligature is often difficult to dissect out of the scar tissue.

Many patients have carried out an 'auto-Palma' by developing huge anterior-wall or presacral side-to-side collaterals. These patients are not helped by a bypass. Only patients who develop a significant rise in the femoral venous pressure during muscular work should be selected for operation. Ring supported PTFE can also be used to bypass occluded

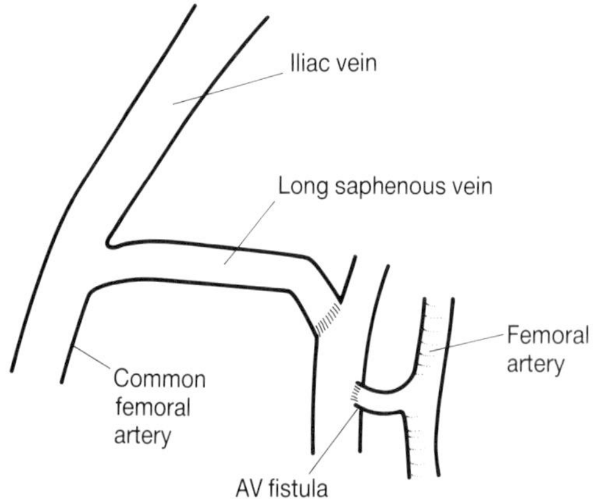

Fig. 21.11 The saphenous vein of the right leg is anastomosed to the common femoral vein of the left leg. An arteriovenous fistula is formed between the femoral artery and the femoral vein below the veno-venous anastomosis.

iliac veins and the lower vena cava, through the retroperitoneum. This type of femorocaval bypass is extremely successful in reducing symptoms and should also be combined with temporary arterio-venous fistulae in both groins.

A number of procedures have been described to repair or transplant valves into deep veins with severe venous reflux. These procedures can rarely be used in limbs with severe post-thrombotic venous damage and are probably best reserved for deep veins with congenital valvular aplasia (although it is possible that some deep veins may achieve perfect recanalization after thrombosis, and valvular repair under these circumstances is also appropriate). There is little firm evidence that these procedures abolish limb swelling and they should at present only be performed as part of a controlled trial.

Klippel Trenaunay syndrome

This rare syndrome usually develops at birth or in childhood. Abnormal veins are associated with a capillary naevus and with bony abnormalities (Fig. 21.12.). There is often a persistent lateral (axial) vein on the outer side of the leg and the deep veins may be aplastic. The capillary naevus may draw attention to the condition. The affected limb is often larger than its fellow and lymphatic abnormalities may coexist. Phlebography confirms that the deep veins are patent. Patients may then have their surface veins excised, but there is a high incidence of postoperative DVT and support stockings are an alternative.

Iliac vein compression syndrome

This is a relatively rare cause of leg swelling, but must be considered in patients presenting with swelling of the left leg. The left common iliac vein may become severely compressed as it passes behind the right common iliac artery. This can be demonstrated by phlebography (Fig. 21.13). The treatment is to carry out a Palma bypass (described above).

Lymphoedema

The diagnosis of lymphoedema must always be considered in any patient with chronic swelling of the lower limb. Lymphoedema is the likely cause if the swelling develops in childhood, if both lower limbs are swollen, if there is similar swelling of one or

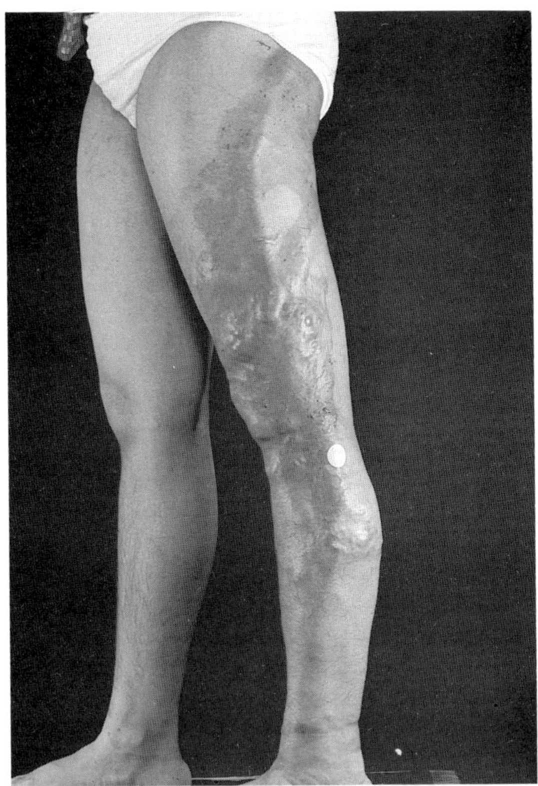

Fig. 21.12 Abnormal veins with a capillary naevus on the leg of a patient with Klippel Trenaunay syndrome.

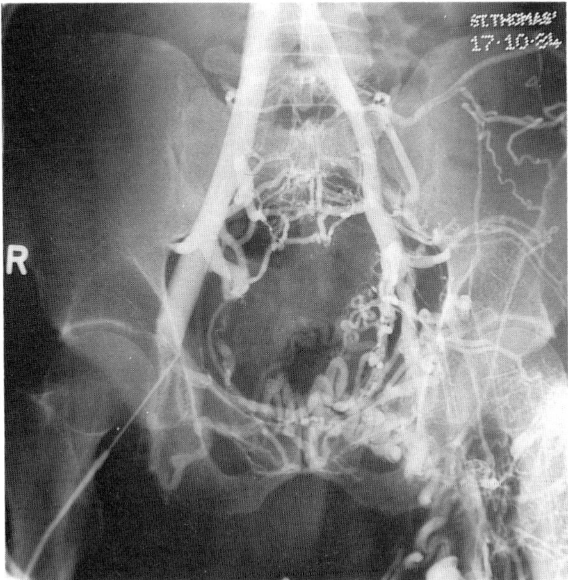

Fig. 21.13 Phlebogram showing compression of the left common iliac vein as it passes behind the right common iliac artery with cross-pelvic collaterals.

other upper limb or the genitalia, or if there is an obvious predisposing cause.

Children who are born with limb swelling are likely to be suffering from lymphatic aplasia (Milroy's disease). The presence of multiple arteriovenous fistulae (Parks–Weber syndrome) must be excluded (see earlier) and a few children will be suffering from gigantism. The swelling associated with AV fistulae or gigantism is the result of overgrowth of all the tissues (muscle and bone) within the limb, and the swelling does not 'pit' on pressure. Lymphoedema always 'pits' provided that adequate pressure is applied for long enough. CT scanning is the definitive test of gigantism, showing that the bones and muscle rather than the subcutaneous tissues are enlarged.

Primary lymphoedema usually develops in young girls shortly after puberty (praecox) and presentation at this age is much more common than Milroy's disease. The swelling is usually mild, confined below the knee and often bilateral. It rarely becomes severe or progresses above the knee. About a third of the patients have a family history of limb swelling.

A small group of patients, with an approximately equal sex-distribution, develop severe whole-limb oedema from the toes to the groin, sometimes also involving the buttock and suprapubic region which may also be swollen. This distribution, often associated with sparing of the foot, indicates the possibility of a proximal lymphatic occlusion. The work of Wolfe indicates that this is often caused by fibrosis in the inguinal or iliac nodes. Some patients with other congenital abnormalities, such as distichiasis (two rows of eyelashes), micrognathia (small jaw), yellow nail syndrome and mixed arteriovenous anomalies, have associated lymphoedema. Patients with congenital cardiac deformities sometimes have an associated aplastic thoracic duct.

Some patients with lymphoedematous limb swelling have vesicles in the skin which frequently burst and leak lymph or chyle (milky looking fluid). These patients usually have large, dilated and incompetent lymphatics which allow the lymph and chyle to reflux back into the limb. This lymphatic abnormality may be associated with lymphatic chylous ascites, chyluria, vaginal lymph leakage and chylothorax.

Lymphoedema occasionally comes on later in life (tarda) when it may be associated with severe obesity. Under these circumstances, the lymph nodes become replaced with fat and subsequently fibrose. A 'secondary' cause must be considered in every elderly patient developing lymphoedema, and for that matter in all patients presenting with a short history of leg swelling. The important causes of 'secondary' lymphoedema are filariasis (which is most common in East Africa), malignant involvement of lymph nodes, surgical block dissection and radiotherapy. Trauma, cellulitis and chronic inflammatory conditions such as eczema and rheumatoid arthritis are less common causes of secondary lymphoedema.

A careful history and examination often suggests the possibility of a cause for the lymphoedema, but blood testing for microfilaria, CT scanning of the pelvis and abdomen and even biopsy to exclude primary or secondary malignancy may be necessary. Contrast lymphography is also sometimes helpful, with secondary deposits being seen as filling defects within dye-filled nodes (Fig. 21.14). False negative examinations can however occur when the whole node is filled with tumour and as a result does not fill with contrast.

Clinical features

Patients usually present with painless, slowly progressive limb swelling, although the onset may be quite sudden on occasions. An attack of cellulitis may be the first indication of the problem and this is then assumed to be the cause of the swelling when in reality it is the effect. Patients with lymphoedema do not clear bacteria from the subcutaneous tissues. In addition they have an increased incidence of fungal infection between the toes, and a reduced immune response. Many patients first notice the swelling after a minor injury or insect bite. Some patients have an obvious predisposing cause such as a block dissection often after mastectomy and axillary clearance. The presence of lipodermatosclerosis and varicose veins on examination suggests a venous aetiology, while lymphoematous limbs have normal-looking skin with square toes. This is because footwear restricts swelling and produces this characteristic appearance. Lymphoedema does pit but requires prolonged digital pressure. The skin is often thickened and covered with papillae and vesicles which may leak lymph. The genitalia and upper limbs may also be oedematous.

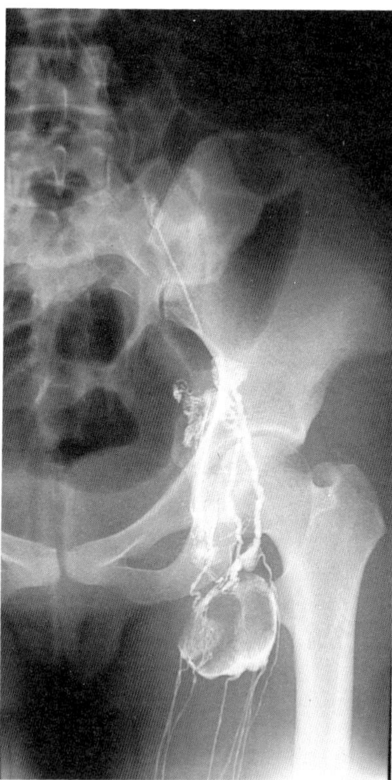

Fig. 21.14 Contrast lymphogram. Secondary deposits of melanoma can be seen as filling defects within dye-filled nodes.

Differential diagnosis

Venous oedema, cyclical oedema, cardiac oedema, renal oedema, hypoproteinaemia, hysterical oedema, gigantism, lipodystrophy and arteriovenous fistulae must all be considered in the differential diagnosis and excluded.

Lymphoedema can usually be confidently diagnosed by isotope lymphangiography. Rhenium sulphur colloid injected subcutaneously into a web space is taken up by the lymphatics and transported to the inguinal, iliac and para-aortic lymph nodes. The percentage of the injected dose reaching the groin nodes within 30 and 60 minutes can be measured. If reduced or negligible counts are detected this signifies the presence of lymphatic disease. Contrast lymphangiography may be required to confirm the diagnosis in difficult cases and to display the anatomical site of obstruction if this is present, as this may influence treatment. Other tests that may be valuable include venography, duplex Doppler, CT scanning of the leg and abdomen to exclude an alternative cause for the oedema and to confirm or refute the presence of lymphatic metastases.

The urea and electrolytes, serum protein levels, liver function tests and a haemoglobin and sedimentation rate should be obtained in all patients as baseline investigations. The presence of microfilarae should be excluded by a nocternal blood sample if patients live or have lived in a part of the world where filaria are endemic. The only other investigation that may be of value is the chromium chloride isotope test which is used to discover the amount of protein that is being lost from the gastrointestinal tract. This can occur in some patients with lymphoedema and is suspected when there are very low albumin levels, especially if the patient has evidence of lymphatic reflux with cutaneous vesicles, chylous ascites, chylothorax or chyluria. Very occasionally lymph node biopsy may be required to exclude malignancy. This is now usually by fine needle aspiration, but lymphoma will usually require a lymph node excision. There is some danger that node excision may make the swelling much worse if patients have hyperplastic lymph glands and primary lymphoedema rather than lymphoma. For this reason it is always advisable to perform contrast lymphography before node biopsy.

Management

Most patients with mild primary lymphoedema should be managed conservatively in the first instance. As there is no cure for lymphoedema, it is important to confirm the diagnosis, usually by an isotope lymphogram. Patients can then be properly counselled. They should be advised to wear elastic support stockings all day (usually only below-knee, but full-length stockings or tights may be required if the thigh and buttock are involved). The stocking should be put on in bed in the morning when the swelling is at its best and taken off last thing at night. The affected leg should be elevated whenever possible, but once the stocking has been put on, walking should not be discouraged. Standing still for prolonged periods and sitting with the leg hanging down should, if possible, be avoided. Massage and repeated applications of tight bandages have been found to be effective but their application is often time-consuming and professional massage is costly. This approach requires an obsessive personality for a good result.

Pneumatic compression devices may be purchased which take over the job of a personal masseuse and some patients who apply these devices overnight find that they are very effective.

It is important to avoid portals of entry for bacteria that can cause cellulitis which can become a recurrent and intractable problem. Athlete's foot (Tinea pedis) is almost always present in patients with lymphoedema, perhaps because of a reduction in their immunological competence. The cracks that form between the toes are an important site for bacteria to enter the subcutaneous tissues. Tinea pedis must be vigorously treated with antifungisides. Local application of zinc undecenoate (Mycota) and Whitfield's ointment may be supplemented by systemic treatment with griseofulvin if the fungus proves difficult to control. Patients must be warned of the dangers of minor injury of the swollen limbs because breaches in the skin can also be a potential site of bacterial egress. It may be advisable to give patients a small stock of amoxycillin, flucloxacillin (Staphylococcus is the usual organism that infects) or augmentin to start prophylaxis after any injury or breach of the skin. This also allows patients who do suffer from recent cellulitis to start treatment at once if they begin to feel shivery and pyrexial. Patients with recurrent attacks of cellulitis without an obvious portal of entry may require long-term low-dose antibiotics.

Drugs

Drugs that reduce oedema include the rutosides, the coumarins and diuretics. There are few controlled trials that support the use of any of these. At present there are no pharmaceutical preparations that unblock blocked lymphatics. Endolymphatic steroids have been tried and produced some benefit in a few patients.

Surgical intervention

Surgical treatment of lymphoedema should be reserved for those patients with massive limb swelling which is interfering with daily living. This probably represents 5% or less of the total population with lymphoedema. Patients must have the results of operation explained to them in detail and preferably be shown some examples of the sort of result that can be expected. It is important not to offer extensive reconstruction (and unsightly scars) to patients with mild lymphoedema who are better treated conservatively. It is equally important to be able to offer surgical treatment to a patient whose life is made miserable by massive limbs which restrict him or her to a chair-bound or house-bound existence.

There are basically two types of operation for lymphoedema. The first is to bypass the sites of occlusion (enteromesenteric bridge and lymphovenous bypass); the second is to excise lymphodematous tissue (reduction operations). Patients who are suitable for lymphatic bypasses have normal limb lymphatics with a proximal occlusion in the femoral or iliac lymph nodes. Bypass operations are only applicable to about 2–5% of all lymphoedematous patients being considered for operation.

Patients with occluded, hypoplastic, aplastic or

ectalic limb lymphatics can only be treated by excision of affected tissue.

Lymphatic bypass operations. Despite many ingenious attempts in the past which have included attempts to attach lymph nodes directly to veins (Nieubulewitz) and to use omentum as a lymphatic conduit (Gillies), there are now only two main methods of bypassing lymphatics. The first is by directly anstomosing lymphatics to veins. The second is to use an enteromesenteric bridge developed by Kinmonth and employed mainly at St Thomas' Hospital.

Lymphatics in the groin are outlined by the injection of patent blue in the foot before being dissected out and directly anastomosed end-to-side with 10/0 or 12/0 sutures to the femoral vein in the groin, using a surgical microscope. This technique is time-consuming and difficult. At least two or three anstomoses should be performed if possible. O'Brien has claimed good results for this technique, but there is little evidence that the limb decreases dramatically in size and most of the improvement is produced by a reduction in 'tension' (i.e. the limb feels less tense or softer). Many of the anastomoses occlude because of the 'low lymph flow' and thrombosis occurring at the site of the anastomosis in the vein. For these reasons the technique is not widely practised.

The enteromesenteric bridging operation was developed by Kinmonth and his colleagues as an alternative to the use of omentum, on the grounds that the ileum has a rich lymphatic plexus which drains its wall. An isolated loop of terminal ileum is made by dividing part of the mesentery and the bowel wall to leave about 5–10 cm of bowel with an intact blood supply and lymphatic drainage. The bowel is resutured behind the pedicle, which can then be brought down to the groin region. The antimesenteric border is opened and the lumen of the bowel fully exposed. Adrenaline in normal saline (1:400 000) is infiltrated beneath the mucosa, which is then removed by sharp dissection and blunt abrasion with a swab. This leaves the rich submucosal lymphatic plexus exposed. A lymph node in the iliac chain is detected by palpation or an inguinal node is exposed through a further incision in the groin. Any lymph node that is found is bivalved and sutured apart. The submucosal surface of the bridge is then sutured over the divided node (Fig. 21.15). The mesenteric pedicle may have to be brought in to the thigh behind the inguinal ligament through the femoral canal.

These enteromesenteric bridges work in between half and three-quarters of selected patients with a proximal lymphatic occlusion, often achieving dramatic results with reductions of 5–10 cm in the size of the limb. However, it must be noted that nearly half the patients obtain little or no improvement despite a major operation. It is as yet impossible to decide with any certainty which patients will benefit! We have performed just over 20 of these operations in about 10 years at St Thomas' Hospital.

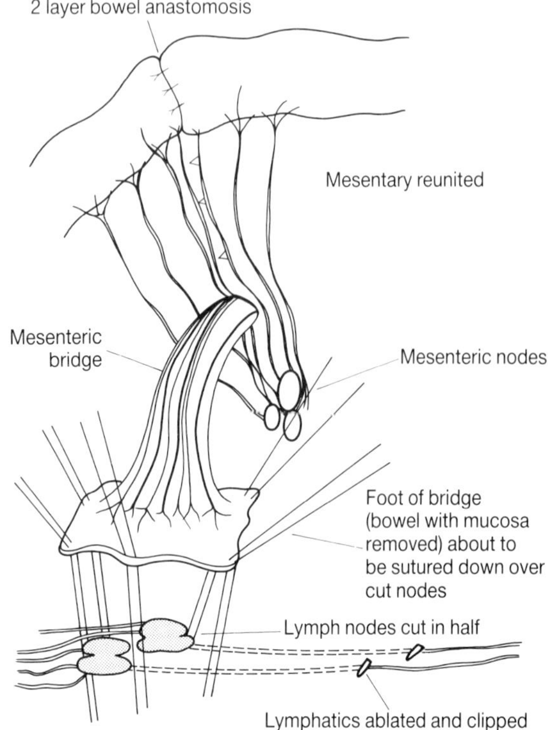

Fig. 21.15 Enteromesenteric bridge operation described by Kinmonth and colleagues.

Reduction operations. Although Sistrunk, Kondoleon and Thomson's operations have been in vogue in the past, there are now only two major types of reduction that are practised.

In Homan's reduction, the limb is suspended from the theatre ceiling using a Steinman pin through the calcaneum, which is attached via a horseshoe connection to a block and tackle. This allows access to all sides of the limb, which is further facilitated by dropping the end of the operating table and rotating it outwards to provide even better access to the medial side (Fig. 21.16). The leg is then exsanguinated with Esmarch bandages and a pneumatic tourniquet. The skin incisions are marked out with indelible ink as shown in the figure. The medial side of the limb is almost always reduced first. Skin flaps are raised from the side of the limb to the front and back as shown. They should not be too thin as this impairs the blood supply. They should not extend too far backwards or forwards as this also puts the flap's viability in doubt. They should have a narrow origin and a wide base. Cross incisions may be placed a hand's breadth below the knee and sometimes at the ankle, although this is often not necessary. Once the flaps have been raised the subcutaneous tissue is excised down to the deep fascia. The incision may be extended up the inner side of the thigh to excise a large wedge of subcutaneous tissue as far as the groin (see Fig. 21.16). A dart may also be taken out of the ankle to produce a nice taper. The flaps are put back in place and excess skin excised from either or both sides. All visible cut ends of blood vessels are picked up and ligated with catgut or polyglycolic acid sutures. The tourniquet is then released and complete haemostasis achieved by diathermy, ligature and under-running of bleeding vessels. Multiple Redivac drains are inserted and the wounds completely closed with interrupted nylon sutures or staples.

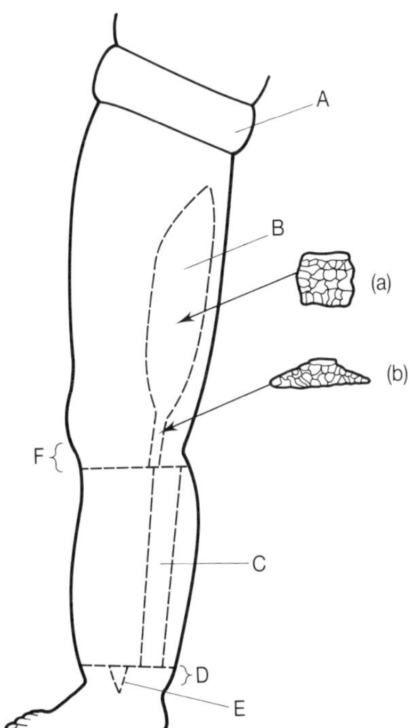

Fig. 21.16 Modified Homan operation for oedema of leg and thigh. A = tourniquet. B = thigh reduction, 'Indian club' shape with handle near knee. Flaps need little or no undermining (a) except at knee (b). C = area of skin excised between anterior and posterior leg flaps. D = two fingers above os calcis. E = dart (cut later in operation). F = three fingers below patella.

The limb is dressed and bandaged over a thick layer of cotton-wool to reduce oozing. The patients are nursed in bed for several days and the dressings are taken down after about 5–7 days. Redivacs can then be removed and mobilization begun. Patients may go home with bandages after about 10 days and can be refitted with stockings in about a month. The lateral side of the leg can be reduced in a similar manner after about 6 months. This type of reduction reduces limb circumference by about 30–50%. It is important to maintain any surgical reduction that has been achieved by the continued wearing of elastic compression stockings or the obsessional application of elastic bandages.

The Charles reduction is a much more radical limb reduction and is reserved for massive limbs, especially those with severe cutaneous changes (lymphatic papillae or warts). Once again the operation is performed with the limb suspended and exsanguinated. The skin and subcutaneous tissue of the calf are completely excised down to the deep fascia. The subcutaneous tissue of the ankle and knee are trimmed and flaps raised to make a nice 'taper' down the limb, avoiding an unsightly 'pantaloon' effect. The raw surface is then covered with split skin grafts taken from the opposite limb or the torso (Fig. 21.17). These may be thinly meshed and are best

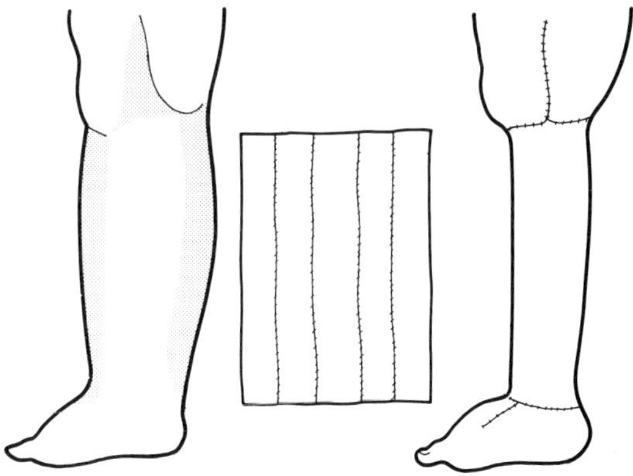

Fig. 21.17 Charles's operation for lymphoedema. Thiersch grafts are brought from healthy areas such as the back and placed over the denuded deep fascia of the leg.

attached by skin staples. The limb is then carefully bandaged and the patient kept on bed-rest for a week. The dressings are removed and the wounds inspected. Additional skin grafts may be applied to any areas where the grafts have not taken. The limbs may then be re-bandaged or left open, depending on the percentage of graft take. The patient is then gently mobilized. The staples can be removed after another week and patients may be discharged from hospital when fully mobile with adequate skin cover. They should continue to wear dressings and bandages until all the wounds have healed, but do not usually require stockings in the long term.

The Charles procedure provides very good limb reduction but the cosmetic appearances may not be acceptable to many young women. It is an ideal approach for a massive limb with cutaneous involvement. The calf reduction is usually perfect, but future reduction procedures may be required on the foot, ankle and thigh. The Homan procedure is better cosmetically but is not so radical, and if the limb is left uncompressed the swelling will recur.

Recommended further reading

1. Browse NL, Burnand KG, Lea Thomas M. *Diseases of the Veins: Pathology, Diagnosis and Treatment.* London: Edward Arnold, 1988.
2. Negus D. *Leg Ulcers: A Practical Approach to Management.* Oxford: Butterworth-Heinemann, 1991.
3. Kinmonth JB. *The Lymphatics: Diseases, Lymphography and Surgery.* London: Edward Arnold, 1972.
4. Kinmonth JB. *The Lymphatics: Surgery, Lymphography and Diseases of the Chyle and Lymph Systems,* 2nd edn. London: Edward Arnold, 1982.
5. May R, Partsch H, Staubesand J, *et al.* (eds). *Perforating Veins.* 1981.
6. May R. *Surgery of the Veins of the Leg and Pelvis.* Georg Thieme, Stuttgart: 1979.
7. Gottlob R, May R. *Venous Valves.* New York: Springer-Verlag, 1986.

22

Varicose veins

Simon G Darke

Although the management of varicose veins might be regarded as somewhat prosaic, it is nonetheless a major component of surgical practice. With increasing sub-specialization in the broad field of general surgery, it is likely that in the future the responsibility for this condition will fall increasingly and ultimately exclusively on the vascular surgeon. This, however, would not seem to be inappropriate. There are fundamental concepts and modalities of investigation that naturally extend themselves from arterial into venous surgery.

Varicose veins affect 10–12% of the adult population.[1,2] A strong familial predisposition is well established.[3,4] As we shall see, the majority of these, when they do seek advice, will require operation. It is not surprising that this demand has doubled in the UK in the last decade.[5]

Presentation

History

A patient may seek advice for one or more of the following main reasons:

1. asymptomatic but concerned that problems might ensue in the future
2. cosmetic
3. mild pain
4. significant pain associated with measurable swelling
5. skin changes and ultimately ulceration.

Other specific points should be sought in the history which may not be spontaneously forthcoming: the presence or absence of a family history; possible previous episodes of deep vein thrombosis and pulmonary embolism, or situations in the past that may have been associated with these such as trauma or operation.

An evaluation of the patient's general health and fitness should be made – as with most clinical situations this is an essential component of the overall assessment.

Examination

Note should be made of the anatomical distribution of any varicosities and the nature and extent of skin changes such as eczema, pigmentation and ultimately ulceration. Measurements with a tape-measure should be taken of the foot, calf and thigh and a comparison made with the opposite side. It is surprising how often there is a significant disparity of which the patient is quite unaware and which is not apparent on casual inspection.

For assessment of the specific morphology of the varicose veins themselves, use of the hand-held unidirectional Doppler device is essential.[6–9] Varicosities arise from either the long or short saphenous system or both. It is very rare for previously unoperated varicose veins to be derived from isolated perforators either at the ankle or higher level independent of one of the saphenous systems. However, this may occur in recurrent varicose veins.

Two essential points need to be determined:

1. From which of the two saphenous systems are the varicosities derived?
2. What is the extent of incompetence in that main trunk, and in particular does this incompetence extend to the junction with the deep system (i.e. the saphenofemoral or saphenopopliteal junction)?

Although these points are self-evident from simple inspection in some patients, this is not always the case. It cannot be emphasized too strongly how important is the use of the Doppler, and the technique is now described.

Doppler examination of primary varicose veins

The patient is examined while standing and holding a convenient support to remain as immobile as possible.

To determine from which of the two saphenous systems the varicosities are derived, a test of 'sonic continuity' is employed. The probe is first of all located over the saphenofemoral junction in the groin by moving it medially from the femoral artery signal until it ceases. Confirmation of the correct position is obtained by manual calf compression which produces an audible signal. The varicosity in question is now tapped sharply with the finger. A signal indicates sonic and anatomical continuity. If there is no signal then it is unlikely that the varicosity is derived from the long saphenous. At the same time the evaluation of reflux at the saphenofemoral junction can be undertaken by once more compressing the calf and then releasing. If no further signal on calf release is heard this implies competence. Occasionally a very short refluxing signal of less than one second may be heard which is not significant. If, however, a further signal similar to that heard on compression follows the release of calf squeezing, this indicates incompetence. Further confirmation can be gained by demonstrating a signal with a patient's cough. Abolition of this refluxing signal by compression of the long saphenous vein in the thigh, either by hand or by tourniquet, further confirms saphenofemoral incompetence – but this is seldom necessary.

A similar procedure is used to assess saphenopopliteal derivation and incompetence. The probe is located over the popliteal vein in the popliteal fossa by first finding the arterial signal and then moving slightly laterally. Confirmation of derivation is again demonstrated by tapping the varicosity. Saphenopopliteal incompetence is established by calf compression and release.

No cough impulse is demonstrable in the short saphenous unless the deep valves are extensively incompetent as well. If this is the case then it has to be conceded that some difficulty may be experienced regarding the discrimination of saphenopopliteal and popliteal vein incompetence. Some distinction can be achieved by manual or tourniquet calf compression of the short saphenous below the saphenopopliteal junction. If this abolishes the refluxing signal it implies that incompetence is confined to the short saphenous. A persistent signal, not abolished by calf compression, indicates deep incompetence. Doubt may still remain as to whether the short saphenous is incompetent as well. However, this area is easily accessible to the duplex scanner. This should be employed in cases of uncertainty because it gives valuable and accurate information on both anatomy and incompetence.[10]

Table 22.1 summarizes my experience of patients with primary varicose veins seen over a 30-month period. This is in a secondary referral practice and represents a relatively pure sample of the situation as it exists within the community. From this it will be seen that of the 466 patients with primary varicose veins without complex disorders of ulcer or excessive pain and swelling, the great majority (all but 46) had saphenous incompetence.

Table 22.2 shows the more specific outcome of the use of Doppler assessment in 100 consecutive limbs with varicose veins.[9] Careful distinction was made between long and short saphenous incompetence.

In common with other reports, the use of Doppler increases the proportion of patients in whom the short saphenous is found to be the source of varicosities (approximately 25%).[10,11]

Table 22.1 Consecutive series of patients with chronic venous disorders over a 30-month period

Total number of patients	594
Patients with primary varicose veins	466
No saphenous incompetence	46
Saphenous incompetence	420
Patients with complex disorders	128 (145 limbs)
48 limbs with ulcer	(26 women, mean age = 56)
52 limbs with ulcer, pain and swelling	(22 women, mean age = 54)
45 limbs with pain and swelling alone	(22 women, mean age = 40)

Table 22.2 Outcome of unidirectional Doppler system analysis of 100 consecutive limbs with varicose veins

	Long saphenous	Short saphenous
Total	85	27
Incompetent	60	25
Competent	25 (29%)	2 (7%)
Recurrent	6 (all incompetent)	8 (all incompetent)
Both systems	6	6

Further investigation

For the majority of patients presenting with primary uncomplicated varicose veins, the foregoing quick, simple and cheap evaluation is all that is required. It is only occasionally that the source of primary varicosities may be in doubt, and under these circumstances venography and varicography may be of value. Radiology is more usefully and frequently applied in the assessment of recurrent varicose veins, which are discussed later.

There are, however, two circumstances under which further investigation with venography is required.

The first is if there is doubt as to whether the patient may have had a previous deep vein thrombosis. A conventional ascending venogram to examine this possibility should be employed in these cases. If this is found to be positive then a dilemma may exist as to whether the superficial varicosities play an important collateral role in terms of venous outflow. The extent of deep vein occlusion on X-ray may give some indication. In order to be certain it is necessary to employ a quantifiable test of venous function; normally some form of plethysmography. Two factors need to be addressed; outflow and reflux with and without a tourniquet to simulate the effects of saphenous excision ligation. Details of these tests are outside the scope of this chapter, but briefly a reduction in reflux with tourniquet indicates significant superficial incompetence. Benefit will be derived from surgery. Diminished outflow with the tourniquet indicates the saphenous and it's associated 'varicosities' to be major collaterals. Surgery is contraindicated.

Secondly, a detailed venography examination becomes mandatory in patients with pain and swelling and advanced skin change. An overview of this is described in Chapter 20. However, there is an interface with this chapter in terms of the impact of saphenous ligation for patients in this category.

Until recently, ascending and descending venography complemented the Doppler assessment mentioned above remains as the optimal means by which a comprehensive evaluation of the venous morphology in complex venous disorders can be obtained.[12] However, it is likely that Duplex Scanning will become the future means of assessing deep valve function. By these means a variety of abnormalities may be defined which may occur in different combinations:

1. primary varicose veins affecting long or short saphenous system
2. incompetence of ankle perforators
3. primary incompetence of the deep system, superficial and deep femoral and popliteal
4. post-phlebitic damage causing a combination of outflow obstruction and valvular destruction.

On this basis patients with venous ulceration can be classified into four broad categories of venous morphology (see Table 22.3).[13]

Management

Compression sclerotherapy

Compression sclerotherapy should be reserved for patients without saphenofemoral or saphenopopliteal incompetence. Injections used in the presence of saphenous reflux carry a recurrence rate of 63% at 3 years[14] and 93% at 6 years.[15] Recent studies with real-time colour duplex further confirm that sclerotherapy under these circumstances is most unlikely to have a durable result.[16] This form of treatment, therefore, is essentially confined to cosmetic treatment for recurrence or persistences after appropriate operation, or for those patients who have not as yet developed major incompetence of the saphenofemoral or saphenopopliteal junction. As indicated in Table 22.1, these patients are in a minority. Even in these it must be recognized that varicose veins are likely to be progressive. Although at the time of initial evaluation there may not be major incompetence demonstrable, the patient should be warned that this may develop in the future. Operation may ultimately become necessary to control the situation.

Compression sclerotherapy is not without its complications. Of these, pigmentation is the most common, occurring in approximately 30% of patients. In the majority this lasts from 6 to 12 months and is probably independent of the type of sclerosant used.[17] The appearance of telangiectasia, so called 'matting',[18] occurs in about 15% of patients treated. It occurs particularly on the thigh.[17] Risk factors for this complication include obesity, oestrogen therapy, pregnancy and a family history. Age and an excess of standing do not influence the outcome.[19] Other complications include urticaria and fainting. One distressing but fortunately uncommon problem is cutaneous necrosis which is more likely to be due to injection of a dermal arteriole rather than extravasation of sclerosant.[17] Injection into a major artery at ankle level can have disastrous consequences but should not occur provided reasonable care is taken.[20] Very rarely, systemic allergic reactions can take place and therefore standard facilities for rescuscitation should be available when this modality of treatment is being undertaken.[17]

Telangiectasia and radicular veins

It is possible to sclerose radicular veins, the blue venules that are seen immediately under the skin, and telangiectasia themselves. In general the same sclerosants that are used for conventional varicosities are employed at one-third of the strength. Size

27 to 30 gauge needles are required and 2 ml syringes of good quality. Magnification with a loop is preferable and good lighting essential.

One technique to minimize the risks of extravasation is to keep a bubble of air in the hub of the needle and to inject this first; thus if the needle is not in the correct position only air is injected into the dermis. However, when intraluminal penetration is achieved a very gratifying result can occur. Compression immediately following injection reduces the subsequent pigmentation. This form of treatment is subject to the same complications as those mentioned above for varicosity injections.

Other forms of treatment for 'thread veins', such as electrolysis, subcutaneous diathermy and lasers have all been described. Their roles have yet to be fully evaluated.

Operation

It will be apparent from what has already been discussed that effective treatment in the majority of patients is going to require operation. However, it is important to remember that the indications are relative. Risks, however small, still exist, particularly in the older patient. If, therefore, we look again at the presenting complaints, it is worthwhile reconsidering the indications and perceived benefits of surgery.

1. *'Asymptomatic but concerned that problems might ensue in the future'*

Advice here will depend on the severity of the varicosities and the age at which the patient presents. Clearly if there is advanced incompetence of a major junction at a relatively young age then the patient has a marked inherent predisposition to varicosities. In these patients there is often a strong family history. The implications are that the condition will progress as the patient has the greater part of a lifespan during which problems may ensue. On this basis surgical intervention is usually justified. The other end of the spectrum is illustrated by a patient in their 60s with only early incompetence and free from skin complications or other symptoms. In these, reassurance and conservative measures are appropriate.

2. *'Cosmetic'*

In these patients the same philosophy as mentioned above applies. In addition, consideration must be given to limitations of surgery in this respect. There are risks of recurrence and need for further treatment. Pigmentation and telangiectasis may occur.

3. *'Mild pain'*

In my view it seems most unlikely that pain occurs in varicosities unless there is demonstrable incompetence at the saphenopopliteal or saphenofemoral junction. This, however, is a difficult hypothesis to prove because pain is a subjective symptom. However, there seems a distinct likelihood that a number of patients underwrite their wish for a cosmetic result by claiming that there is coexistent pain. It is as well to appreciate this fact.

4. *'Significant pain associated with measurable swelling'*

This can be a common complaint and is reported as occurring in 60–70% of patients.[21] Pain and swelling can be expected to be relieved by appropriate operation.[22] This represents a legitimate indication for surgical intervention provided no major contra-indication exists.

5. *'Skin changes and ultimately ulceration'*

This is the most rewarding area in which an operation is indicated. Reference has been made to the different groups of morphology. Patients in group 2 in whom the only detectable abnormalities are saphenous and perforator incompetence should be treated by saphenous ligation and stripping. This will achieve a 95% durable healing rate. In this group of patients, subfascial ligation of perforators is seldom necessary.[13,23]

It is interesting to speculate why all patients with significant varicose veins do not develop skin changes. This is probably a function of the duration and degree of saphenous incompetence,[24] and the coexistence of ankle perforator incompetence.[25]

Patients in group 3 with a combination of saphenous and primary deep incompetence appear to benefit from saphenous ligation, but there is evidence that this is less durable and effective than for patients in group 2. In group 3 patients, subfascial perforator ligation may also be required.[25]

Technical operative notes

Saphenofemoral incompetence

Dissection of the groin for accurate saphenofemoral disconnection should carry no specific problems. It is, of course, prudent to remove all tributaries from the common femoral vein because these are undoubtedly a potential site for recurrence; although in all probability this as a cause of recurrence is overstated.[26,27]

Major technical errors are fortunately rare but

have potentially serious consequences. Of these, mistaken ligation of the common femoral vein is the most usual. It is thus important to identify the junction of the saphenous with the common femoral vein beyond any doubt before any major vessels are ligated. In this respect it is helpful to remember that this junction lies high in the groin, usually in the skin crease.

The next question is whether or not the long saphenous trunk should be stripped. The role that this plays in the pathogenesis of recurrent varicose veins is discussed further below and has recently been reviewed.[26,27] Retention of the saphenous trunk undoubtedly significantly increases the risk of recurrent varicose veins.[15,28] Unless there are very compelling reasons for its retention, therefore, this should be stripped. Legitimate reasons for trunk preservation include risks of exacerbating congenital lymphoedema, and anticipation that it be required for future coronary or femorodistal arterial bypassing. For completeness, it is worth noting that some authors recently advocated the use of limb exsanguination and tourniquet control for distal varicosity avulsions. It is claimed that this reduces blood loss and improves the early cosmetic result.[29,30]

Saphenopopliteal junction

This procedure should not be undertaken by an unsupervised inexperienced surgeon. It is made difficult by the wide variation not only in anatomy but in the source of varicosities. The dissection is deep and requires negotiation of a number of important structures, principally the popliteal vessels and nerves.

An appreciation of anatomy is crucial. In approximately two-thirds of limbs there is a dual popliteal vein. Furthermore, in the formation of these two veins there is considerable variation. In practical terms one is usually much larger than the other and thus the site of the saphenous junction self evident. The popliteal veins are in turn formed from the six venae concomitantes of the tibioperoneal vessels and the much larger gastrocnemius and soleal veins. Of practical importance, the gastrocnemius veins tend to drain directly into the popliteal vein at or above the knee joint. The remainder form below this level.[31]

To these considerations must be added the inconsistencies of the siting of the saphenopopliteal junction itself. In only 75% is this in the popliteal fossa. Of those terminations outside this area, two-thirds are higher up in the superficial or deep veins of the thigh and the remainder are in the veins below the knee.[32,33]

Finally, it is important to recognize that it is not just the short saphenous vein itself that may be incompetent and the source of varicosities. In one study the gastrocnemius vein was involved in 70% (usually the medial vein). The 'popliteal area vein', a variable and anatomically ill-defined vessel, is another significant source.[33]

In view of this complex variation it is essential that operation is preceded by preoperative ultrasound examination. At the very least this consists of an extension of the unidirectional hand-held Doppler to which reference has already been made. By moving the probe up the limb, each small advance associated by a squeeze and release of the calf, the point at which the incompetent saphenous enters into competent popliteal is identified and marked.[34] If any doubt exists, in particular in recurrent problems, a colour-coded duplex gives comprehensive information into the anatomy and the areas and origin of incompetent vessels.[10] On-table venography[35] is a time-consuming, costly and less easy to interpret.

Table 22.3 Distribution of types of venous morphology: consecutive series of patients with 232 limbs with venous ulceration

	Number of limbs	Females
Type 1: Calf perforator incompetence alone	9 (3.9%)	6
Type 2: Calf perforator incompetence and saphenous incompetence	91 (39.2%)	54
Type 3: Primary deep venous incompetence (often with associated saphenous and perforator incompetence)	81 (34.9%)	24
Type 4: Post-phlebitic damage	51 (22.0%)	24

Recurrent varicose veins

Persistence or re-emergence of varicose veins after previous operation is of the order of 20–25% some five to ten years after surgery. These figures are roughly comparable whether derived from series subsequently followed up[14,15,21,36–38] or from new patients re-evaluated.[26]

This high recurrence rate is disappointing for surgeon and patient alike and has important resource implications. An understanding of the underlying morphology is necessary for the especial reasons of attempting to minimize recurrence and treating it effectively when it does occur. Three principal types of recurrence are recognizable.

Type 1

This is recurrence without further or new incompetence in the saphenopopliteal junction (as evaluated by hand-held Doppler described above). The group constitutes about 25% of patients.[26] The source of the problem is usually a thigh perforator often connected to a residual or accessory long saphenous vein. This should be removed, the perforator identified and tied and multiple avulsions undertaken. Varicography may be helpful in identifying the source of the problem.

Type 2

There is evolution *de novo* in a second saphenous system (usually the short saphenous). Some of these cases may be 'persistence' due to incomplete evaluation at the time of the original surgery. This group constitutes 10% of the total.

Type 3

The remainder (65%) have recurrent saphenofemoral incompetence as judged by hand-held Doppler. These patients require comprehensive ascending and descending venography and varicography to define the source of the problem. In the majority there is a reconstitution of the junction due to neovascularization between the femoral vein and the retained saphenous trunk.[39] Alternatively there may be a thigh perforator above which there is no competent valve (hence the Doppler signs of reflux). Associated deep vein incompetence tends to be a feature of these patients.[26] Any remaining saphenous trunk should be stripped with multiple avulsions. Religation of the groin can be difficult due to scarring and multiple fragile tortuous recurrent channels. A vertical incision just medical to the femoral artery gives access to the common femoral vein in virgin territory just below the inguinal ligament. The recurrences are then cleared from above downwards. Some authors suggest that further recurrence might be minimized by applying a Dacron patch over the denuded femoral vein.[40]

Occasionally 'recurrence' is due to collateral development as a consequence of previous deep vein thrombosis. Constant awareness of this possibility should be kept in mind. If any doubt exists, then venography should be undertaken prior to any decision regarding surgery.

References

1. Coon WW, Willis PW, Keller JB. Venous thromboembolism and other venous disease in the Tecumseh Community Health Study. *Circulation* 1973; **48:** 839–46.
2. Widmer LK, Hall T, Mactin H. Epidemiology and sociomedical importance of peripheral venous disease. In: *Treatment of Venous Disorders*. Lancaster: MTP Press, 1977: 3–12.
3. Widmer LK, Kaufmann, Hartman G, *et al.* Organisation der Bosler Studie. Arteries, Venen, under herz Knarkheiker. *Schweiz Med Ugschr* 1976; **97:** 499–520.
4. Reagan B, Folse R. Lower limb venous dynamics in normal person and children of patients with varicose veins. *Surg Gynae Obst* 1971; **132:** 15–22.
5. Campbell WB. Varicose veins. *Br Med J* 1990; **300:** 763–4.
6. McIrvine AJ, Corbett CRR, Aston ND, *et al.* The demonstration of saphenofemoral incompetence: Doppler ultrasound compared with standard clinical tests. *Br J Surg* 1984; **71:** 506–8.
7. Hoare MC, Nicolaides AN, Miles CR, *et al.* The role of primary varicose veins in venous ulceration. *Surgery* 1982; **92:** 450–3.
8. Chan A, Chisholm I, Royle JP. The use of directional Doppler ultrasound in the assessment of saphenofemoral incompetence. *Aust NZ J Surg* 1984; **53:** 399–402.
9. Mitchell DC, Darke SG. The assessment of primary varicose veins by Doppler ultrasound: the role of sapheno-popliteal incompetence and the short saphenous system in calf varicosities. *Eur J Vasc Surg* 1987; **1:** 113–15.
10. Vasdekis SN, Clarke GH, Hobbs CJ, Nicolaides AN. Evaluation of non-invasive and invasive methods in the assessment of short saphenous vein termination. *Br J Surg* 1989; **76:** 929–32.
11. Sheppard M. The incidence, diagnosis and management of sapheno-femoral incompetence. *Phlebology* 1986; **1:** 23–32.
12. Darke SG, Andress MR. The value of venography in the manaement of chronic venous disorders of the lower limb. In: *Diagnostic Techniques and Assessment Procedures in Vascular Surgery*, Greenhalgh RM (ed). London: Grune & Stratton, 1985: 421–46.
13. Darke SG, Penfold C. Venous ulceration and saphenous ligation. *Eur J Vasc Surg* 1992; **6:** 4–9.
14. Hobbs JT. Surgery and sclerotherapy in the treatment of varicose veins. *Arch Surg* 1974; **109:** 793–6.
15. Jakobsen BH. The value of different forms of treat-

ment for varicose veins. *Br J Surg* 1979; **66:** 182–4.
16. Bishop CCR, Fronek HS, Fronek A, *et al.* Real time colour duplex scanning after sclerotherapy of the greater saphenous vein. *J Vasc Surg* 1991; **14:** 505–10.
17. Goldman MP. Compression sclerotherapy and its complications. In: *Venous Disorders*, Bergan JJ, Yao JT (eds). Philadelphia: WB Saunders, 1991: 233–49.
18. Duffy DM. Small vessel sclerotherapy: an overview. In: *Advances in Dermatology Vol. 3*. Chicago: Year Book Medical Publishers, 1988: 221–43.
19. Davis LT, Duffy DM. Determination of incidence and risk factors for post sclerotherapy telangiectatic matting of the lower extremity: a retrospective analysis. *J Dermatol Surg Oncol* 1990; **16:** 327–30.
20. Sadick N. Treatment of varicose and telangiectatic leg veins with hypertropic saline: a comparative study of heparin and saline. *J Dermatol Surg Oncol* 1990; **16:** 24–8.
21. Lofgren EP. Treatment of long saphenous varicosities and their recurrence at long-term follow-up. In: *Surgery of the Veins*, Bergan JJ, Yao JST (eds). New York: Grune & Stratton, 1985: 285–300.
22. Speakman MJ, Collin J. Are swelling and aching of the legs reduced by operation on varicose veins? *Br Med J* 1986; **293:** 105–6.
23. Sethia KK, Darke SG. Long saphenous incompetence as a cause of venous ulceration. *Br J Surg* 1984; **71:** 754–5.
24. Sutton R, Darke SG. Stripping the long saphenous vein: peroperative retrograde saphenography in patients with and without ulceration. *Br J Surg* 1986; **73:** 305–7.
25. Darke SG. 1993. In preparation.
26. Darke SG. Recurrent varicose veins and short saphenous insufficiency. In: *Venous Disorders*, Bergan JJ, Yao JST (eds). Philadelphia: WB Saunders, 1991: 217–32.
27. Darke SG. Chronic venous insufficiency – should the long saphenous vein be stripped? In: *Vascular Surgery: Current Questions*, Barros D'Sa AAB, Bell PRF, Darke SG, Harris PL (eds). Oxford: Butterworth-Heinemann, 1991: 207–18.
28. Munn SR, Morton JB, MacBeth WAAG, McLeish AR. To strip or not to strip the long saphenous vein? A varicose vein trial. *Br J Surg* 1981; **68:** 426–8.
29. Corbett R, Jayakumar KN. Clear up varicose vein surgery: use of tourniquet. *Ann Roy Coll Surg Eng* 1989; **71:** 57–8.
30. Thompson JF, Royle GT, Farrands PA, *et al.* Varicose vein surgery using a pneumatic tourniquet: reduced blood loss and improved cosmosis. *Ann Roy Coll Surg Eng* 1990; **72:** 119–22.
31. Williams AF. The formation of the popliteal vein. *Surg Gynae Obst* 1953; **97:** 769–72.
32. Dodd H. The varicose tributaries of the popliteal vein. *Br J Surg* 1965; **52:** 350–4.
33. Moosmann DA, Hartwell SW. The surgical significance of the subfascial course of the lesser saphenous vein. *Surg Gynae Obst* 1964; **113:** 761–6.
34. Gilliland EL, Gerber CJ, Lewis JD. Short saphenous surgery: pre-operative Doppler ultrasound marking compared with on-table venography and operative findings. *Phlebology* 1987; **2:** 109–14.
35. Hobbs JT. Per-operative venography to ensure accurate sapheno-popliteal vein ligation. *Br Med J* 1980; **223:** 1578–9.
36. Sheppard M. A procedure for the prevention of recurrent sapheno-femoral incompetence. *Aust NZ J Surg* 1978; **48:** 322–6.
37. Royle JP. Recurrent varicose veins. *World J Surg* 1986; **10:** 944–58.
38. Berridge DC, Makin GS. Day case surgery: a viable alternative for surgical treatment of varicose veins. *Phlebology* 1987; **2:** 103–8.
39. Glass GM. Prevention of recurrent sapheno-femoral incompetence after surgery for varicose veins. *Br J Surg* 1989; **76:** 1210.
40. Glass GM. Neovascularisation in recurrence of the varicose great saphenous vein following transection. *Phlebology* 1987; **2:** 81–91.

23

Ischaemia of the upper limb

JHH Webster

Ischaemia of the arm is very much less common than in the leg. In a review by McColl of 4452 major amputations for vascular disease or diabetes, just 12 arms were amputated.[1] A further important difference is that atherosclerosis is not the predominant cause of ischaemia as it is in the leg.

Atherosclerosis

This typically affects the proximal part of the subclavian or brachiocephalic artery, and is likely to be part of a pattern of widespread atherosclerosis. It may cause claudication of the forearm, but because of the profuse collateral circulation around the shoulder, the absence of distal pulses or reduced blood pressure may only be discovered as a chance finding on examination of a patient for some other reason.

If the atherosclerotic occlusion occurs in the subclavian artery *proximal* to the origin of the vertebral artery, then it may cause symptoms of subclavian steal, where dizziness or fainting are induced by use of the arm (Fig. 23.1).

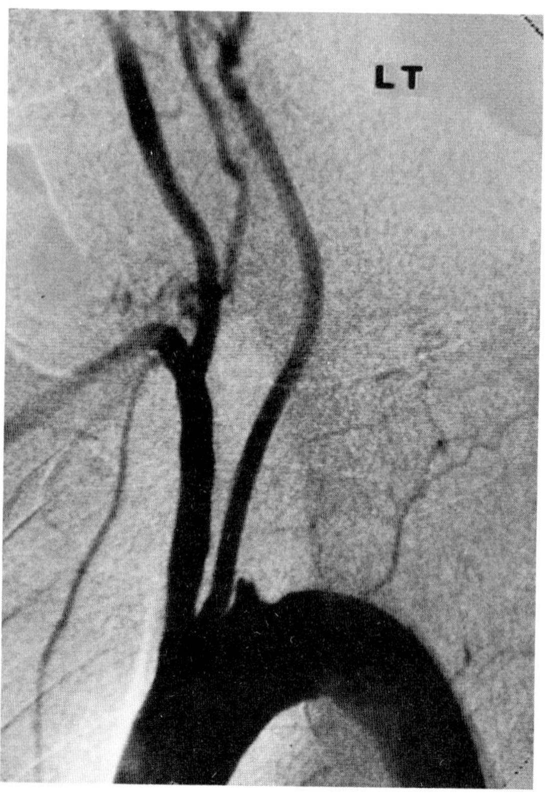

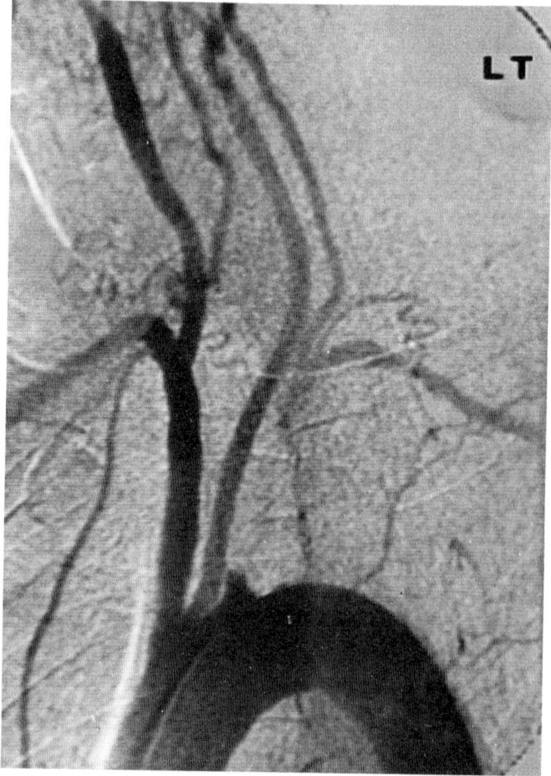

Fig. 23.1 (Left) Occlusion just beyond origin of left subclavian artery. (Right) Retrograde flow down vertebral artery when exercising the arm.

Major ischaemic changes due to atherosclerosis in the arm or forearm are unusual, except as a terminal event in the very old.

Investigation

Doppler examination of the subclavian artery will confirm the diagnosis, and if the patient's symptoms justify it, an arteriogram will show the site and extent of the disease.

Treatment

Direct operation (e.g. by endarterectomy) is very difficult to perform on the proximal subclavian artery and is particularly dangerous on the left side. Some form of crossover graft is best used, either from the opposite subclavian or brachial artery, or from the ipsilateral common carotid. The normal common carotid can allow full flow into a graft to the arm without any disturbance of the cerebral circulation. The graft chosen for these bypasses can be either autogenous saphenous vein or a prosthetic material. It is often easier to use vein as the subclavian artery can be extremely thin and friable and may be very difficult to suture to a prosthetic graft.

Embolism

Emboli to the main arteries of the arm typically come from clots within the heart. There are two common sites for the embolus to lodge, the proximal brachial artery at the takeoff point of the circumflex humeral artery, and the bifurcation of the brachial artery at the elbow. The site of the embolus should be easy to determine by palpation of the pulses. It is important to remember that the collateral circulation in the arm is so profuse that many patients may recover spontaneously over 24–48 hours.

Treatment

Anticoagulation with heparin is essential and the clinical condition of the limb must be carefully monitored. If pain, loss of sensation or loss of movement do not recover rapidly, embolectomy should be performed. If possible this should be done through a transverse incision in the artery, and a 3FG embolectomy catheter is particularly useful. The arteriotomy should be closed with great care using a 6/0 Prolene suture. The place of intra-arterial fibrinolytic therapy is still being evaluated in the arm because of the problems of placing the arterial catheter.[2]

Raynaud's phenomenon

This is dealt with in Chapter 16. Particularly urgent attention should be paid to *unilateral* Raynaud's phenomenon which is usually due to microemboli from a post-stenotic subclavian aneurysm and may progress to irreversible ischaemia *very rapidly*. A patient with unilateral Raynaud's should have duplex scanning and arteriography urgently. An appropriate subclavian artery reconstruction, with or without thoracic outlet decompression, should be performed as soon as possible. This may involve urgent referral to a specialist vascular centre.

Trauma

The two commonest forms of external trauma causing ischaemia are traction injuries around the shoulder, and supracondylar fractures of the humerus.

Shoulder injuries

The subclavian artery may be torn or crushed in these injuries. Various fractures may also occur, but the important associated injury, if it occurs, is to the brachial plexus.

If there is an associated Horner's syndrome, irrecoverable neurological damage has occurred. Unless there is unequivocal evidence that the plexus is intact, the damaged artery should not be explored. Such an exploration should only be done in a specialist vascular unit. It will involve a sternal split to gain proximal control and will be both difficult and dangerous.

Supracondylar fracture of the humerus

The backward angulation of the fracture may tear or contuse the distal brachial artery. Following reduction of the fracture careful observation of the distal circulation must be maintained. The presence of a pulse heard on Doppler at the wrist is not sufficient.

The development of Volkmann's contracture in the muscles of the forearm is related to small-vessel thrombosis and increasing tissue tension due to bleeding from the fracture. If there is any doubt at all about the circulation in the forearm, the damaged artery should be explored and wide fasciotomies of the forearm performed.

Iatrogenic trauma

Inadvertent, intra-arterial injection of hyperosmolar, acid or alkaline or thrombogenic solutions, may cause extensive distal thrombosis. Perfusion of the arterial system of the arm with large quantities of colloid or crystaloid solution may exsanguinate the arm irreversibly. Alcoholic solutions such as hibitane in spirit can cause irreversible histological fixation of the tissues. The essence is to avoid such injuries. Intravenous injection and intravenous drips in the anticubital fossa, especially under emergency conditions, should be avoided. Extreme care must be taken to check arterial lines in the arm.

Treatment

If an incorrect arterial injection is suspected, the line must be immediately flushed with heparin, and then saline, and the line removed. The arm must be closely monitored and, if there is any doubt about the circulation in the hand, a stellate ganglion block or a surgical upper thoracic sympathectomy should be considered.

Frostbite

In this variety of thermal injury, tissue death by cellular freezing and subsequent bursting is unlikely to be extensive in a temperate climate. However, the cold will cause prolonged vasospasm and this will be followed by prolonged reactive hyperaemia and oedema. These can be minimized by sympathectomy, if it can be performed at a very early stage of severe frostbite. Prostacyclin infusion also appears to be of considerable help in hastening demarcation of dead tissue. Surgical debridement or amputation should be delayed as long as possible, in the absence of infection, to allow exact definition of the lines of demarcation.

Arteritis

Buerger's disease

This is a genetically influenced condition with hypersensitivity to tobacco. It is much commoner in men than women. Typically both arteries and veins are involved in both the legs and arms and it is commonly associated with patches of thrombophlebitis. Painful ulceration of the digits occurs, and as the disease affects the small arteries, any loss of pulses will spread from distal to proximal. The appearances of spiral collaterals on arteriography are no longer considered to be diagnostic. There is an excellent review of the pathophysiology of Buerger's disease by Eastcott.[3]

Treatment

This disease cannot be treated unless the patient stops smoking, and there is anecdotal evidence that 'passive smoking' is also of importance. Some patients may also need sympathectomy.

Upper thoracic sympathectomy. The patient is placed in the half-lateral position and a transverse incision made in the lower part of the axillary skin. The incision is deepened into the third intercostal space, which is opened. Rib resection is not necessary. A small rib spreader is inserted and the lung is retracted with a small (paediatric size) lung retractor. The upper thoracic sympathetic chain is visible as a white nodular line running vertically down the neck of the ribs. The mediastinal pleura is incised along the line of the chain, and three or four ganglia are removed by cutting the rami communicantes. The chest is closed with a drain. Long fine instruments are essential for this operation, as also are metal haemostatic clips and an applicator.

Increasingly this operation is being performed endoscopically and this approach may now be considered definitive.[4] Damage to the stellate ganglion is almost impossible surgically as it cannot be seen, and should not occur with the endoscopic procedure.

Upper thoracic sympathectomy through the root of the neck ('cervical sympathectomy') or from the back by resection of ribs have become operations of only specialist indication, in rare circumstances.

Takayashu's disease

This is almost the opposite of Buerger's disease. It occurs almost exclusively in young women from South East Asia, and there is a sizeable population of patients in Provence.

In this disease, a progressive fibrous obliteration of the aortic arch and its branches develops, which leads to the rather old-fashioned name of 'pulseless disease' disease. The loss of pulses in the arm gives rise to forearm claudication, and ultimately cerebral ischaemia is likely. The condition may spread down the aorta and lead to occlusion of the visceral and renal arteries.

Treatment
This depends on the degree of vascular involvement. In cases diagnosed early, steroids, given for several years, may be helpful. In more advanced disease, arterial bypass, between normal, noninflamed arterial segments, may be necessary. Though technically difficult, the results of these procedures can occasionally be gratifying.

Nonspecific arteritis

Painful necrotic lesions may rarely develop anywhere in the hand or the arm and the pulses will be normal. Very occasionally the temporal artery may be tender and can be biopsied. The ESR is likely to be raised and various haematological abnormalities may occasionally be found.

Surgical treatment can only be by sympathectomy. This is essentially a medical condition. Physicians may advise immune suppression or plasmapheresis.

Thoracic outlet compression syndrome (TOCS)

This covers a group of conditions in which the neurovascular bundle (subclavian artery, subclavian vein and lower trunk of the brachial plexus) are compressed as they cross the first rib. Various causes of compression have been identified:

1. scalenus anterior
2. scalenus medius (these muscles may be hypertrophic, have abnormal attachment or have various fibrous bands which encase the nerve or vessel)
3. pressure on the first rib by the clavicle. This may be associated with an obviously hypertrophied subclavius muscle) many of these patients play a great deal of sport or perform DIY)
4. cervical rib.

It is important to realize that most cervical ribs are asymtomatic and that, even if the patient has TOCS, a cervical rib may not necessarily be the cause of the compression. Although removal of the cervical rib may relieve the compression,[6] experience strongly suggests[7–9] that the only accurate method of assessing the cause of compression is by direct palpation after the neurovascular bundle has been dissected, preferably through the axilla.

The TOCS occurs predominantly, but by no means exclusively, in young women. Increasingly a history of trauma is identified as initiating the symptoms.[5]

The symptoms will vary according to which structure is being compressed so there may be any combination of pain, paraesthesia, exercise pain, emboli in the fingers, or blueness and swelling from venous compression. Simple clinical examination may demonstrate a bruit over the subclavian artery which may vary with the position of the arms, but various static postural tests which have been described are now no longer considered reliable. The most valuable dynamic clinical test is the Roos test where the fists are rapidly clenched with the shoulder braced back. If there is thoracic outlet compression this test will reproduce the symptoms in almost every case. The symptoms often become intolerable after a short time during this test, and at this stage a subclavian artery bruit may be heard that was not present at rest.

Investigation

If the symptoms are essentially neurological, every effort must be made to exclude cervical spine lesions, and multiple re-examination is particularly valuable. Nerve conduction studies are normal in the TOCS, but may be of great help in excluding ulna nerve compression at the elbow or carpal tunnel syndrome. If there is any evidence of vascular abnormality, arteriography and venography, if necessary, should be performed with the arm in different positions during examination (Figs 23.2 and 23.3).

If the artery is abnormal and there are emboli in the fingers, surgical treatment becomes a matter of urgency.

Surgical treatment

This remains controversial. There are two main approaches.

Supraclavicular approach
This allows exposure of the vessel and division or resection of scalenus anterior. A cervical rib can also be removed, but the exposure is cramped and limited, and the nerve trunk is at appreciable risk.

Transaxillary approach
This has very many advantages and has been ex-

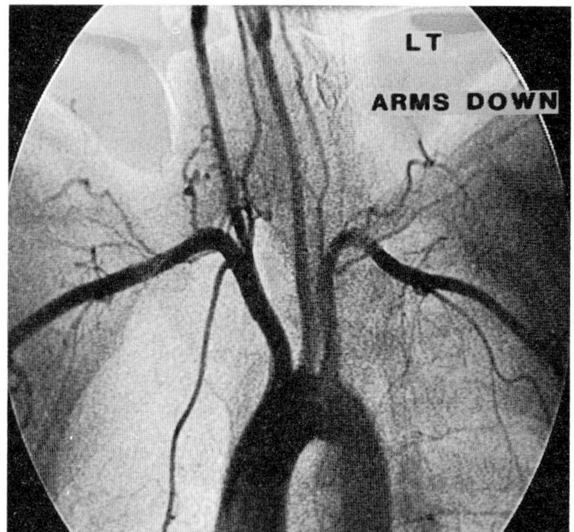

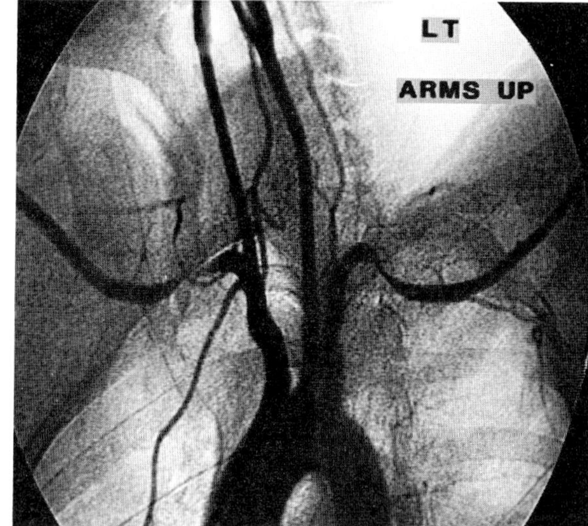

Fig. 23.2 Postural compression of the subclavian artery over the first rib.

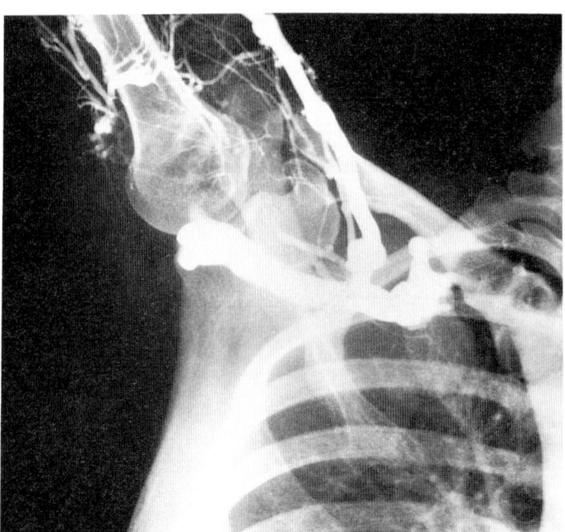

Fig. 23.3 Compression of the subclavian vein by an abnormal first rib.

tensively publicized and advocated by Roos[7,10] and Cooley and Wurash.[11]

With the patient in the half-lateral position, and the arm held by an assistant, an incision is made in the lower part of the axilla. The incision is deepened on to the chest wall (not into the axillary contents), and the lateral thoracic vessels ligated and divided. As the first rib is reached by gentle dissection, the superior thoracic vessels are ligated and divided, and when the assistant lifts the arm, the neurovascular bundle is lifted clear of the chest wall. The first rib together with a cervical rib can be completely excised together with as much of the muscles as seems desirable. The neurovascular bundle can then be completely dissected free and there is no longer any floor against which compression can occur. If the artery needs reconstruction, the axilla is closed and a supraclavicular incision now allows extremely easy access to the vessels. This can be improved still further, if necessary, by a separate incision below the clavicle splitting pectoralis major.

Provided that the diagnosis is *correct*, that irreversible vascular damage has not occurred, and that complete decompression is achieved, 75% of patients can expect excellent relief of symptoms. However, some symptoms (usually neurological) remain in the remaining 25%. The technical details of these operations are well described by Roos[10] and by Sanders.[5]

References

1. McColl I. DHSS report: *Review of Artificial Limb and Appliance Centre Services*. London: HMSO, 1986.
2. Berridge DC, Gregson RHS, Makin GS, Hopkinson BR. Tissue plasminogen activator in peripheral arterial thrombolysis. *Br J Surg* 1990; **77:** 179–82.
3. Eastcott HHG. *Arterial Surgery*. London: Pitman Medical, 1969: 94–110.
4. Weale FE. In: *Current Operative Surgery – Vascular Surgery*, Crawford, Jamieson (eds). London: Baillière Tindall, 1985: 74–9.
5. Sanders RJ. *Thoracic Outlet Syndrome: A Common Sequela of Neck Injuries*. Philadelphia: JB Lippincott, 1991.

6. Brown SCW, Charlesworth D. Results of excision of a cervical rib in patients with the thoracic outlet syndrome. *Br J Surg* 1988; **75:** 431–3.
7. Roos DB. The place for scalenectomy and first rib resection in thoracic outlet syndrome. *Surgery* 1982; **92:** 1077–85.
8. Parry E. The thoracic outlet compression syndrome. *Aust NZ J Surg* 1981; **51:** 84–91.
9. Thompson JF, Webster JHH. First rib resection for vascular complications of thoracic outlet syndrome. *Br J Surg* 1990; **77:** 555–7.
10. Roos DB. In: *Current Operative Surgery – Vascular Surgery*, Crawford, Jamieson (eds). London: Baillière Tindall, 1985: 133–46.
11. Cooley DA, Wukash DC. In: *Techniques in Vascular Surgery*. Philadelphia: WB Saunders, 1979: 45–90.

24

Renal artery disease

Ali Bakran and Peter L Harris

Disease of the renal artery (RAD) is considerably under-diagnosed. This is mainly due to lack of specific symptoms related to the condition. It presents clinically as hypertension, or in a small proportion of cases, renal failure.

The classic experiments of Goldblatt[1] demonstrating that renal artery constriction produced hypertension in the dog, first implicated renal artery stenosis as a potent cause of hypertension. Clinical confirmation was demonstrated when nephrectomy or repair of renal artery stenosis (RAS) resulted in relief of hypertension. Subsequently, the relationship between RAD and renovascular hypertension became more clearly defined by the Co-operative Study on Renovascular Hypertension,[2] and is considered to be the commonest correctable cause of hypertension in man. Also, since the end-point of a stenosis is occlusion, untreated bilateral renal artery disease will lead to renal hypoperfusion, renal dysfunction and eventually renal failure.

Whilst there are several causes of renal artery disease (Table 24.1), the commonest are atherosclerosis in approximately 60% of cases and fibromuscular dysplasia in almost 40%. These two disease processes are quite different in aetiology although they share common features in clinical presentation. Attention will be focused on the relationship between them and their association with renovascular hypertension.

Table 24.1 Causes of renal artery disease

Common
Atherosclerosis
Fibromuscular dysplasia
Infrequent
Renal artery aneurysm
Arteriovenous fistula
Rare
Renal artery thrombosis
Renal artery embolism
Takayasu's arteritis
Neurofibromatosis

Epidemiology of renovascular hypertension

The exact prevalence of renovascular hypertension is unknown. Hypertension is thought to afflict up to 10–15% of the adult population, perhaps up to 40 million people in the USA. It has been variously estimated that less than 1% to 15% of the hypertensive population is due to renovascular disease, although the more likely figure is between 1% and 5%. Even so, this will mean that approximately one million Americans[3] and 200 000 people in the UK will suffer from this condition.

Pathology

Atherosclerotic renal artery disease is often part of a generalized arterial disease involving the coronary, carotid and peripheral arteries. The location of the atheromatous plaques is usually at the renal artery ostium, as part of aortic disease, or within the first 1–2 cm of the artery (Fig. 24.1). One-third of the lesions are bilateral and 35% have concomitant aneurysmal or occlusive disease involving the infrarenal aorta. If the lesions are left untreated there is a high probability of progression to complete occlusion, which may occur in 10–17% of cases over a 2–3 year period. Also, 40% of patients with unilateral disease develop contralateral stenosis within 52 months.[4,5]

In contradistinction to atherosclerosis, fibromuscular dysplasia usually affects the distal two-thirds of the renal artery with extensions into the segmental branches in 20%, and is characterized by the impression of a 'string of beads' on angiography (Fig. 24.2). Ninety per cent of adult cases are caused by medial and perimedial fibroplasia, mainly affecting women in their 40s and 50s. Morphologically, appearances range from a solitary focal stenosis to multifocal stenoses caused by thick fibromuscular bands with intervening aneurysmal outpouchings. Progressive

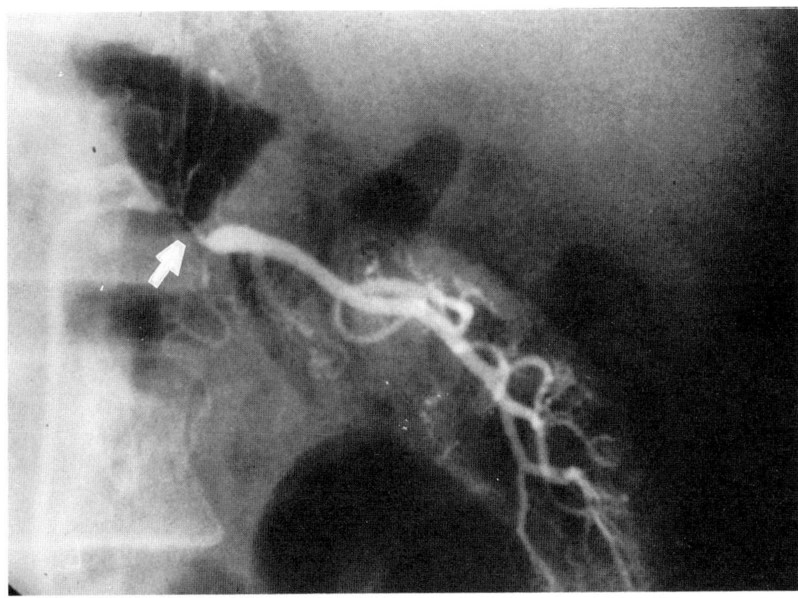

Fig. 24.1 Selective arterogram showing renal artery stenosis (arrowed) with a poststenotic dilatation.

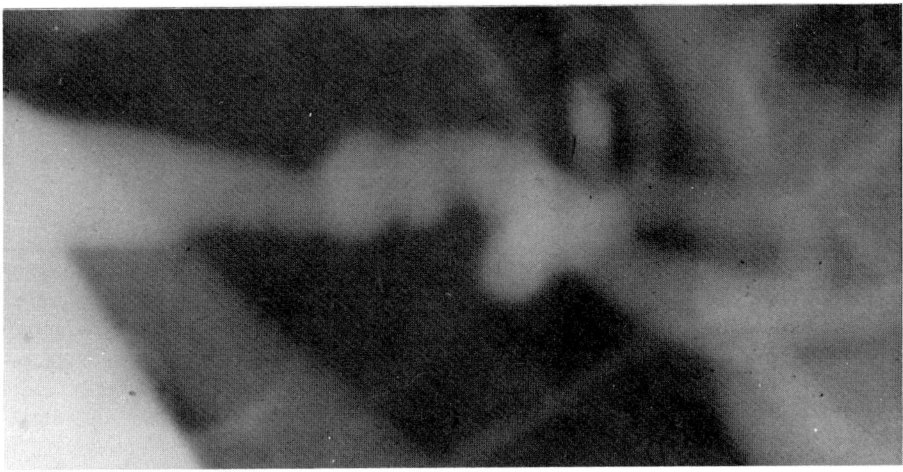

Fig. 24.2 'String of beads' appearance of fibromuscular hyperplasia.

occlusion of the renal artery is rare in medial fibroplasia but is more common in perimedial fibroplasia. Intimal fibroplasia is a condition which mainly affects children and may also lead to arterial occlusion.

Clinical presentation and characteristics

It must be emphasized that although renal artery stenosis and renovascular hypertension have become synonymous, this is not necessarily the case. Indeed, in a post-mortem study, almost 50% of patients normotensive in life had moderate or severe disease in one or both renal arteries.[6] Other authors have reported unsuspected renal artery stenosis in normotensive patients undergoing arteriography for peripheral vascular disease.[7]

Renal artery disease is an anatomical diagnosis based on angiographic demonstration of a stenotic lesion. Renovascular hypertension, however, implies cure or improvement of hypertension following revascularization of the affected kidney(s) or nephrectomy, and thus is a retrospective diagnosis after treatment. There are no specific features which distinguish patients with essential hypertension and renovascular hypertension,[2] although certain characteristics should prompt a high index of sus-

Table 24.2 Clinical characteristics suggesting renovascular hypertension

- **Hypertension**
  Starting at a young age (<20 years) or after 50 years
  Recent onset or short duration
  Accelerating or malignant
  Diastolic BP >105 mmHg
  Difficult to control with medical therapy
  No family history
- Abdominal and/or flank bruit, particularly systolic/diastolic
- Severe retinopathy
- Elevated blood urea/creatinine

picion (Table 24.2). The finding of an abdominal bruit is a particularly significant feature.

There is also considerable overlap of features between patients with atherosclerotic and fibromuscular dysplastic renovascular disease. However, patients in the latter category tend to be younger, predominantly female, with hypertension starting at an earlier age, and with no family history of hypertension, whereas the older male patient with other signs of arterial disease is likely to have atherosclerotic renal artery disease.

Interestingly, it is not uncommon nowadays to diagnose significant RAS following a deterioration in renal function after treatment of hypertension with an angiotensin converting enzyme (ACE) inhibitor. Following development of RAS, increased renin is released by the juxtaglomerular apparatus in the ischaemic kidney. Renin converts circulating angiotensinogen to angiotensin I, which is further degraded to angiotensin II by the angiotensin converting enzyme in the lungs. Angiotensin II is a powerful peripheral vasoconstrictor and also acts on the adrenal glands to release aldosterone, thereby producing sodium and water retention. Both mechanisms increase the systemic blood pressure. ACE inhibitors will prevent this cycle and cause a fall in blood pressure with a consequent under-perfusion of the kidney, a fall in glomerular filtration rate, poorer renal function and a rise in blood urea and serum creatinine. Fortunately, in most instances, stopping the ACE inhibitor results in a return of renal function. Subsequent angiography usually confirms RAS.

Diagnosis of renal artery stenosis

Screening tests for renal artery disease are unfortunately notoriously inaccurate. There was enthusiasm initially in the use of intravenous urography (IVU), which usually reveals the delayed appearance of hyperconcentrated contrast medium in a small kidney in comparison with the normal kidney. However, there are considerable false-positive and false-negative rates (±20%). It is now generally accepted that the IVU is insufficiently sensitive as a screening test.[8]

Radioisotope renography using ^{131}I orthoiodohippurate,[99] Tc-labelled diethylenetriaminepentacetic acid (DTPA) and, latterly, mercaptoacetyltriglycine (MAG_3) have all been used successfully to diagnose unilateral RAS.[9] There needs to be a greater than 60% stenosis before there is any change on scintigraphy. More recently, scanning before and after addition of an ACE inhibitor has enhanced the effectiveness of these studies. The effect of an ACE inhibitor on the kidney with RAS is detected by a fall in measured individual kidney glomerular filtration rate, a prolongation of parenchymal transit time or as a change in differential function. As RAS approaches 100%, however, the kidney shrinks in size, renal function is severely impaired and the ACE inhibitor effect is less evident. Unfortunately, the specificity of tests suffer from false-positive examinations resulting from any unilateral renal disease with attendant compromised renal function. Sensitivity is affected by false-negatives in patients with bilateral symmetrical disease or mild RAS. Overall, whilst some claim a sensitivity of 94% and specificity of 95%, the value of ACE inhibitor renography remains uncertain.

Even less invasive than isotope renography is Doppler ultrasound, with or without colour coding. A low-frequency transducer (3 MHz) is used to measure flow velocities in renal arteries compared with that in the aorta (renal–aortic ratio). The peak systolic and end diastolic velocity in the renal artery is a measure of relative flow resistance. In very experienced hands, comparison with angiography suggests that Doppler can detect down to 40% stenosis with possible sensitivity of 83% and specificity of 97%.[10] However, few can match these results and colour duplex ultrasound is not recommended at present as a screening method for detection of RAS.

In view of the interrelationship between RAS and renin release from the ischaemic kidney, measurement of renin levels in peripheral blood or in the draining renal vein would seem most appropriate as a screening method for RAS, or in evaluating the significance of the stenosis in the causation of hypertension or renal failure. Indeed, comparison of renin levels in the two renal veins (the renal-vein renin ratio or RVRR) is widely employed and a ratio of

>1.5 is considered to be diagnostic. Unfortunately, several factors bedevil accuracy of this measurement. Abnormal RVRR need not indicate hypersecretion of renin or lateralization of renal disease and results may be normal in bilateral RAD. In order to make the values more reliable, strict test conditions – including controlled sodium intake, withdrawal of all antihypertensive drugs, and the addition of frusemide or ACE inhibitor[11] – must be imposed. A cure rate of 95% following operation is said to occur in patients with a truly positive result, but 35% of patients with a negative RVRR also responded.[12] Thus, the renal-vein renin ratio cannot be used as an absolute criterion for diagnosis of renovascular hypertension nor for decision regarding treatment. Peripheral-vein renin values are too inconsistent to diagnose renovascular hypertension.

Bilateral ureteric catheterization provides detailed quantitative information on renal function in each kidney. The test is invasive, technically difficult to perform, requires inpatient study and is complicated by urinary tract infection, dysuria and haematuria, but it may reliably predict the functional importance of RAS. A haemodynamically significant stenosis produces reduction in urine output, clearances of creatinine, inulin and p-aminohippurate and sodium concentration whilst the concentration of creatinine, inulin and PAH is enhanced.[13] Most centres, however, have abandoned this technique.

Intravenous digital subtraction angiography (DSA) was hailed as a suitable screening procedure. Unfortunately, initial enthusiasm has been tempered by disappointment since images are not as good as those obtained with conventional arteriography, although experienced operators can produce excellent results. Improved images can be obtained by placing a catheter in the superior or inferior vena cava but clearly this is more invasive. As a screening method it has advantages over IVU or isotope renography since bilateral RAS and stenosis in those with a single kidney can be detected. However, patients with limited cardiac function will require intra-arterial DSA. The intravenous route also tends to underestimate the degree of stenosis and does not detect stenoses in peripheral parts of renal arteries or accessory renal arteries. Fibromuscular dysplastic lesions in particular may be missed. Nevertheless, whilst sensitivity of 100% and specificity of 93% with a predictive value of 83% have been claimed,[14] the high rate of technically unsatisfactory examinations and poor resolution makes this method less than optimal.

Although there are encouraging reports indicating the usefulness of magnetic resonance imaging[15] as an investigative tool, conventional arteriography remains the 'gold standard' for the diagnosis of RAD, though it cannot be condoned as a screening procedure. Not only is the site, extent and likely nature of the arterial lesion defined, but also the presence of aneurysmal dilatation, collateral circulation and post-stenotic dilatation. The functional significance of the RAD can be confirmed by demonstrating a pressure gradient across the lesion. This appears to be one of the most reliable signs of significant RAD although little used so far.[16]

In summary, therefore, no single test is by itself diagnostic of significant RAS. The most accurate anatomical diagnosis is made by conventional angiography, although DSA, especially when using a central vein, can be a useful screening test. The physiological importance of such a stenosis still requires validation. Captopril renography, renal-vein renin ratio and a significant pressure gradient across the stenosis are helpful in making this decision. An investigation and management strategy is outlined in Fig. 24.3.

Management of RAS

The two indications for treatment of renal artery stenosis are firstly to control hypertension and secondly to preserve or improve renal function. Renovascular hypertension can be successfully managed medically, radiologically and by surgery. However, only angioplasty and surgery can preserve or improve renal function.

Medical management

The panoply of antihypertensive medication has enabled physicians to control even the severest of hypertensive disease. However, two main concerns remain: progression of renal artery disease and the haemodynamic effects of blood pressure reduction on renal function. Hypotensive agents preserve renal function only insofar as they may halt progress of hypertensive damage in the contralateral kidney and, indeed, ACE inhibitors may even promote the risk of occlusion in the stenosed renal artery.

Hunt and Strong[17] showed that when medical and surgically treated patients were compared over a 7-year period, there was a 70% mortality in the medically treated group compared with a 30% mortality in those treated surgically. Most of the deaths were due to myocardial infarction or stroke and only

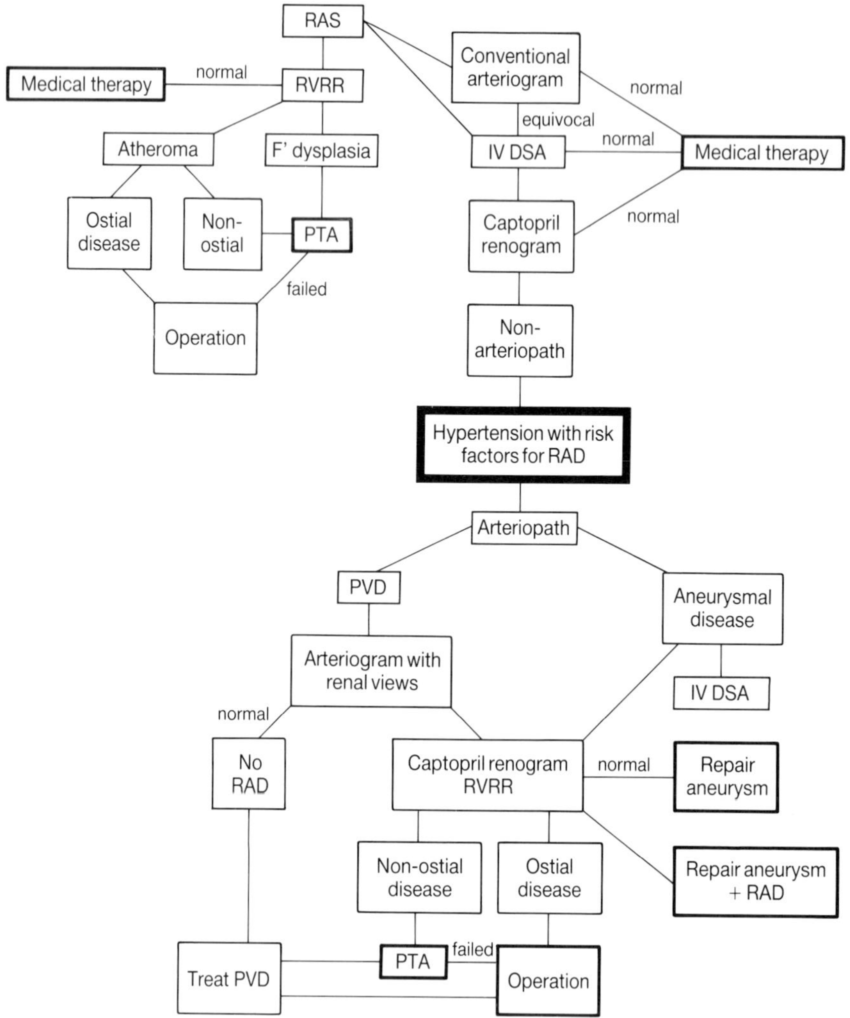

Fig. 24.3 Algorithm for investigation and management of renal artery disease.

a minority died of renal failure. It has also been shown that 10–17% of stenotic renal arteries will occlude within a few years[4] and a significant proportion will have deteriorating renal function. In view of this, nonmedical management of RAS is justified.

There will remain, however, patients who are medically unfit due to generalized atherosclerotic cardiac and cerebrovascular disease and who have failed angioplasty, who should be managed conservatively. It is particularly important to underline again that unless the renal artery disease is shown to be haemodynamically significant, medical management alone is indicated, but close monitoring of such patients for progression of disease is mandatory.

The whole range of drugs, including beta-blockers, diuretics, alpha-blockers, calcium channel blockers, peripheral vasodilators and ACE inhibitors, may be used singly or in combination. However, beta-blockers, since they suppress renin release, and ACE inhibitors, since they produce a reduction in angiotensin II levels, are most appropriate. Long-term monitoring of renal function is essential.

Percutaneous transluminal angioplasty

Considerable experience has been gained with percutaneous transluminal angioplasty (PTA) for renovascular disease since the introduction of this technique by Grüntzig in 1978.[18] The technical results, short-term and long-term clinical efficacy and complications are gradually being documented. Technical success rates of 80–90% have been reported and appear also to be associated with high therapeutic success, resulting in a drop in blood pressure and improvement in renal function.[19]

The best result with long-term durability after PTA is in patients with fibromuscular dysplasia and it is now the treatment of choice for this condition. In patients with atheromatous disease, however, results are not nearly so good.[20] A significant factor is that ostial lesions are more difficult to dilate since these are extensions of aortic plaques as opposed to plaques arising within the renal artery. However, encouraging results with PTA even in these lesions have been published recently. Rigorous follow-up is essential and repeat angioplasty is performed when appropriate.[16] Renal artery angioplasty with stenting of ostial lesions has been performed more recently. However, technical success does not necessarily equate to long term benefit. Careful follow-up data are required before this can be recommended.

The advantages of PTA are a short hospital stay, low mortality and low cost, although there may be a 10–12% complication rate, including renal artery thrombosis and renal artery dissection. Overall, success is somewhat better with surgery in experienced hands, but this must be balanced against the higher mortality and nephrectomy rate. Surgery, however, remains an option after failed angioplasty, and PTA itself appears not to jeopardize subsequent surgical revascularization.[21]

In view of the significant morbidity associated with PTA, it should only be undertaken by interventional radiologists having close links with an experienced surgical team.

Surgical reconstruction

The important distinction between renal artery disease and renovascular hypertension has already been made and thus no surgical attempt to repair a stenosis should be made without careful evaluation of its significance. Most patients are now controlled by medical management and are only referred for operation if hypertension becomes resistant to treatment and PTA has failed. In the patient with fibromuscular dysplasia, operation is not only required if the branch renal arteries are involved. Patients with atherosclerotic disease often have ostial disease which may not respond to PTA, and then surgical revascularization would be appropriate. In addition, a proportion of these patients will have a combination of aneurysmal and renal artery disease which can be best dealt with simultaneously.

Before surgical repair, a general evaluation of the patient for cardiovascular and cerebrovascular disease is necessary since myocardial infarction and stroke are a significant cause of postoperative death. Ideally after a careful history and physical examination, routine blood tests, chest X-ray, ECG, echocardiography, dipyridamole thallium scanning and carotid duplex ultrasound should be organized. One particular symptom which should not impede surgical treatment is recurrent pulmonary oedema which is associated with renovascular hypertension and is not due to the severity of the underlying cardiac insufficiency.[22] Patients are often on a combination of antihypertensive therapy including a diuretic and will require careful rehydration, either before or during the surgery, in order to avoid postoperative hypotension.

The surgical options for treatment of renovascular hypertension are shown in Table 24.3. Nephrectomy is only considered in the exceptional case with severe arteriolar nephrosclerosis, noncorrectable renal artery disease, after a failed revascularization procedure, or severe renal atrophy (kidney <9 cm).

As for all major vascular cases, an arterial pressure line, central venous pressure line, Swann–Ganz catheter, urethral catheter and wide-bore peripheral venous line should be inserted after general anaesthesia. Heparin and mannitol are given prior to application of the aortic clamp.

Surgical approach

A subcostal incision with extension down the other side (rooftop) for bilateral operations or a midline incision giving access to the distal iliac artery would seem to cover all eventualities. The right renal artery can be best approached by reflecting the

Table 24.3 Surgical options in renovascular hypertension

- Nephrectomy
- Aortorenal bypass
- Thromboendarterectomy
- Extra-anatomical bypass:
  - hepaticorenal
  - splenorenal
  - iliacorenal
- Autotransplantation, with or without extracorporeal repair

ascending colon, hepatic flexure and second part of the duodenum medially, exposing the renal vein and inferior vena cava (IVC). The artery lies behind the renal vein, and needs to be followed under the IVC to the aorta. The proximal part of the artery is reached at its junction with the aorta, medial to the IVC. The left renal artery can also be found after mobilizing the splenic flexure, descending colon, and pancreas forward, but this is often not necessary. It can be approached more directly at its origin from the aorta, by elevating the left renal vein after ligating adrenal, gonadal and lumbar vein branches.

The most frequently performed revascularization procedure for RAS is aortorenal bypass,[23] although this is not appropriate if the aorta is heavily diseased. Autogenous saphenous vein is most often used, although an arterial autograft (such as the internal or external iliac artery) has theoretical advantages. However, the internal iliac artery is often too short and frequently atherosclerotic, whilst external iliac artery excision would require a replacement with a Dacron graft. The saphenous vein dilates with time, becoming aneurysmal, but there have not been any reported cases of rupture. PTFE or Dacron grafts are acceptable alternatives if autogenous material is not available.

The aorta is dissected sufficiently to allow a side clamp to be applied, and an elliptical-shaped aortic segment excised. The aortic anastomosis is completed using a fine suture, a small arterial clamp is applied to the vein graft and the aortic clamp released prior to ligation of the renal artery at its junction with the aorta. The ends of the renal artery and saphenous vein should be spatulated and joined end-to-end again using a fine running suture. On the right, the bypass graft may be placed anterior or posterior to the IVC, depending on ease of access and degree of mobilization of the renal artery. Provided the distal anastomosis can be completed within 30 minutes, no cooling of the kidney is required. Bilateral repair can be executed by making a side-to-side anastomosis between the aorta and saphenous vein followed by end-to-end anastomosis to each renal artery. Aortic cross-clamping would, of course, be necessary.

Aortorenal thromboendarterectomy[24] is the next commonest method of repair of RAS and is particularly useful in bilateral disease. It is critically important that the endarterectomy is started in the aorta and then extended into the renal arteries. The distal intima usually feathers out but may require tacking down. A completion angiogram is necessary to confirm that there is no intimal flap.

If the aorta is severely diseased or has been the site of previous surgery, other methods of revascularization are available. An alternative on the right side is a hepaticorenal bypass graft,[25] and on the left a direct splenorenal graft.[26] A splenectomy is not necessary if the middle portion of the splenic artery is used. Iliacorenal and mesentericorenal grafts have also been described. It is essential to confirm patency of the coeliac and superior mesenteric arteries for these approaches.

Aortic replacement and simultaneous renal revascularization is associated with higher operative mortality (6–30%) compared with renal artery reconstruction alone and should only be performed for aortic aneurysmal or severe occlusive disease. The procedures of choice are thromboendarterectomy followed by aortic replacement, or aortic replacement followed by a bypass from the inserted Dacron graft to the renal artery.

One further option frequently preferred by surgeons with experience of renal transplantation is autotransplantation of the kidney to the iliac vessels. Clearly, the iliac arteries have to be free of disease. The kidney is mobilized completely, sacrificing the capsular collateral blood supply but leaving the ureter intact. To prevent ischaemic damage, the kidney is perfused with cold hyperosmolar perfusion fluid (e.g. hypertonic citrate) as in renal transplantation. The renal vein is anastomosed to the iliac vein, and the renal artery can be joined to the internal iliac, external iliac or the common iliac artery.

When *in situ* repair cannot be performed, as in fibromuscular dysplasia involving the branch renal arteries, extracorporeal 'bench' surgery and then autotransplantation is necessary. The freedom of a bloodless surgical field, protection from warm ischaemia, the facility to utilize microvascular techniques with optical magnification and optimum illumination, are major advantages.[27]

Complications of reconstruction

Hypertension may persist despite a good revascularization procedure, relief of hypertension depending to some extent on the length of history prior to surgery. It may also result from stenosis or thrombosis of the repaired artery. The latter occurs in 5% of cases and may be the result of a technically inadequate anastomosis, or kinking of anastomosed vessels. Postoperative hypotension due to hypovolaemia must be avoided by adequate pre- or intraoperative replacement of fluids, since this can result in thrombosis of the renal artery and even lead to a stroke.

Haemorrhage from the operative bed may require re-exploration after adequate replacement of clotting factors and reversal of systemic heparinization.

Re-stenosis of the renal artery can occur weeks, months or years after operation. Angioplasty is probably the treatment of choice.

Acute renal failure may develop if there is prolonged clamping of the renal arteries. Episodic perfusion of the kidney with cold Hartmann's solution will prevent the damaging effects of warm ischaemia during *in-situ* revascularization. Rather than oliguria, polyuric failure may occur. Both types of renal failure will recover provided adequate perfusion to the kidney is maintained, even if temporary haemofiltration or haemodialysis is required. An isotope scan will confirm the patency of the renal circulation non-invasively.

Results

Results of renal revascularization will mirror the experience of the operator in this rather specialized field. The major centres with considerable expertise claim an 85–90% cure or improvement in hypertension associated with atherosclerotic renovascular disease. Morbidity and mortality have been reduced markedly and thrombosis/re-stenosis rates of less than 5% and mortality less than 2% are claimed.[28] There is a mortality of up to 12% if aortic and renal reconstruction are performed together.[29] Graft failure due to thrombosis has been as high as 18–45% in the past[30] and probably reflects poor patient selection and inexperience of the surgeon. Surgery for fibromuscular dysplasia also has a success rate of 90% in cure or improvement of hypertension.[8] Surgical mortality in this group is low since patients are younger and fitter.

Renal artery occlusion

Whilst acute occlusion of a renal artery usually leads to infarction of the kidney, acute thrombosis of a previously stenosed renal artery does not. Collateral blood supply is often sufficient to maintain viability, although with considerably impaired or loss of renal function. The resulting ischaemia will also maintain renovascular hypertension. If the contralateral kidney is normal, there may be no clinical symptoms or change in renal function. However, if the other renal artery is diseased or occluded, a fall in renal function and oliguria supervenes.

No treatment or nephrectomy alone may be indicated in the former case, especially in the elderly high-risk patient; but in the latter, attempt at revascularization is required urgently. PTA has been successful in the recently occluded renal artery but surgical revascularization is most often necessary. The patient must be thoroughly prepared and may need haemodialysis temporarily. The presence of a good nephrogram, in a normal-shaped kidney of size >9 cm, and filling of a main renal artery distal to the occlusion on angiography, are helpful signs in deciding whether to proceed to reconstruction.

Renal artery aneurysm

Renal artery aneurysms occur in approximately 0.7% of the population and consist of four types: saccular, fusiform, dissecting and intrarenal. The majority are asymptomatic but may cause hypertension or, rarely, rupture. Renal-vein renin assay may assist in deciding the clinical significance of the aneurysm and hence the need for repair. Aneurysms exceeding 2 cm in size probably justify repair although evidence is sketchy. *Ex vivo* repair using saphenous vein or an internal iliac arterial graft is most suitable. Intrarenal aneurysms are best treated by arterial embolization or partial nephrectomy.

Other causes of renal artery disease

Renal arteriovenous fistulae are uncommon and are found incidentally on angiography during the search for other disease. The majority are acquired following renal biopsy although a small number are congenital, traumatic or neoplastic in origin. Symptoms of high-output cardiac failure and hypertension may be produced, together with pain and haematuria. The commonest sign is a flank bruit and arteriography is diagnostic. Treatment should only be offered if clinical symptoms arise. Embolization or surgical ligation of the feeding artery may be performed.

Renal artery thrombosis may result from polycythaemia, tumour, trauma or intimal fibroplasia. The commonest cause, however, remains acute thrombosis of a previously stenosed artery. There may be no symptoms associated with this event if the contralateral kidney is normal, although flank pain, malaise and headache may occur.[31] Serum creatinine often rises and anuria/oliguria may ensue if there is occlusion in a single functioning kidney. Treatment by thrombolysis with or without PTA or surgical revascularization is possible, although seldom performed since the diagnosis is often missed.

Emboli to the renal artery usually originate in the heart as a consequence of atrial fibrillation, myocardial infaction or bacterial endocarditis. Symptoms are often vague and reflect the consequences of acute renal infarction – flank pain, loin tenderness, nausea and vomiting and haematuria. Bilateral emboli will cause acute renal failure with anuria/oliguria. Diagnosis is rarely made early enough to prevent renal infarction, although intra-arterial thrombolysis and surgical embolectomy have both been successful.

Takayasu's disease is an inflammatory arteriopathy which initially affects the major trunks of the aortic arch but may also involve the renal artery, producing stenosis. Systemic signs are nonspecific: headache, malaise, myalgia and fever. The ESR is usually raised and can be used to monitor the response to treatment with long-term oral steroids. Arterial bypass from a noninvolved artery to the normal renal artery distal to the inflamed segment may be indicated if steroid therapy fails.

Neurofibromatosis is inherited through recessive genes and is characterized mainly by cutaneous neurofibromas and *café au lait* spots. Renal artery stenosis is the usual cause of hypertension although phaeochromocytoma and coarctation of the aorta may coexist. The proximal renal artery is affected and may not respond to PTA but surgical revascularization remains an option. This condition may occur in young children.

Conclusions

The prevalence of renal artery disease is higher than is frequently acknowledged. The two commonest causes are atherosclerosis and fibromuscular dysplasia. The screening tests available are not individually conclusive and so a combination of tests is required before the definitive diagnosis can be established. Conventional arteriography remains the 'gold standard' for diagnosis. A pressure gradient across the stenosis together with a renal-vein renin ratio of >1.5 is usually diagnostic of significant disease and is best able to predict success following revascularization.

Neither PTA nor surgery should be performed without confirming the functional significance of a renal artery lesion. PTA is well established as a successful form of treatment for renovascular hypertension and is now the treatment of choice in patients with fibromuscular dysplasia and nonostial renal artery disease, although long-term durability is uncertain. Provided that it is performed on appropriately selected cases, reconstructive surgery has low morbidity and mortality with long-term success. However, in order to achieve this goal, reconstruction for renovascular disease should be restricted to those centres with experience in this specialized branch of vascular surgery.

Recommended further reading

1. Stanley JC, Ernst CB, Fry WJ. *Renovascular Hypertension*. Philadelphia: WB Saunders, 1984.
2. Novick AC. Surgical correction of renovascular hypertension. *Surg Clin North Am* 1988; **68:** 1007–25.

References

1. Goldblatt H, Lynch J, Hanzal RF, Summerville WW. Studies on experimental hypertension. I: The production of persistent elevation of systolic blood pressure by means of renal ischaemia. *J Exp Med* 1934; **59:** 347–78.
2. Simon N, Franklin SS, Bleifer KH, Maxwell MH. Clinical characteristics of renovascular hypertension (Co-operative Study of Renovascular Hypertension). *JAMA* 1972; **220:** 1218.
3. Maxwell MH. Epidemiology and clinical manifestation of renovascular hypertension. In: *Renovascular Hypertension*, Stanley JC, Ernst CB, Fry WJ (eds). Philadelphia: WB Saunders, 1984: 100–3.
4. Wollenweber J, Sheps SG, Davis GD. Clinical course of atherosclerotic renovascular disease. *Am J Med* 1968; **21:** 60–70.
5. Schreiber MJ, Pohl MA, Novick AC. The natural history of atherosclerotic and fibrous renal artery disease. *Urol Clin North Am* 1984; **11:** 383–92.
6. Holley KE, Hunt JC, Brown AL, Kincard OW, Sheps SG. Renal artery stenosis: a clinico-pathologic study in normotensive and hypertensive patients. *Am J Med* 1964; **37:** 14–22.
7. Eyler WR, Clark MD, Garman JE, Rian RL, Meininger PE. Angiography of the renal areas, including a study of renal artery stenosis in patients with or without hypertension. *Radiology* 1962; **78:** 879–92.
8. Grim CE, Luft FC, Weinberger MH. Sensitivity and specificity of screening tests for renal vascular hypertension. *Am J Intern Med* 1979; **91:** 617–22.
9. Mann SJ, Pickering TG, Sos TA, Uzzo RG, Sarkar S, Fiend K, Rackson ME, Laragh JH. Captopril renography in the diagnosis of renal artery stenosis: accuracy and limitations. *Am J Med* 1991; **90:** 30–40.
10. Taylor DC, Kettler MD, Moneta GL, Kohler Tr, Kazmers A, Beach KW, Strandness DE. Duplex scanning in the diagnosis of renal artery stenosis: a prospective evaluation. *J Vasc Surg* 1988; **7:** 363–9.

11. Rudrick MR, Maxwell MH. Diagnosis of renovascular hypertension: limitations of renin assay. In: *Controversies in Nephrology and Hypertension*, Narins RG (ed). New York: Churchill Livingstone, 1984: 123–60.
12. Russel RP. Renal hypetension. *Surg Clin North Am* 1974; **54:** 349–61.
13. Stamey TA, Nudelman IJ, Good PH, Schwentker FN, Hendricks F. Functional characteristics of renovascular hypertension. *Medicine* 1961; **40:** 347–94.
14. Dunnick NR, Svetkey LP, Cohan RH. Intravenous digital subtraction renal angiography: use in screening for renovascular hypertension. *Radiology* 1989; **171:** 219–22.
15. Vock P, Terrier F, Wegmuller H, Mahler T, Gertsch P, Souza SP, Dumoulin CL. Magnetic resonance angiography of abdominal vessels: early experience using the three-dimensional phase contrast technique. *Br J Radiol* 1991; **64:** 10–16.
16. Weibull H, Bergqvist D, Jonsson K, Hulthen L, Mannhem P, Bergentz SE. Longterm results after percutaneous transluminal angioplasty of atherosclerotic renal artery stenosis: the importance of intensive follow up. *Eur J Vasc Surg* 1991; **5:** 291–301.
17. Hunt JC, Strong CG. Renovascular hypertension: mechanisms, natural history and treatment. *Am J Cardiol* 1973; **32:** 562–74.
18. Grüntzig A, Kuhlman U, Vetter W, Lulolf K, Meyer B, Siegenthaler W. Treatment of renovascular hypertension with percutaneous transluminal dilatation of a renal artery stenosis. *Lancet* 1978; **i:** 801–2.
19. Sos TA, Pickering TG, Sniderman K, Saddekni S, Case DB, Silane MF, Vaughan ED, Laragh JH. Percutaneous transluminal renal angioplasty in renovascular hypertension due to atheroma or fibromuscular dysplasia. *N Engl J Med* 1983; **309:** 274–9.
20. Dean RH, Callis JT, Smith BM, Meacham PW. Failed percutaneous transluminal renal angioplasty: experience with lesions requiring operative intervention. *J Vasc Surg* 1987; **6:** 301–7.
21. Martinez AG, Norvick AC, Hayes JM. Surgical treatment of renal artery stenosis after failed percutaneous transluminal angioplasty. *J Urol* 1990; **144:** 1094–6.
22. Pickering TG, Devereux RB, James DG. Recurrent pulmonary oedema in hypertension due to bilateral renal artery stenosis: treatment by angioplasty or surgical revascularization. *Lancet* 1988; **ii:** 551–2.
23. Dean RH. Management of renovascular hypertension due to atherosclerosis. In: *Vascular Surgery*, Rutherford RB (ed). Philadelphia: WB Saunders, 1989: 1245–53.
24. Wylie EJ, Stoney RJ, Ehrenfeld WK. Renovascular atherosclerosis. In: *Manual of Vascular Surgery Vol. 1*, Wylie EJ, Stoney RJ, Ehrenfeld WK (eds). New York: Springer Verlag, 1980: 233–57.
25. Chibaro EA, Libertino JA, Novick AC. Use of the hepatic circulation for renal revascularization. *Ann Surg* 1984; **199:** 406–11.
26. Brewster DC, Darling RC. Splenorenal arterial anastamosis for renovascular hypertension. *Ann Surg* 1979; **189:** 353–8.
27. Novick AC. Management of intrarenal branch arterial lesions with extracorporeal microvascular reconstruction and auto transplantation. *J Urol* 1981; **126:** 150–4.
28. Stanley JC, Ernst CB, Fry WJ. Surgical treatment of renovascular hypertension: results in specific patient subgroups. In: *Renovascular Hypertension*, Stanley JC, Ernst CB, Fry WJ (eds). Philadelphia: WB Saunders, 1984: 363–71.
29. Dean RH, Keyser JE, Dupont WD, Nadeau JH, Meacham PW. Aortic and renal vascular disease: factors affecting the value of combined procedures. *Ann Surg* 1984; **200:** 336–44.
30. Foster JH, Maxwell MH, Franklin SS. Renovascular occlusive disease: results of operative treatment. *J Am Med Assoc* 1975; **231:** 1043–8.
31. Weibull H, Bergqvist D, Andersson I, Choi DL, Jonsson K, Bergentz S-E. Symptoms and signs of thrombotic occlusion of atherosclerotic renal artery stenosis. *Eur J Vasc Surg* 1990; **4:** 159–65.

25

Risk management in vascular surgery

Nigel Keddie

Risk management evolved in the USA as a positive response to an escalation in medicolegal claims. It has emerged as a constructive approach not only to reduce claims but also to improve standards of care by making clinicians more aware of common sources of risk to patients. A vital part of risk management in all areas is the reporting of untoward incidents followed by constructive discussion of their cause purely to learn how to ensure that they do not recur. In this chapter the vascular surgical cases reported to the Medical Defence Union in the UK will be described and guidelines given to minimize the risk of these problems recurring (Table 25.1). It must be stressed that these cases reported to the Union are inevitably selected, but 80% of British hospital doctors are members so it is considered that the cases are representative of the problem as a whole.

Table 25.1 Claims arising from vascular surgery in the year before Crown Indemnity (1990)

Varicose veins	11
Amputations	17
Abdominal aortic aneurysm*	12
Deep vein thrombosis	9
Angiography:	10
cerebral damage (2)	
cardiac arrest (1)	
ischaemia:	
lower limbs (5)	
upper limb (1)	
buttock (1)	
Angioplasty:	2
stroke (1)	
arterial rupture (1)	
Arterial injury:	5
laparoscopic (2)	
laminectomy (1)	
fracture dislocation of knee (1)	
aortic stab wound (1)	
Postoperative haemorrhage	3
Paraplegia	2
Impotence	1
Brachial plexus damage	1
Sepsis	3
Death	3

*other than ruptured aneurysm

Varicose veins

Vast numbers of patients are treated for varicose veins, often by relatively inexperienced surgeons. So it is hardly surprising that many claims arise from this source (Table 25.2).[1]

Complications of operative treatment

Vein and artery damage

Femoral vein damage still occurs, usually when an inexperienced surgeon is performing saphenofemoral ligation without adequate supervision.[2] It is

Table 25.2 Problems arising from the treatment of varicose veins

Operative treatment
Femoral vein damage
Femoral artery damage
Nerve damage:
lateral popliteal nerve
long saphenous nerve
short saphenous nerve
Wound infection
Unsatisfactory scars:
size, site, number
keloid
tattooing
Recurrent saphenofemoral incompetence
Deep vein thrombosis ± pulmonary embolism
Injection treatment
Extravasation of sclerosant:
skin necrosis
unsightly pigmentation
Incorrect site:
lateral popliteal nerve
posterior tibial artery

essential to know how to deal with the problem. The wound should be packed to control bleeding and ideally a senior colleague with experience of vascular surgery contacted. Tears at the saphenofemoral junction can often be repaired without any long-term ill-effects; but if the femoral vein is ligated in error, or worse if a segment is excised or stripped out, it is much more difficult. Prosthetic grafts have been used to replace segments of the femoral vein with good short-term results, but it is not known if there will be a long-term patency. If the long saphenous vein is used to replace the segment of damaged femoral vein, the diameter is inadequate to provide a lasting good result. A tube of appropriate diameter can be constructed using long saphenous vein to replace the damaged segment and this seems to give the best long-term results. In cases reported to the MDU, a distal arteriovenous fistula has sometimes been created to increase the flow rate (the external pudendal artery being used); but this does not appear to improve long-term patency unless the vein graft used is comparable in size to the femoral vein.

Femoral artery damage should not occur but occasionally does.[3] The critical point is to recognize it and get immediate expert help. The greatest risk is when a femoral vein injury causes profuse bleeding and ill-advised efforts are made to apply clamps which may damage the artery. Firm packing is the way to handle excessive bleeding in the groin. After a few minutes, gently removing the pack and the careful use of a sucker usually allows accurate identification of the source of the bleeding. In a unique case the stripper was erroneously inserted into the posterior tibial artery and brought out through the femoral artery, followed by stripping of the arterial tree in the lower limb. There were disastrous consequences.

Nerve damage

During venous operations around the knee or lower, the lateral popliteal nerve may be damaged in various ways. The result is expensive, indefensible claims. The nerve is occasionally clamped, divided and ligated over the neck of the fibula in mistake for a vein. As soon as this error is recognized, referral to an expert in nerve suture is essential so that primary repair can be performed as quickly as possible. Other cases have followed exploration of the popliteal fossa when ligating the short saphenous vein. When it is clear that no operation has been performed near the nerve, then compression from bandaging may be the cause of the damage. Spontaneous recovery can be expected in this case.

Numerous claims are made for injury to the long saphenous nerve, mostly complicating stripping of the long saphenous vein from ankle to groin. The nerve may be carefully separated at the ankle but has a variable relation to the vein in the leg and so can be avulsed by stripping. The patient develops numbness across the lower limb and top of the foot, as well as quite unpleasant burning pain. The short saphenous nerve may be damaged during avulsion of veins in the popliteal fossa or lateral calf or by incisions over its course.

Use of the vein stripper is controversial.[4,5] I abandoned it many years ago. Others use it from knee to groin only, or strip from above down (although trials examining the direction of stripping have not provided consistent results). The results of long saphenous vein stripping are better than simple ligation so far as the long-term relief of varicose veins is concerned, but at the price of possible injury to the long saphenous nerve.

Wound infection

Claims for wound infection are successfully defended on the basis that this is an unavoidable complication in a small percentage of patients. Perhaps the time has come when patients should be warned of this possibility.

Unsatisfactory scars

Many young women have treatment for varicose veins, mainly for cosmetic reasons. These patients must be fully counselled about the outcome of varicose vein operations. All efforts must be made to minimize scarring. Incisions should be as short as possible, in the line of the natural skin creases, and closed with Steristrip or subcuticular sutures where closure is necessary. The number of incisions should be kept to a minimum to deal with the veins satisfactorily. Patients still need to be warned that they *will* have scars and that these may be quite numerous for scattered varicosities. Keloid scarring is rare and fortunately settles with time, but the patient needs careful handling during this time. Tattooing of the skin occasionally occurs in scars made through marking ink and is indefensible. Some surgeons find that 'redheads' pigment their scars more readily than others.

In recent years there have been a number of claims for recurrent saphenofemoral incompetence, the allegation being made that tributaries of the long saphenous vein were missed at the original operation. These claims can be defended when an experienced surgeon performed the initial procedure, and recent evidence has demonstrated that saphenofemoral ligation may well fail to prevent retrograde flow in the long saphenous vein even shortly after surgery (see Chapter 22).

Injection therapy

This produces its own batch of claims. Extravasation of sclerosant is the common problem and is very difficult to defend. Claims arise for skin and soft tissue necrosis and ulceration, or for areas of subcutaneous induration and brown discolouration followed by permanent pigmentation.

Rarely claims arise from injection of sclerosant into the lateral popliteal nerve; apart from permanent functional damage, severe persistent pain may follow this indefensible problem. One claim arose from inadvertent injection of sclerosant into the posterior tibial artery with ischaemic damage to several toes and the forefoot.[6]

Deep vein thrombosis

DVT, with or without pulmonary embolism, can occur after operation or injection therapy. Routine prophylaxis with heparin or similar preparations should be considered for all operations, but it is not feasible to cover injection sclerotherapy where the patient is treated as an outpatient and he or she is fully mobile immediately after the injection.

This complication is defensible provided appropriate prophylaxis is given to cover the operation. Oestrogen-containing oral contraceptives must be discontinued for at least a full cycle before operation. It is probably not necessary to do this before injection therapy. Some surgeons would recommend that the pill is not prescribed to patients with varicose veins. There is no evidence yet that hormone replacement therapy increases the risk of thromboembolism postoperatively.

Arterial surgery

The volume of arterial surgery performed has increased dramatically over recent years and claims have also inevitably increased. Certain problems keep on reappearing.

Arterial injuries

Because these are not common they are either missed or not treated with an appreciation of the urgency of the situation. All casualty officers know about arterial bleeding, but arterial obstruction due to trauma is the problem that leads to claims. These cases are usually associated with upper or lower limb fractures or dislocations and demand urgent action if the limb is to be saved. Pulses must be checked in all cases of limb injury, and if absent a specialist vascular surgical opinion urgently obtained. 'Spasm' should not be diagnosed as intimal tearing is the more likely cause of arterial occlusion. Fasciotomies are essential to reduce muscle damage to a minimum. In stab wounds the weapon should be left *in situ* if possible, until the patient is anaesthetized and prepared for exploration of the wound.

Major arterial or venous injuries can occur during laparoscopy leading to expensive claims if they are not handled properly.

Late effects of arterial injury, usually iatrogenic (following angiography or surgical trauma), are arteriovenous fistula with distal ischaemia and false aneurysm.[7] Claims are rarely defensible.

Angiography and angioplasty

Radiologists and vascular surgeons work together very closely and the surgeon must be available to deal with any complications of angiography. The very controversial topic of informed consent arises in the context of angiography. Where should the line be drawn? There is some evidence that complications are more frequent amongst those who have been warned most fully about them. Claims have been made for all of the recognized hazards: haematoma (groin, scrotal or retroperitoneal), dissection, thrombosis, embolism.

Angioplasty, too, has brought a crop of claims in its wake. Embolism is the commonest problem and demands urgent intervention. Arterial rupture may occur with disastrous consequences for the limb if not prompty treated.

Sympathectomy

'Cervical' sympathectomy, by the classical approach through the supraclavicular fossa, has resulted in several claims for brachial plexus damage, arterial injuries, pneumothorax or Horner's syndrome. These have occurred in very experienced hands on occasions. The transaxillary approach through the second intercostal space is much safer and gives excellent exposure.

Following lumbar sympathectomy, claims for impotence still occur. Chemical sympathectomy is the most usual reason for claims, and experts advising claimants state that it is essential to use an image intensifier. Claims for nerve damage and ureteric injury have been made. Rarely spinal cord damage has been caused.

Excision of cervical ribs or the first rib may be associated with claims for brachial plexus injury or subclavian artery damage.

Lower-limb ischaemia

Delays in diagnosis of ischaemia symptoms are a common source of claims, usually against general practitioners. Failure to recognize diabetes is another frequent problem in patients with painful or infected feet. If amputation has to be performed, allegations of dilatory or inadequate treatment may be difficult to refute.

Abdominal aortic aneurysm

Failure to diagnose a leaking abdominal aortic aneurysm is becoming a common cause for claims, as back pain is not recognized as being due to this cause, and atypical presentations delay the diagnosis (see Chapter 11). In two recent cases allegations were made that the surgeon who operated had inadequate vascular surgical experience and the CEPOD report was quoted by the plaintiff's solicitor. Another claim arose from the death of a patient during transfer to a vascular unit. One other claim alleged that lack of proper vascular surgical instruments contributed to an unsuccessful repair of a ruptured aortic aneurysm.

Claims following arterial reconstructive surgery

Informed consent and realistic expectations are essential. *Limb loss* is the most frequent cause for claims, especially if there have been delays in diagnosis and treatment.

Impotence and *paraplegia* must be mentioned as hazards in thoracoabdominal surgery.

Colonic necrosis is a rare cause of allegations of negligence in aortic surgery.

Graft sepsis has caused claims, particularly where secondary haemorrhage occurs and amputation is required. Delay in diagnosis is the common problem, 'warning bleeds' having been ignored.

Nerve damage during removal of the long saphenous vein for reversed saphenous vein grafting can be a source both of unpleasant symptoms and of claims.

Many of the problems referred to are defensible, others warrant early settlement. Each case has to be considered on its merits. Claims can be extremely frustrating, an example being that for a meatal stricture following urethral catheterization after a successful operation for a ruptured abdominal aortic aneurysm! This can easily be avoided by the use of suprapubic catheterization.

References

1. Keddie NC. Medico-legal problems from the treatment of varicose veins. *J Med Def Un* 1987; winter edn: 8–9.
2. Welch GH, Gilmour DG, Pollock JG. Femoral vein division during Trendelenberg operation. *J Roy Coll Surg Edin* 1985; **30:** 203–4.
3. Liddicoat JE, Bekassy SM, Daniell MB, De Bakey, ME. Inadvertent femoral artery 'stripping': surgical management. *Surgery* 1975; **77:** 318–20.
4. Darke SG. Chronic venous insufficiency: should the long saphenous vein be stripped? In: *Vascular Surgery*, Barros D'Sa AAB, Bell PRF, Darke SG, Harris PL (eds). London: Butterworth-Heinemann, 1991: 207–18.
5. McMullin GM, Coleridge Smith PD, Scurr JH. Objective assessment of high ligation without stripping the long saphenous vein. *Br J Surg* 1991; **18:** 1139–42.
6. Cockett FB. Arterial complications during surgery and sclerotherapy of varicose veins. *Phlebology* 1986; **1:** 3–6.
7. Natali J, Benhamou AC. Iatrogenic vascular injuries. *J Cardiovasc Surg* 1979; **20:** 169–75.

26

Arteriovenous malformations

Averil O Mansfield

Arteriovenous malformations (AVM) are congenital abnormalities of blood vessels which are almost invariably present at birth. Vascular abnormalities which present a few weeks later are usually haemangiomata with a far greater likelihood of spontaneous regression and therefore a better prognosis. It is for this reason that the history of onset is so important.

Nature of the lesions

The sponge-like collection of vessels is a variation of normal development of the vascular tree but its persistence beyond birth is pathological. Communications between arteries and veins occur at a more proximal level than those normally seen at the capillary level. The more distally that these communications occur, the smaller the volume of flow through them. Proximal large-vessel communications will carry a high blood flow, and owing to short-circuiting of the capillary circulation there is a requirement for a greater cardiac output. In some lesions the communications between arteries and veins appear to be far fewer (or perhaps nonexistent) and the abnormality is largely or totally venous. These arteriovenous communications are often multiple, whereas a single communication is more likely to be traumatic or iatrogenic in origin. The large number of communications within the lesions is responsible for the high flow and high cardiac output. It also makes them difficult to treat.

Presentation

The lesions may occur virtually anywhere. Those occurring within the chest, abdomen or brain are only detected when complications arise.

The majority are visible as the result of swelling, discolouration or sometimes bleeding (Fig. 26.1). If they appear late in life then a malignant lesion should be excluded, usually by biopsy. Highly vascular tumours such as sarcomas or secondaries from a renal tumour must always be considered in the differential diagnosis. The face, neck and limbs are common sites for AV malformations. Those on the face can be particularly distressing for the patient.

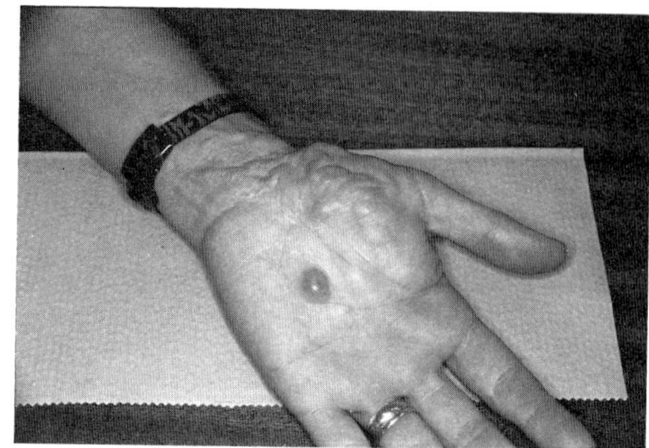

Fig. 26.1 Typical appearance of arteriovenous malformation in the hand. It was highly pulsatile.

Pain can be severe in some patients and nonexistent in others. It is quite often the reason for the request for treatment. Occasionally pain is due to pressure on local structures such as the brachial plexus.

Bleeding may occur spontaneously or as the result of trauma. If there is a major arterial component bleeding can be severe, and if the lesion has been previously undetected it can complicate procedures such as dental extraction. There is always anxiety in the high-flow arterial lesions that major haemorrhage will occur spontaneously and be life-threatening. Fortunately this is rare. Bleeding can also occur from the low-flow venous lesions but this is virtually never life-threatening and is easily controlled by elevation or by direct pressure.

Cardiac failure is the most feared complication. It can cause death, occasionally rapidly. Fortunately it is rare and the presence of high-output failure is not always associated with symptoms. Prevention of this complication is one of the main reasons for offering treatment to the otherwise asymptomatic patient.

The history

The age of onset of the lesion must be determined, often from the parents. Any change in the nature of the lesion should be recorded, for example in colour, size or symptoms. It is particularly important in women to record any changes that might have occurred at the menarche or during pregnancy. Local changes such as bleeding, increased limb length and ulceration should be recorded, as should any history of cardiac problems. All previous interventions and their results should be noted.

Examination

Apart from recording the site, size and consistency of the lesions, their effect on local tissues and organs should be documented.

The effect of elevation and dependency on the lesion will be helpful in deciding whether it is primarily arterial or venous. If it is arterial it will not diminish on elevation, whereas in venous lesions there may be a dramatic increase in size on dependency. In lesions involving a limb, the lengths of the affected limb and the normal limb should be recorded (Fig. 26.2).

Gentle palpation should be used to search for a palpable thrill and this should be followed by auscultation for the classical machinery murmur.

Photographic recording of the lesion will prove helpful for later comparison.

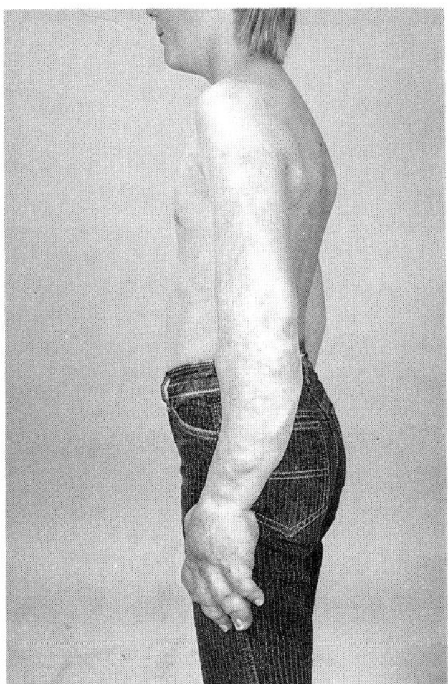

Fig. 26.2 Venous malformation of arm with overgrowth of arm and hand.

Doppler examination

This is the most important step in examination. The type of lesion can usually be determined quite accurately by using the pocket Doppler. This should be a standard step in the initial examination. With minimal experience it is possible to detect the high-flow arteriovenous signals and to distinguish them from low-flow lesions and from those without any arterial signal.

Investigations

Apart from a biopsy when malignancy cannot otherwise be excluded, investigations are not necessary in order to make the diagnosis. The diagnosis is based on clinical examination, and further investigations are then part of treatment. Often these patients do not require treatment and so further tests beyond the Doppler examination are not needed.

Whenever possible, investigations of an invasive type should be delayed until adult life when arterial catheterization will become both easier and safer.

Plain X-ray

Radiography is of limited value but may reveal the extent of soft tissue swelling and calcification due usually to phleboliths within the lesion. Phleboliths are normally only seen in venous lesions. A chest X-ray is important in arterial lesions in order to monitor heart size.

Ultrasound and duplex Doppler

These noninvasive investigations can be ordered at any age and may be used to determine involvement of deeper tissues and to assess flow. Examination of the venous system can largely be made by duplex Doppler, and in particular the patency or otherwise of the deep venous system can be determined. This is important in vascular malformations of the legs where the deep veins can sometimes be absent. Operating on the prominent superficial veins in this circumstance can result in clinical deterioration.

Venography

This is still useful in order to visualize the venous system when surgical intervention is planned.

CT scanning

CT is valuable for establishing the extent of a lesion beyond that which is visible. When contrast is given it will provide a clear picture of the vascularity of the lesion.

Magnetic resonance imaging

MRI is probably the investigation of choice to determine the extent and depth of a lesion (Fig. 26.3). It is particularly valuable in deciding to what extent the lesion involves muscles and other tissues. When excision is planned it is very important to know at the outset whether the lesion extends deep into other planes, as damage that would ensue from complete excision may well be regarded as unjustified. The depth of lesions as evidenced in this way is often surprising.

MRI has the great advantages of being noninvasive and having no exposure to radiation. The latter is important in patients who may, by the nature of their problem, be exposed to frequent X-rays.

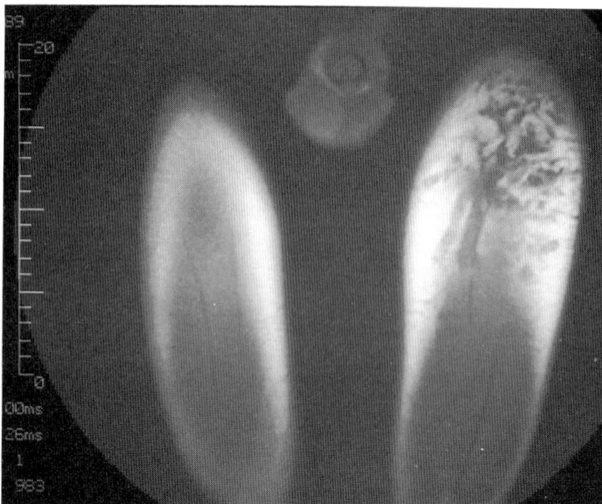

Fig. 26.3 Magnetic resonance scan clearly delineates extent and depth of a lesion in the upper thigh.

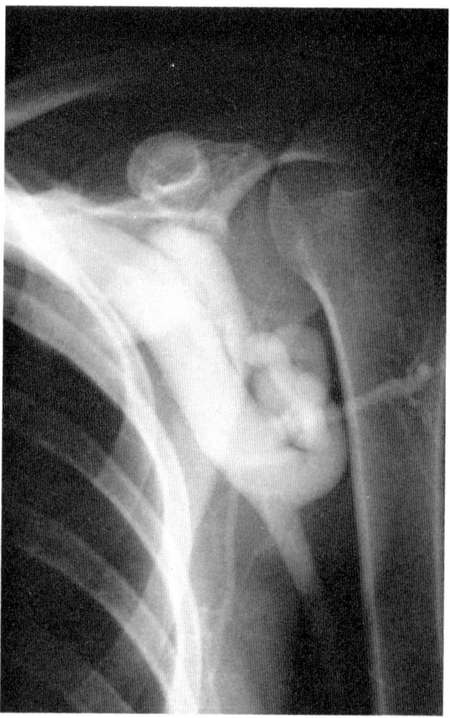

Fig. 26.4 Angiogram showing typical dilatation of the proximal feeding artery.

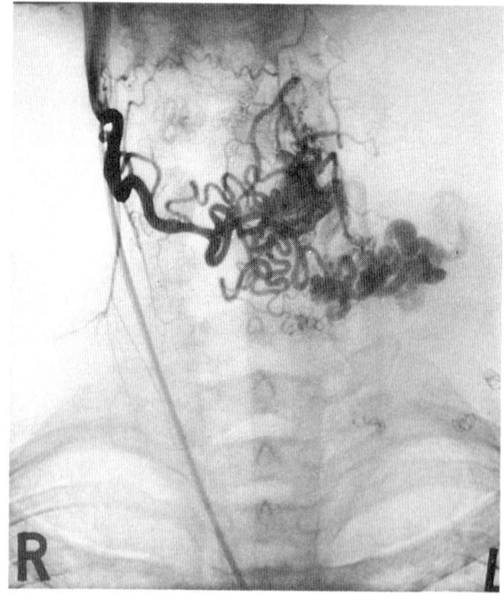

Fig. 26.5 Angiogram of a lesion in the left side of the neck reveals large blood supply from the right side. This is a typical appearance of the vessels in an arteriovenous malformation.

Angiography

This is employed in lesions that are largely arterial and which require treatment (Fig. 26.4 and 26.5). As previously stated, it should not be employed for diagnosis and should be delayed as long as possible to avoid angiography in children. The route of injection should be arterial because intravenous studies are confusing.

A catheter study is carried out usually from the groin and selective arterial injections are required. When a lesion is arising mainly from one artery it is essential to investigate all alternative sources of supply. Treatment must be directed at all of these sources, otherwise the lesion will rapidly be revascularized from alternative vessels.

The mainstay of treatment is embolisation, and so consideration of the direction of flow once the principal supply is blocked is important particularly when there is an adjacent vital structure such as the eye, brain or a digit. Angiography is usually the immediate prelude to therapeutic embolisation. It does not normally require anaesthesia unless it *has* to be carried out in children, and it can be helpful to have an awake patient who may be able to indicate that a problem has arisen.

Management

This can vary widely, ranging from counselling to complex excisional surgery employing cardiopulmonary bypass.

The basic approach is to use the minimal intervention compatible with control of symptoms and prevention of complications. It is very helpful to see these patients in the outpatient clinic with an interventional radiologist so that management can be agreed and planned together from the outset. Patients and families will require considerably more time for the initial consultation than for routine vascular consultations. Many parents have a sense of guilt that has its basis in the folklore surrounding these malformations, believing that they appear as the result of some event during pregnancy. There is no basis for that belief. There is also great concern that the lesions are familial, but again there does not appear to be any basis for this anxiety. In more than 400 patients seen in my clinic, only one patient was known to have a close relative with a malformation.

Most parents and patients hope that modern medicine will have a cure for the problem and are often disappointed to learn that treatment may not be advised or that it should be delayed until the child is older. It is also difficult to explain to the majority of patients in whom treatment is advised that the basis of treatment is control rather than cure.

Treatment may involve disciplines other than vascular surgery and radiology. A cardiologist may be needed to assess the heart, an orthopaedic surgeon may be required for the management of limb length, a plastic surgeon may be able to help with treatment of disfigurement, and a faciomaxillary surgeon can deal with common oral and facial lesions. It is helpful to establish a good relationship with doctors in these disciplines who have at least an interest, and better still, experience in management of these lesions.

The role of surgery

It must always be kept in mind that the appearance of vascular tumours and secondary deposits may be similar to an arteriovenous malformation. Secondaries from thyroid and kidney are remarkably vascular and both have been seen masquerading as AVMs. Sarcomas have presented in the same way and have proved difficult to diagnose with certainty. These possibilities must be kept firmly in mind, and when the possibility arises that a malignant tumour may be present a biopsy must be undertaken. This is particularly important to remember when an apparent AVM appears at an unusual time in life (i.e. unrelated to birth, puberty or pregnancy).

Biopsy

This must be a representative sample from the lesion and may be difficult because of bleeding. Some assistance may be obtained from preoperative embolisation simply to lessen haemorrhage.

Excision

If it is possible and safe, this is an attractive proposition in the hope of preventing the need for further treatment. Such an opportunity is, however, rare. More often partial excision is achieved, which involves removing the area that is most disfiguring.

Ligation of feeding arteries

This should be avoided whenever possible because arterial access is forever lost and alternative routes of supply soon develop. However, if bleeding is life-threatening then the necessary procedure should be undertaken immediately.

Skeletonization

This involves an attempt to ligate all the supplying vessels coming off the adjacent main artery. It has now been superseded by therapeutic embolisation (see below). It is *not* recommended.

Amputation

This is occasionally necessary and may range in extent from a digit to a limb. It is only required on the rare occasion when other methods of control have failed to control pain, bleeding or ulceration.

Provision of access for embolisation

When a feeding vessel has been ligated in the past

it is sometimes impossible to obtain a route of access for therapeutic embolisation, and so this has to be provided in the form of a vein bypass or direct repair of the vessel. I have, for example, had to reconstruct the lingual artery when this had been previously ligated in an attempt to control a lesion in the tongue. The vascular supply had rapidly been restored to the tumour from collaterals but access had been removed.

Plastic and reconstructive surgery

This is often required for lesions on and around the face where disfigurement can be extreme. Embolisation to lessen operative bleeding is usually required first.

Orthopaedic surgery

This usually involves procedures to control overgrowth of a limb.

Intratumoural ligation

Sutures are inserted deep into the lesion and ligated either externally or subcutaneously. This results in a cobblestone appearance which is rather ugly, but the procedure can be life-saving.

Cardiopulmonary bypass

This may be considered for the very extensive lesions where the only hope of control is extensive excision during a period of total circulatory arrest.

Therapeutic embolisation

This is the mainstay of management in those with a dominant arterial component. It usually requires a catheter to be inserted into the femoral artery (or other suitable access vessel) and manipulated by the radiologist into the lesion.

The principle of the treatment is to fill the lesion from within. It has become evident that the easier option of closing off feeding vessels will provide short-term gain while preventing subsequent treatment, as does ligation. It is important to choose material for embolisation which will not pass straight through the lesion and produce a pulmonary embolus.

Great care has to be taken when planning embolisation to anticipate the resulting flow changes which might jeopardize an adjacent organ. Hands and feet are particularly difficult to treat because of the risk of blocking the digital artery with embolic material. Patients should be warned of this possibility if treatment is to be embarked upon. The overlying skin may also become ischaemic if embolisation succeeds in rendering the lesion relatively bloodless.

The treatment usually has to be repeated at least once and sometimes several sessions are required. The patient is carefully followed up and further treatment given if control is being lost.

A variety of materials are used for embolisation and the choice is beyond the scope of this chapter.

Venous malformations

Lesions that have few if any arterial communications are impossible to treat with embolisation. It may, however, be possible to inject sclerosants. This is best undertaken in the radiology department, when a preliminary injection of contrast helps to ensure that the sclerosant does not stray into other structures that could be damaged.

It is sometimes possible to remove some of the offending veins. However, an extensive operation may be required and the outcome is often unsatisfactory in the long term.

Recommended further reading

1. Rosen RJ, Riles TS, Berenstein A. Congenital vascular abnormalities. In: *Vascular Surgery*, 3rd edn, Rutherford RB, (ed). Philadelphia: WB Saunders, 1989: 1049–61.
2. Sumner DS, Eastcott HHG, Rich NM, Merland JJ, Riche MC. Ateriovenous fistulae. In: *Arterial Surgery*, 3rd edn, Eastcott HHG (ed). Edinburgh: Churchill Livingstone, 1992: 521–59.
3. Halliday AW, Mansfield AO. Arteriovenous malformations: current management approaches. *Br J Hosp Med* 1989; **42:** 196–202.
4. Halliday AW, Smith EJ, Jackson J, Allison DJ, Mansfield AO. Indications for surgery for arteriovenous malformations. *Br J Surg* 1992; **79:** 36–102.

27

Overview of data relevant to decision-making in vascular surgery

JA Michaels and RB Galland

In order to make choices about appropriate treatment it is necessary to know something of the natural history of untreated disease and the likely outcomes of the alternative methods of management. The intention of this chapter is to provide an overview of the data which are relevant to such decisions in vascular surgery. The information is provided in graphical and summary form for ease of reference, and readers should refer to the quoted sources for a more detailed description of the data. Where there are suitable review articles available these have been referenced rather than all of the original source material.

Interpretation of published data

In interpreting published data there are a number of possible pitfalls which should be considered. These are discussed with particular reference to those problems seen in relation to the vascular surgical literature.

Sources of data and patient selection

Epidemiological studies show that there is considerable variation in the incidence of vascular disease which depends upon a number of environmental factors. For this reason, great care must be taken when interpreting data relating to the incidence, natural history and outcome of vascular disease. When looking at any such results the first point to consider is the population to which the data relate. Patients who are identified as having peripheral vascular disease in a population-based screening study will constitute a very different group from those presenting to general practitioners, who will in turn differ again from those seen in hospital practice. Thus, conclusions about outcome which rely upon comparisons with data published elsewhere must be treated with great caution. This is particularly true of publications relating to selected groups of patients where the criteria of selection are not apparent.

A good example of this can be seen in the reported mortality rates for the treatment of elective and ruptured aortic aneurysms. In the case of ruptured aneurysm there is considerable selection taking place in that only a proportion of those suffering from this complaint will be diagnosed, and many of these will not survive to reach hospital or undergo operation.[1] Thus, the mix of cases seen in an urban district general hospital will be considerably different from that seen in rural practice or in a large centre for tertiary referral. Such differences may be expected to result in variation in outcome, so that adequate interpretation is impossible without detailed information regarding case-mix.[2] A recent study has demonstrated that the incidence of aneurysms in one area of Scotland has increased from 55 to 63.6 per 100 000 of population over the age of 55 years,[3] and there would appear to be a similar trend in the USA.[4] This has been associated with a similar increase in the incidence of ruptured aneurysm, out of proportion to the ageing population. It may be that these changes are, at least in part, the effect of a changing pattern of identification of aneurysms. Thus, the associated changes in complications and mortality may be influenced by alterations in the case-mix of patients undergoing operation.

There are large geographical differences in practice as regards aneurysm screening[5,6] and indications for elective aneurysm repair.[4] If screening is successful in identifying small asymptomatic aneurysms, then those centres with an active screening programme and an aggressive policy towards the treatment of small aneurysms may be expected to be dealing with a selected population for both elective and ruptured aneurysms.

Definitions

In order to make realistic comparisons it is necessary to be sure that we are all talking the same language. However, it is perhaps surprising how often the definition of a particular disease or outcome will vary between publications. Claudication is usually defined in terms of walking distance but critical ischaemia is less easily defined. Recent publications have attempted to agree a uniform definition,[7] although there are other definitions available and this remains controversial.[8]

The definition of abdominal aortic aneurysm also varies between publications,[9] with various absolute measures of diameter being used or definitions which depend on the size relative to the suprarenal aorta. These differences can be of practical importance when it comes to evaluation of published results as they affect the apparent incidence of the disease. A recent trial demonstrated a 300% difference in incidence depending on the definition used.[10]

There are also discrepancies in the definition of 'ruptured' aneurysms, with several series failing to distinguish between emergency operations carried out for painful but unruptured aneurysms and those for true ruptured aneurysms. Thus, results may be distorted if there are differences in the proportion of patients with 'suspected' rupture or associated shock.[11]

Measurements

The reporting of the incidence of disease and the outcome of treatment depends on a number of clinical, radiological and laboratory measurements. There are often several ways in which a particular outcome may be measured. For example, graft patency is one of the most frequently used measures of outcome and may be assessed clinically by pulse status and symptoms, or by various investigations including ankle brachial pressure index (ABPI), duplex ultrasonography and angiography. Since it is well established that clinical measures may underestimate graft occlusion, it is important that the method used to assess patency is taken into account when clinical results are compared.

Most of the current literature regarding abdominal aortic aneurysms is based on the measurement of aneurysm size by ultrasonography, although older papers may use other methods of measurement.[12] Thus, care must be taken when interpreting data based on measurements made by other means such as CT scan[13] and direct measurements made at the time of operation or post-mortem.[14]

Similarly, recent developments in carotid surgery have meant that the measurement of the degree of stenosis is vital in clinical decision-making (see Chapter 19). However, such measurements may vary considerably depending on whether they are estimated by duplex ultrasound, conventional angiography or magnetic resonance angiography.[15,16]

Sampling and censoring of data

A common source of error in the interpretation of data comes in the assumption that failure to demonstrate significant differences between patient groups indicates that there is no clinically significant difference between the outcomes. This is only the case if the sample size is sufficiently large to exclude a type II error.[17] The importance of even small differences in operative mortality or limb loss, and the high general mortality amongst patients with vascular disease, may make it difficult to collect sufficiently large series to eliminate such errors. Even in very large studies, long-term patency results may be suspect if follow-up is incomplete, since it is difficult to be sure that patients lost to follow-up do not skew the results.

It is also difficult to ensure adequate randomization in surgical trials since there may be many influences upon treatment choice. For example, in a very large randomized trial comparing vein and PTFE for infrainguinal grafts there were considerable differences between centres as regards their ability to find usable vein for grafting, and those patients who were excluded from the trial due to lack of suitable vein had substantially different outcomes from those who were randomized to prosthesis.[18]

Reporting of results

There is clearly a tendency for large teaching centres to report clinical results and for good results to be published in preference to poor ones. This produces a marked 'reporting bias'. When large cross-sectional studies have been carried out based on an entire region or country, they often show that most publications produce an optimistic view of results.[19]

Results can sometimes be reported in such a way that they appear misleading. For example, there are inconsistencies in the way that the results of interventional radiological treatments are reported,[20] such as when cumulative patency is based on the initial successes rather than on all patients undergoing treatment. It is always important to consider whether there are factors causing prior selection of the group of patients for whom the results are reported, as may be the case if only a small proportion of ruptured aneurysms undergo operation.

Appropriate measures of outcome

The outcome of vascular surgery may be presented in a number of ways using a variety of different measures as discussed above. It is important that the measure used is appropriate to the question being asked. 'Success' of angioplasty may be reported in terms of reduction of the radiological stenosis to less than 50%. This may be a suitable measure for comparing the effect of different radiological methods, but clinical results are often more important. It has been demonstrated that, under some circumstances, the clinical results of an exercise programme may be better than those of angioplasty,[21] although this clearly has no effect on the degree of stenosis!

Perhaps the most common omissions from published data are satisfactory measures of outcome in terms of quality of life. Those who work with vascular patients are aware that some may have a far better quality of life with an amputation than with chronic rest pain or persistent ulceration.[22,23] Thus, limb salvage and graft patency constitute very crude measures of outcome which may correlate poorly with the benefit of treatment.

Prevalence and natural history of vascular disease

The vascular surgeon deals primarily with aneurysmal or occlusive vascular disease affecting the arteries to the lower limbs (Fig. 27.1).[24,25] These cases are usually manifestations of generalized cardiovascular disease, so that the epidemiology and association of such disease may be deduced from a knowledge of atherosclerosis in general.[26]

Occlusive disease

Occlusive disease increases in incidence with age, is commoner in men and is more often seen in developed countries (see Chapter 5). The most common symptom of occlusive disease, claudication, is seen in about 2% of a mixed population with an average age of 66 years.[27] However, population studies based on pressure indices demonstrate a substantially higher prevalence of asymptomatic disease.[28]

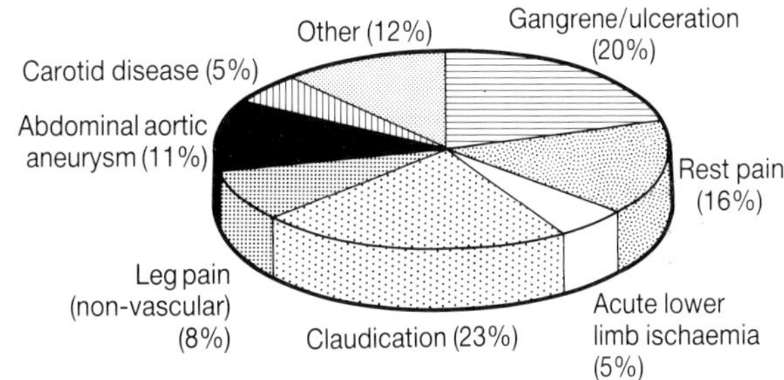

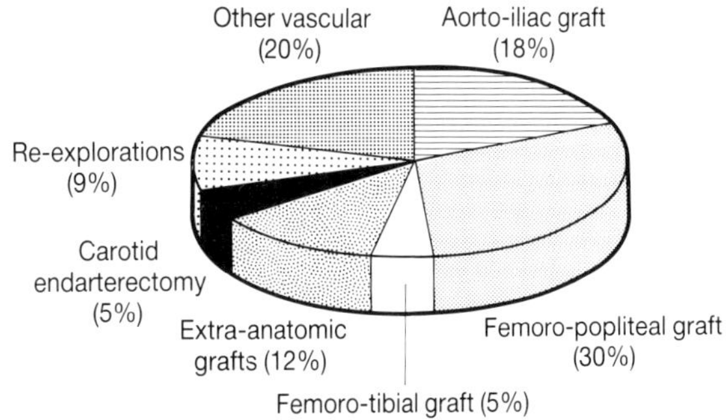

Fig. 27.1 The case-mix of patients treated by a vascular surgeon in a single health region. (a) Referral diagnosis of patients seen in a peripheral vascular clinic. (b) Nature of vascular surgical operations carried out.

Many patients with occlusive disease are elderly and have other manifestations of cardiovascular disease or cardiovascular risk factors (Fig. 27.2).[29,30] Approximately 65% of patients with claudication have occlusive disease which is primarily in the

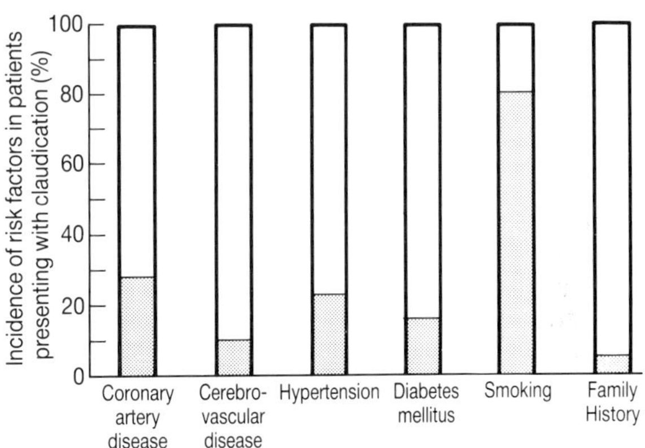

Fig. 27.2 The incidence of coexisting disease and risk factors in patients presenting with symptoms of occlusive peripheral vascular disease.

femoropopliteal segment.[31] Some subgroups have a different distribution with over half of claudicants under 40 years having aortoiliac disease.[32] In most patients the condition will remain stable or improve without active treatment, and many will die within a few years of diagnosis. A relatively small proportion will progress to need amputation or vascular reconstruction (Fig. 27.3).[30]

As would be expected, the major causes of death in these patients are other manifestations of cardiovascular disease (Fig. 27.4),[33] of which ischaemic heart disease is by far the most common. There is some evidence that aggressive identification and treatment of occult coronary artery disease may have a substantial effect on long-term survival (Fig. 27.5).[34]

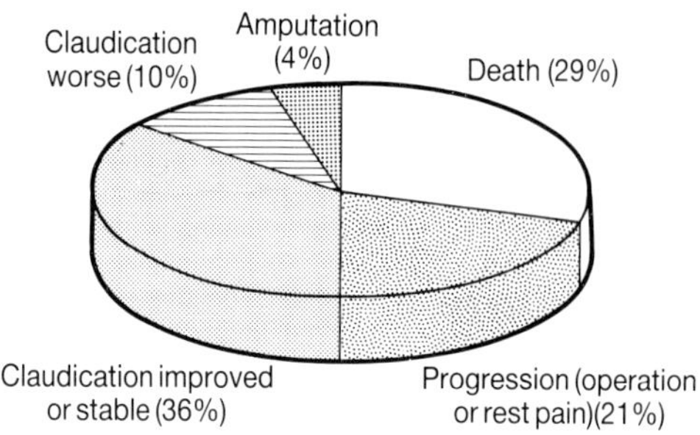

Fig. 27.3 The outcome at 5 years for all patients presenting with claudication.

Aneurysmal disease

Abdominal aortic aneurysms

The prevalence of aneurysmal disease is rather lower than that of occlusive disease and the exact prevalence depends partly on the definition of aneurysm that is used.[10] Screening of an unselected male population at age 65 shows a prevalence of 3.4%.[35] However, selected groups may have a significantly different prevalence, with the disease being less common in women and more common in those with symptoms of occlusive peripheral vascular disease,[36,37] hypertension,[38] popliteal aneurysms[39] and first-degree relatives of those with abdominal aneurysms[40] (see Fig. 27.6).

The natural history of untreated abdominal aortic aneurysms is gradual enlargement and rupture. The rate of growth is related to size, with a proportion of smaller aneurysms remaining static for many years whilst larger aneurysms expand at an increasing rate. The average expansion rate has been reported at 0.2–0.5 mm a year.[41,42] Rupture rate is also related to size. There have been occasional reports of rupture at less than 4 cm diameter, whilst rupture rates exceeding 25% a year are reported for much larger aneurysms.[42,43] The majority of abdominal aortic aneurysms are confined to the infrarenal aorta and iliac vessels, with fewer than 5% extending above the renal vessels.[44] A similar proportion of aortic aneurysms are inflammatory in nature.[45]

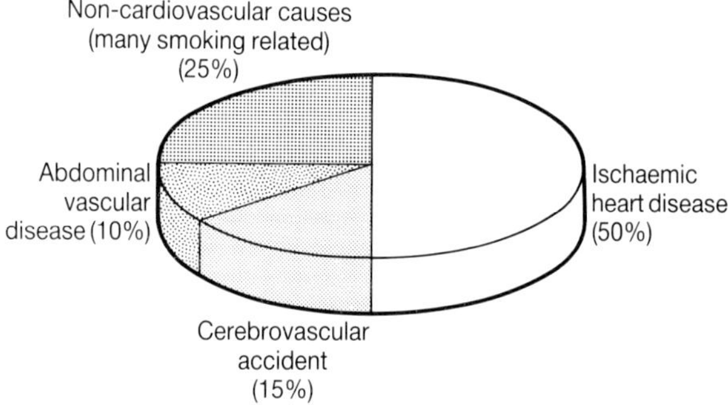

Fig. 27.4 Causes of death in patients with peripheral vascular disease.

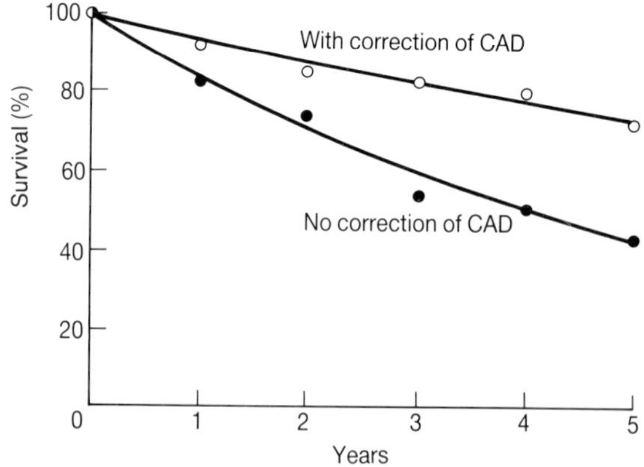

Fig. 27.5 Survival of age-matched patients with peripheral vascular disease with and without correction of occult coronary artery disease.

Other peripheral aneurysms

The vascular surgeon is called upon to deal with aneurysms in other sites. Other than abdominal aortic aneurysms, true aneurysms occur most commonly in the popliteal, femoral and neck vessels.

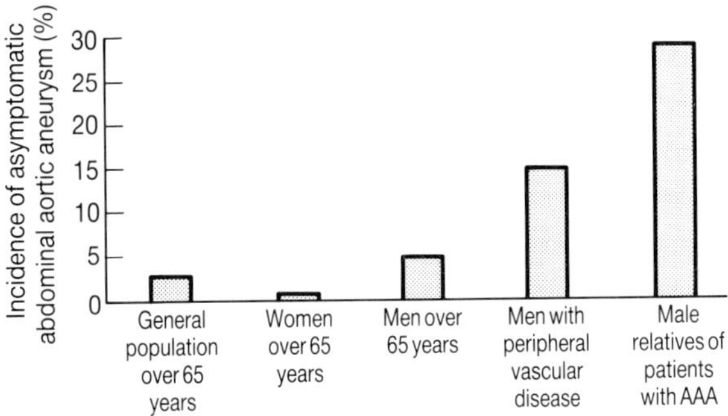

Fig. 27.6 The prevalence of abdominal aortic aneurysms in selected groups of the population as discovered by ultrasound screening.

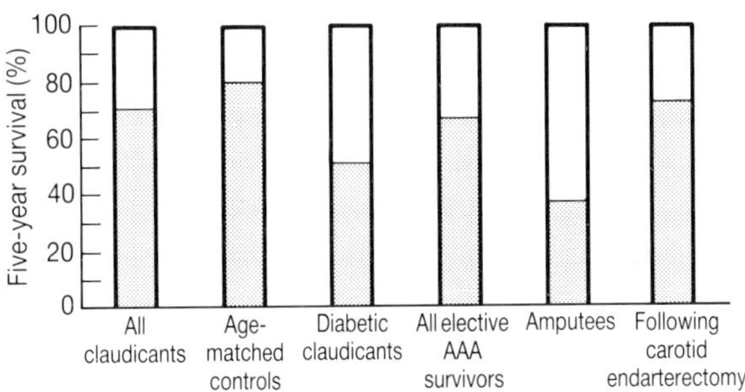

Fig. 27.7 Survival of patients with different manifestations of cardiovascular disease.

False aneurysms are becoming more common and are said to occur over a prolonged period following up to 15% of aortoiliac grafts.[46] They also occur after about 6% of cardiac catheterizations, although most resolve spontaneously.[47]

Carotid disease

It is only in recent years that noninvasive testing has made it possible to measure the degree of carotid stenosis accurately without the risks of invasive angiography. Accurate data are beginning to emerge relating the outcome of carotid reconstruction to the degree of stenosis (see Chapter 19). It is not always possible to be sure of the extent to which carotid stenosis is responsible for cerebrovascular symptoms. Asymptomatic carotid disease is common in patients with other manifestations of atherosclerosis, and those with tight stenoses (over 80%) have a 3–4% a year risk of developing cerebrovascular symptoms.[48] Carotid stenosis is found on the corresponding side in 72% of patients with hemispheric TIAs and approximately 45% of those with nonhaemorrhagic stroke. Although contralateral asymptomatic stenosis is not uncommon, it causes a comparatively low incidence of subsequent cerebrovascular events.[49] Carotid stenosis of over 50% is found in 17%, and over 80% in 5.9% of those over 65 years undergoing coronary artery surgery.[50]

Overall mortality

As discussed above, most of the conditions with which the vascular surgeon deals are manifestations of a generalized disease. Thus, it is not surprising that these groups of patients have a mortality that is higher than a matched population (Fig. 27.7).[22,51–56]

Results of reconstructive vascular surgery

Operative mortality

The high incidence of coexisting disease, particularly ischaemic heart disease, makes vascular patients a high-risk population in respect to any intervention. Thus the mortality of any vascular operation is a measure, not only of the nature of the operation and skill of the surgical and anaesthetic team, but also of the population on whom the operation is performed. For example, the fact that the relatively simple procedure of femoral embolectomy has a very high mortality[55] is related mainly to the general condition of the patients in whom the condition occurs.

It is, however, clear that the benefits of certain operations depend on achieving sufficiently good results as regards operative mortality and morbidity. Most large series from major vascular centres report operative mortality for abdominal aortic aneurysm repair to be less than 5%.[57] However, some studies suggest that in a less selective cross-section of hospitals the mortality may be well over 10%.[19,58] Similarly, the combined rate of operative mortality and stroke following carotid endarterectomy is reported as 2–3% in many centres[59] but is much higher in some settings.[60] These differences are important in the justification of elective aneurysm repair[43] and carotid endarterectomy.[61]

Operative complications

The most frequent early complications following vascular surgery are haemorrhage, myocardial infarction, cerebrovascular accident and renal failure. Fig. 27.8 shows the incidence of fatal and nonfatal myocardial infarct after various categories of vascular

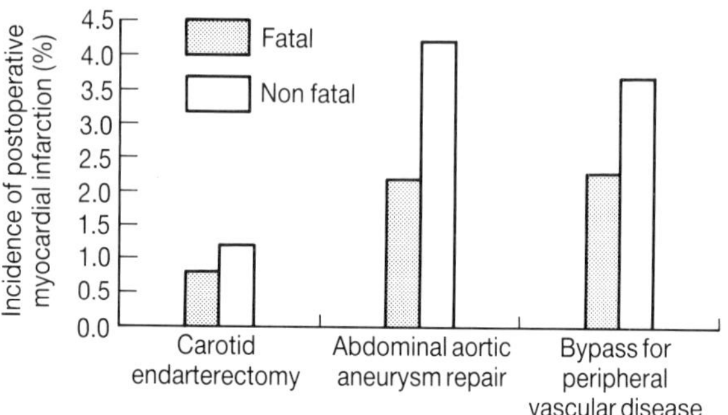

Fig. 27.8 Incidence of fatal and non-fatal myocardial infarction following various categories of vascular surgery.

surgery.[62] The early reoperation rate for haemorrhage or graft occlusion is approximately 5% following major aortic surgery. For complex distal salvage surgery the figure may be considerably higher.[63]

Graft patency

The rate of graft occlusion depends on several factors, the most important being the material and site of the graft. Autologous vein is usually considered to be the 'gold standard' as regards long-term patency.[64] Randomized trials have failed to show any significant difference between reversed veins and those used *in situ*.[65] Prosthetic materials have an occlusion rate which is 50% or more above that of vein in the early years after grafting.[18] This difference becomes increasingly marked with more distal grafts (Fig. 27.9).[64]

In vein grafts and small-calibre prosthetic grafts the rate of occlusion is highest in the early months following reconstruction.[66,67] This may be partly related to technical failures and to stenoses occuring at the anastomoses or within the graft. Recent studies have shown that duplex ultrasonography will often identify stenotic areas prior to occlusion and that treatment of these may improve overall patency.[68]

Later graft occlusion is likely to be more closely related to progression of the disease process within the graft or disease above or below the graft. Thus, it is not surprising that, in addition to the graft material, patency is closely related to the state of the runoff vessels, continued smoking[69] and other risk factors for vascular disease.[70] The patency following thrombectomy or graft revision is somewhat less than that of the primary surgery.[71] The high flow and large calibre of aortoiliac grafts make graft occlu-

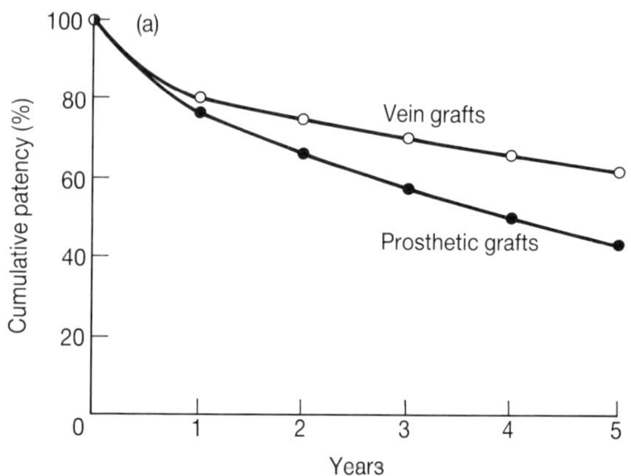

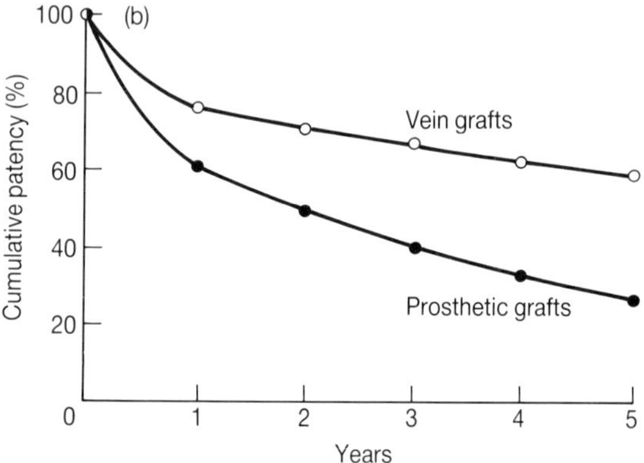

Fig. 27.9 Early patency rates versus graft material for (a) above-knee and (b) below-knee femoropopliteal bypass grafts.

sion less likely, and 5-year patency rates are around 90% with 70% patency at 10 years.[52]

When first introduced, extra-anatomic bypasses were usually reserved for limb salvage in unfit patients. Thus, it is not surprising that early series reported poor overall results and poor long-term patency rates. There is some evidence to suggest that, although the procedure is safer in high-risk patients, the long-term results are less satisfactory than for conventional alternatives.[72] However, some recent results have been more encouraging, particularly with femorofemoral bypass grafts, and some series report good long-term results.[73] Axillofemoral grafts tend to have much lower patency, particularly if they are unilateral,[54] but may have particular indications such as the presence of intra-abdominal sepsis.[74]

Peroperative stroke, (usually due to early thrombosis) is an uncommon but catastrophic complication of carotid endarterectomy and occurs in approximately 1% of cases in large series.[75] Late stroke or transient ischaemic attacks have been reported to occur in only 3% of cases over a 5-year period, but the figure is very dependent on case-mix.[53] They are not necessarily associated with occlusion or re-stenosis.[76] The rate of late re-stenosis after carotid endarterectomy may also be subject to apparent variation due to differences in the definition of 're-stenosis'.[77]

Limb salvage

When grafts are carried out for 'limb salvage' in patients with critical ischaemia, it may be expected that limb salvage would equate with graft patency. However, for a number of reasons, this is not the case. It is occasionally necessary to amputate a limb with a working graft because of infection, extensive tissue loss or inadequate revascularization. More commonly, a graft will occlude without the need for amputation. This may be due to the fact that limb loss was not inevitable at the time of reconstruction or may relate to the development of collateral circulation or the healing of ulceration. As mentioned above, there are several possible definitions of chronic critical ischaemia. Whichever definition is used, the amputation rate in patients without a successful vascular reconstruction is about 70%.[8] Overall, reported limb salvage rates for infrainguinal grafts are generally about 15–25% above those of graft patency.[78,79]

Other complications

Graft infection is a particular problem in prosthetic grafts.[80] The overall incidence is reported to be between 1% and 6% with the highest rates seen in prosthetic grafts involving anastomoses in the groins. It is more common in emergency operations, obese patients and those requiring re-exploration for early complications.[81] It may be a devastating complication with a high rate of limb loss and mortality reported from 25% to 75%, often related to haemorrhage or the development of aortoenteric fistulae.[82]

Anastomotic aneurysms are reported to occur at the anastomosis in up to 5% of prosthetic grafts[46,83] and are sometimes related to infection. Aneurysms may also occur within the graft[84] but are becoming less common with modern graft materials.

Amputation

Statistics from the Department of Health suggest that there are approximately 5000 major amputations of the lower limb per year in the UK.[85] Approximately 90% of these are carried out for peripheral vascular disease and patients have an average age in the early 70s (see also Chapter 10). The total number is static over the past few years despite an increasing incidence of peripheral vascular disease and an ageing population.[86] However, it is difficult to comment on this without adequate data regarding the rate of reamputations and the number of patients with ischaemic limbs who die without amputation.

The level of amputation is important as the quality of life and chance of mobilization is much better with a more distal amputation.[87] Several large centres have been able to achieve a ratio of 3:1 for below-knee to above-knee amputations.[88] However, collected statistics suggest that, overall, more than half of amputations in the UK are above the knee.[85]

The operative mortality for amputation is high, again reflecting the severe generalized disease that is seen in patients requiring amputation. Collected data from published papers suggest that mortality is 2% for below-knee and 9% for above-knee amputations.[51] However, collected hospital statistics in the UK suggest that the 30-day mortality of a below-knee amputation is above 10% and that of an above-knee amputation is over double this figure.[89] These differences may be due to a variety of factors, including patient selection, publication bias and differences in the definition of operative mortality. Long-term mortality remains high and approximately 50% of amputees will have died within 3 years of their amputation.[51]

The extent of rehabilitation following amputation varies with the age and health of the patient as well as the level of amputation. One study showed that approximately 30% of above-knee and 65% of below-knee amputees will be sufficiently rehabilitated to walk on an artificial limb outside their own home,[90] although a more recent study suggested that if all amputees are considered, only about 5% achieve an acceptable degree of rehabilitation.[91]

Angioplasty

Percutaneous transluminal balloon angioplasty (PTBA) and associated minimally invasive techniques are a rapidly developing area of vascular surgery.[92,93] Increasing experience and technological advances are leading to widening indications for the procedure. The best results are seen in short stenoses of larger vessels, whilst the results of dilatation of long occlusions below the inguinal ligament are less promising. Immediate successful dilatation is achieved in over 90% of short iliac stenoses[94] with average long-term patency of 60–70% at 5 years. Some series have suggested that external iliac lesions fare worse than those of the common iliac (47% versus 59% five-year patency)[95] and that the results for critical ischaemia are worse than for claudication (50% versus 80% five-year patency).[96] Good results have been reported in occluded iliac vessels although some series report a significant complication rate due to distal embolisation.[97]

Most large series report similar initial technical success in femoropopliteal stenoses and occlusions of less than 5 cm in length. In these lesions, the 3-year patency is approximately 60% in claudicants and 40% in those with critical ischaemia.[98] By contrast, the radiological success rate is reported as 50–70% of femoral occlusions over 10 cm in length, with half of these having re-occluded in 6 months and a 5-year patency of only about 20%.[95] Current results of tibial vessel dilatation are disappointing, with very poor early results.[95]

Balloon angioplasty is a relatively minor procedure and complications are rare. Local groin complications of haemorrhage, false aneurysm or arteriovenous fistula may occur in up to 9% of procedures, especially those involving the coronary vessels,[47] but they rarely require surgical intervention.[98] About 1% of patients develop acute deterioration of symptoms due to distal embolisation or acute thrombosis.[92]

Technology for minimally invasive treatment is developing rapidly and there are many new devices using mechanical, ultrasonic or laser methods of recanalization. Results comparable with those of PTBA have been reported for laser angioplasty,[99] although randomized trials have not yet shown it to be an improvement on conventional balloon angioplasty.[100] Mechanical atherectomy would appear to be less promising, with a high rate of complications and reocclusion.[101,102]

Thrombolysis

Thrombolysis with streptokinase has been used for peripheral arterial occlusions since the 1960s.[103] Systemic thrombolysis by intravenous injection has a limited success rate, with recanalization achieved in under 40% of cases. There is also a high complication rate, with up to 20% incidence of morbidity or major complication, mainly due to haemorrhage or stroke. The results of intra-arterial low-dose streptokinase are more promising, with successful lysis being achieved in up to 80% of cases, depending on case selection.[104] The rate of success is best in short, recent thromboses or emboli,[105] but some have reported acceptable results with more long-standing occlusions when combined with angioplasty.[106] It has also been used for the treatment of graft thromboses with acceptable short-term results,[107] although long-term patency has been disappointing with only 37% remaining patent at one year.[108]

Complications would appear to be far less frequent than with systemic thrombolysis, with major haemorrhagic complications in about 4% and 2–3% mortality.[103] Of those vessels successfully reopened, good long-term results have been achieved with various series reporting patency of 70% at one year,[109] 81% at two years[104] and 63% at five years.[110] Other thrombolytic agents, especially rtPA, may produce quicker and more effective lysis,[111] although it is currently more expensive and there are insufficient data to determine the relative safety at present.

Vascular surgical work-load

There is an increasing trend towards specialization in all branches of surgery and in many countries vascular surgery is already recognized as a separate subspecialty with its own training and accreditation.[112] This is not yet the case in the UK where the majority of those carrying out vascular surgery are general surgeons with a specialist interest who also have commitments to provide a general surgical service. At present there are approximately 4–5 such surgeons per million of population in the UK whilst there are several times this number in most of Europe and North America.

There is some evidence that the results of some operations are better if carried out by specialist surgeons.[1,2,60,113,114] However, there is little information regarding variation in case-mix in these studies and the conclusions are based on series from the USA where there is a relatively higher number of surgeons. In one of these studies, only three of 26 surgeons carrying out aneurysm repair were doing more than four procedures per year.[1]

Estimates produced by the Vascular Surgical Society in 1987 suggested that an average district general hospital in the UK serving a population of

250 000 would require one or two surgeons with a major vascular interest.[115] This arrangement produces a problem in the management of vascular surgical emergencies.[116] These account for approximately a third of the vascular work-load, and over half of vascular surgeons in the UK are currently on duty for emergency every other night or more.[117] In addition to this, over half of the general surgeons without a special interest in vascular surgery are carrying out small volumes of emergency vascular reconstructions.[118]

It is estimated that there are approximately 800 to 1200 new vascular referrals per million of population per year in the UK. This generates between 200 and 320 elective vascular reconstructions and between 160 and 240 emergency vascular operations per year.[115] These figures are based on audits of practice in the UK and are probably low compared with most other western countries.[119,120] In addition to this, recent trends towards more active attempts at limb salvage, evidence of the value of carotid surgery and the effect of an ageing population make it likely that the demand for vascular surgery will increase substantially over the next few years.

References

1. Johansson G, Swedenborg J. Ruptured abdominal aortic aneurysms: a study of incidence and mortality. *Br J Surg* 1986; **73:** 101–3.
2. Ouriel K, Geary K, Green RM, Fiore W, Geary JE, DeWeese JA. Factors determining survival after ruptured aortic aneurysm: the hospital, the surgeon, and the patient. *J Vasc Surg* 1990; **11:** 493–6.
3. Naylor AR, Webb J, Fowkes FG, Ruckley CV. Trends in abdominal aortic aneurysm surgery in Scotland (1971–84). *Eur J Vasc Surg* 1988; **2:** 217–21.
4. Hollier LH, Taylor LM, Ochsner J. Recommended indications for operative treatment of abdominal aortic aneurysms: report of a subcommittee of the Joint Council of the Society for Vascular Surgery and the North American Chapter of the International Society for Cardiovascular Surgery. *J Vasc Surg* 1992; **15:** 1046–56.
5. Bergqvist D, Bengtsson H. Should screening for abdominal aortic aneurysms be advocated. *Acta Chir Scand* 1990; **555** (Suppl): 89–97.
6. Russell JGB. Is screening for abdominal aortic aneurysm worthwhile? *Clin Rad* 1990; **41:** 182–4.
7. Second European Consensus Document on chronic critical leg ischemia. *Eur J Vasc Surg* 1992 (Suppl).
8. Tyrrell M, Wolfe JHN. Critical leg ischaemia: an appraisal of clinical definitions. *Br J Surg* 1993; **80:** 177–80.
9. Collin J. When is an aneurysm an aneurysm? *Curr Prac Surg* 1990; **2:** 65–7.
10. Moher D, Cole CW, Hill GB. Epidemiology of abdominal aortic aneurysm: the effect of differing definitions. *Eur J Vasc Surg* 1992; **6:** 647–50.
11. Eriksson I, Hallén A, Simonsson N, Åberg T. Surgical classification of abdominal aortic aneurysms. *Acta Chir Scand* 1979; **145:** 455–8.
12. Brewster DC, Darling RC, Raines JK, *et al.* Assessment of abdominal aortic aneurysm size. *Circulation* 1977; **56:** 164–9.
13. Krupski WC, Bass A, Thurston DW, Dilley RB, Bernstein EF. Utility of computed tomography for surveillance of small abdominal aortic aneurysms. *Arch Surg* 1990; **125:** 1345–50.
14. Darling RC, Messina CR, Brewster DC, Ottinger LW. Autopsy study of unoperated abdominal aortic aneurysm: the case for early resection. *Circulation* 1977; **56:** 161–4.
15. Moneta GL, Edwards JM, Chitwood RW, *et al.* Correlation of North American Symptomatic Carotid Endarterectomy Trial (NASCET) angiographic definition of 70% to 99% internal carotid stenosis with duplex scanning. *J Vasc Surg* 1993; **17:** 152–9.
16. Wesbey GE, Bergan JJ, Moreland SI, *et al.* Cerebrovascular magnetic resonance angiography: a critical verification. *J Vasc Surg* 1992; **16:** 619–28.
17. Frieman JA, Chalmers TC, Smith H, Kuebler RR. The importance of beta, the type II error and sample size in the design and interpretation of the randomized control trial: survey of 71 'negative' trials. *N Engl J Med* 1978; **299:** 690–4.
18. Veith FJ, Gupta SK, Ascer E, *et al.* Six-year prospective multicenter randomized comparison of autologous saphenous vein and expanded polytetrafluoroethylene grafts in infrainguinal arterial reconstructions. *J Vasc Surg* 1986; **3:** 104–14.
19. Pilcher DB, Davis JH, Ashikage T, *et al.* Treatment of abdominal aortic aneurysm in an entire state over 7½ years. *Am J Surg* 1980; **139:** 487–94.
20. White RA, Cavaye DM. Letter: Angioplasty restenosis: need for accurate definitions and controls. *J Vasc Surg* 1992; **16:** 797–8.
21. Creasy TS, McMillan PJ, Fletcher EWL, Collin J, Morris PJ. Is percutaneous transluminal angioplasty better than exercise for claudication? Preliminary results from a prospective randomised trial. *Eur J Vasc Surg* 1990; **4:** 135–40.
22. Hosie KB, Kockelberg R, Newbury ER, Callum KG, Nash JR. A retrospective review of the outcome of patients over 70 years of age considered for vascular reconstruction in a district general hospital. *Eur J Vasc Surg* 1990; **4:** 313–15.
23. Albers M, Fratezi AC, De LN. Assessment of quality of life of patients with severe ischemia as a result of infrainguinal arterial occlusive disease. *J Vasc Surg* 1992; **16:** 54–9.

24. Michaels JA, Galland RB. Case mix and outcome of patients referred to the vascular service at a District General Hospital. *Ann Roy Coll Surg Engl* 1993; **75:** 358–61.
25. Michaels JA, Browse, DJ, McWhinnie DL, Galland RB, Morris PJ. The provision of vascular surgical services in the Oxford Region. *Br J Surg* (in press).
26. Fowkes FGR. Epidemiology of atherosclerotic arterial disease in the lower limbs. *Eur J Vasc Surg* 1988; **2:** 283–92.
27. Criqui MH, Fronek A, Barrett-Conner E, Klauber MR, Gabriel S, Goodman D. The prevalence of peripheral arterial disease in a defined population. *Circulation* 1985; **71:** 510–15.
28. Widmer LK, Greensher A, Kannel WB. Occlusion of the peripheral arteries: a study of 6400 working subjects. *Circulation* 1964; **30:** 836–42.
29. Lyons C. An interdistrict audit of vascular surgery. *Qual Assur Hlth Care* 1991; **3:** 293–302.
30. McDaniel MD, Cronenwett JL. Basic data related to the natural history of intermittent claudication. *Ann Vasc Surg* 1989; **3:** 273–7.
31. Cronenwett JL, Warner KG, Zelenock GB, *et al.* Intermittent claudication: current results of non-operative management. *Arch Surg* 1984; **119:** 430–6.
32. Hallett JW, Greenwood LH, Robison JG. Lower extremity arterial disease in young adults: a systematic approach to early diagnosis. *Ann Surg* 1985; **202:** 647–52.
33. Dormandy J, Mahir M, Ascady G, *et al.* Fate of the patient with chronic leg ischaemia: a review article. *J Cardiovasc Surg Torino* 1989; **30:** 50–7.
34. Hertzer NR. Associated coronary disease in peripheral vascular patients. Louis, Missouri: Quality Medical Publishing Inc, 1991: 45–9.
35. Collin J, Araujo L, Lindsell DD. Screening for abdominal aortic aneurysms. *Lancet* 1987; **i:** 736–7.
36. Shapira OM, Pasik S, Wassermann JP, Barzilai N, Mashiah A. Ultrasound screening for abdominal aortic aneurysms in patients with atherosclerotic peripheral vascular disease. *J Cardiovasc Surg Torino* 1990; **31:** 170–2.
37. Galland RB, Simmons MJ, Torrie EPH. Prevalence of abdominal aortic aneurysm in patients with occlusive peripheral vascular disease. *Br J Surg* 1991; **78:** 1259–61.
38. Twomey A, Twomey E, Wilkins RA, Lewis JD. Unrecognised aneurysmal disease in male hypertensive patients. *Int Angiol* 1986; **5:** 269–73.
39. Dawson I, van-Bockel JH, Brand R, Terpsta JL. Popliteal artery aneurysm: long term follow up and results of surgical treatment. *J Vasc Surg* 1991; **13:** 398–407.
40. Collin J, Walton J. Is abdominal aortic aneurysm familial? *Br Med J* 1989; **299:** 49.
41. Collin J. Epidemiological aspects of abdominal aortic aneurysm. *Eur J Vasc Surg* 1990; **4:** 113–16.
42. Cronenwett JL, Sargent SK, Wall MH, *et al.* Variables that affect the expansion rate and outcome of small abdominal aortic aneurysms. *J Vasc Surg* 1990; **11:** 260–9.
43. Michaels JA. The management of small abdominal aortic aneurysms: a computer simulation using Monte Carlo methods. *Eur J Vasc Surg* 1992; **6:** 551–7.
44. Taylor LM, Porter JM. Basic data related to clinical decision-making in abdominal aortic aneurysms. *Ann Vasc Surg* 1986; **1:** 502–4.
45. Pennel RC, Hollier LH, Lie JT. Inflammatory aortic aneurysms: a thirty year review. *J Vasc Surg* 1985; **2:** 859–69.
46. Sieswerda C, Skotnicki SH, Barentsz JO, Heystraten FMJ. Anastomotic aneurysms: an underdiagnosed complication after aorto-iliac reconstruction. *Eur J Vasc Surg* 1989; **3:** 233–8.
47. Kresowik TF, Khoury MD, Miller BV, *et al.* A prospective study of the incidence and natural history of femoral vascular complications after percutaneous transluminal coronary angioplasty. *J Vasc Surg* 1991; **13:** 328–33.
48. Shanik GD, Moore DJ, Leahy A, Grouden MC, Colgan MP. Asymptomatic carotid stenosis: a benign lesion? *Eur J Vasc Surg* 1992; **6:** 10–15.
49. Taylor LM, Porter JM. Basic data related to carotid endarterectomy. *Ann Vasc Surg* 1986; **1:** 264–6.
50. Berens ES, Kouchoukos NT, Murphy SF, Wareing TH. Preoperative carotid artery screening in elderly patients undergoing cardiac surgery. *J Vasc Surg* 1992; **15:** 313–21.
51. De-Frang RD, Taylor LM, Porter JM. Basic data related to amputations. *Ann Vasc Surg* 1991; **5:** 202–7.
52. Naylor AR, Ah SA, Engeset J. Aortoiliac endarterectomy: an 11-year review. *Br J Surg* 1990; **77:** 190–3.
53. Bernstein EF, Kaplan JH, Scala TE, Koziol JA, Dilley RB. CHAT analysis of the influence of specific risk factors on late results after carotid endarterectomy. *J Vasc Surg* 1992; **16:** 575–85.
54. Keller MP, Hoch JR, Harding AD, Nichols WK, Silver D. Axillopopliteal bypass for limb salvage. *J Vasc Surg* 1992; **15:** 817–22.
55. Clason AE, Stonebridge PA, Duncan AJ, Nolan B, Jenkins AM, Ruckley CV. Morbidity and mortality in acute lower limb ischaemia: a 5-year review. *Eur J Vasc Surg* 1989; **3:** 339–43.
56. Rosenbloom MS, Flanigan DP, Schuler JJ, *et al.* Risk factors affecting the natural history of intermittent claudication. *Arch Surg* 1988; **123:** 867–70.
57. Mutirangura P, Stonebridge PA, Clason AE, *et al.* Ten-year review of non-ruptured aortic aneurysms. *Br J Surg* 1989; **76:** 1251–4.
58. Buck N, Devlin HB, Lunn JN. *Report of a Confidential Enquiry into Perioperative Deaths (CEPOD).* London: Nuffield Provincial Hospitals Trust, 1987.

59. Brien HW, Yellin AE, Weaver FA, Carroll BF. A review of carotid endarterectomy at a large teaching hospital. *Am Surg* 1991; **57:** 756–62.
60. Gibbs BF, Guzzetta VJ. Carotid endarterectomy in community practice: surgeon specific versus institutional results. *Ann Vasc Surg* 1989; **3:** 307–12.
61. Winslow CM, Solomon DH, Chassin MR, Kosecoff J, Merrick NJ, Brook RH. The appropriateness of carotid endarterectomy. *N Engl J Med* 1988; **318:** 721–7.
62. Yeager RA. Basic data related to cardiac testing and cardiac risk associated with vascular surgery. *Ann Vasc Surg* 1990; **4:** 193–7.
63. Cheshire NJ, Noone MA, Wolfe JH. Re-intervention after vascular surgery for critical leg ischaemia. *Eur J Vasc Surg* 1992; **6:** 545–50.
64. Michaels JA. Choice of material for above-knee femoropopliteal bypass graft. *Br J Surg* 1989; **76:** 7–14.
65. Harris PL, Veith FJ, Shanik GD, Nott D, Wengerter Kr, Moore DJ. Prospective randomized comparison of *in situ* and reversed infrapopliteal vein grafts. *Br J Surg* 1993; **80:** 173–6.
66. Quinones BW, Prego A, Ucelay GR, Vescera CL, Moore WS. Failure of PTFE infrainguinal revascularization: patterns, management alternatives, and outcome. *Ann Vasc Surg* 1991; **5:** 163–9.
67. Dalman RL, Taylor LJ. Basic data related to infrainguinal revascularization procedures. *Ann Vasc Surg* 1990; **4:** 309–12.
68. London NMJ, Sayers RD, Thompson MM, *et al.* Interventional radiology in the maintenance of infrainguinal graft patency. *Br J Surg* 1993; **80:** 187–93.
69. Krupski WC. The peripheral vascular consequences of smoking. *Ann Vasc Surg* 1991; **5:** 291–304.
70. Prendiville EJ, Yeager A, O'Donnell TJ, *et al.* Long-term results with the above-knee popliteal expanded polytetrafluoroethylene graft. *J Vasc Surg* 1990; **11:** 517–24.
71. Bergamini TM, Towne JB, Bandyk DF, Seabrook GR, Schmitt DD. Experience with *in situ* saphenous vein bypasses during 1981 to 1989: determinant factors of long-term patency. *J Vasc Surg* 1991; **13:** 137–47.
72. Ricco JB. Unilateral iliac artery occlusive disease: a randomized multicenter trial examining direct revascularization versus crossover bypass (Association Universitaire de Récherche en Chirurgie). *Ann Vasc Surg* 1992; **6:** 209–19.
73. Fahal AH, McDonald AM, Marston A. Femorofemoral bypass in unilateral iliac artery occlusion. *Br J Surg* 1989; **76:** 22–5.
74. Bacourt F, Koskas F. Axillobifemoral bypass and aortic exclusion for vascular septic lesions: a multicenter retrospective study of 98 cases (French University Association for Research in Surgery). *Ann Vasc Surg* 1992; **6:** 119–26.
75. Edwards WH, Edwards WJ, Jenkins JM, Mulherin JJ. Analysis of a decade of carotid reconstructive operations. *J Cardiovasc Surg Torino* 1989; **30:** 424–9.
76. Bernstein EF, Torem S, Dilley RB. Does carotid restenosis predict an increased risk of late symptoms, stroke, or death? *Ann Surg* 1990; **212:** 629–36.
77. Civil ID, O'Hara PJ, Hertzer NR, Krajewski LP, Beven EG. Late patency of the carotid artery after endarterectomy: problems of definition, follow-up methodology, and data analysis. *J Vasc Surg* 1988; **8:** 79–85.
78. Shah DM, Darling RC, Chang BB, Kaufman JL, Fitzgerald KM, Leather RP. Is long vein bypass from groin to ankle a durable procedure? An analysis of a ten-year experience. *J Vasc Surg* 1992; **15:** 402–7.
79. McCarthy WJ, Pearce WH, Flinn WR, McGee GS, Wang R, Yao JS. Long-term evaluation of composite sequential bypass for limb-threatening ischemia. *J Vasc Surg* 1992; **15:** 761–9.
80. Johnson JA, Cogbill TH, Strutt PJ, Gundersen AL. Wound complications after infrainguinal bypass: classification, predisposing factors, and management. *Arch Surg* 1988; **123:** 859–62.
81. Pons VG, Wurtz R. Vascular graft infections: a 25-year experience of 170 cases. *J Vasc Surg* 1991; **13:** 751–3.
82. Olah A, Vogt M, Laske A, Carrell T, Bauer E, Turina M. Axillo-femoral bypass and simultaneous removal of the aorto-femoral vascular infection site: is the procedure safe? *Eur J Vasc Surg* 1992; **6:** 252–4.
83. Edwards JM, Teefey SA, Zierler RE, Kohler TR. Intra-abdominal para-anastomotic aneurysms after aortic bypass grafting. *J Vasc Surg* 1992; **15:** 344–50.
84. Sommeling CA, Buth J, Jakimowicz JJ. Long-term behaviour of modified human umbilical vein grafts: late aneurysmal degeneration established by colour-duplex scanning. *Eur J Vasc Surg* 1990; **4:** 89–94.
85. Department of Health and Social Security. *Review of Artificial Limb and Appliance Centre Services.* London: HMSO, 1986.
86. Stern PH. Occlusive vascular disease of lower limbs; diagnosis, amputation surgery and rehabilitation: a review of the Burke experience. *Am J Phys Med Rehabil* 1988; **67:** 145–54.
87. Michaels JA. The selection of amputation level: an approach using decision analysis. *Eur J Vasc Surg* 1991; **5:** 451–7.
88. McCollum PT, Spence VA, Walker WF. Amputation for peripheral vascular disease: the case for level selection. *Br J Surg* 1988; **75:** 1193–5.
89. Department of Health and Social Security, Office of Population Censuses and Surveys. *Hospital Inpatient Enquiry.* London: HMSO, 1983–5.

90. Couch NP, David JK, Tilney NL, Crane C. Natural history of the leg amputee. *Am J Surg* 1977; **133:** 469–73.
91. Houghton AD, Taylor PR. Thurlow S, Rootes E, McColl I. Success rates for rehabilitation of vascular amputees: implications for preoperative assessment and amputation level. *Br J Surg* 1992; **79:** 753–5.
92. Ahn SS, Eton D, Moore WS. Endovascular surgery for peripheral arterial occlusive disease. A critical review. *Ann Surg* 1992; **216:** 3–16.
93. Michaels JA. Percutaneous arterial recanalization. *Br J Surg* 1990; **77:** 373–9.
94. van-Andel GJ, van-Erp WFM, Krepel VM, Breslau PJ. Percutaneous transluminal dilatation of the iliac artery: long term results. *Radiology* 1985; **156:** 321–3.
95. Johnston KW, Colapinto RF, Baird RF. Transluminal dilatation. *Arch Surg* 1982; **117:** 1604–10.
96. Zeitler E, Richter EI, Roth FJ, Schoop W. Results of percutaneous transluminal angioplasty. *Radiology* 1983; **146:** 57–60.
97. Colapinto RF, Stronell RD, Johnson KW. Transluminal angioplasty of complete iliac obstructions. *AJR* 1986; **146:** 859–62.
98. Adar R, Critchfield GC, Eddy DM. A confidence profile analysis of the results of femoropopliteal percutaneous transluminal angioplasty in the treatment of lower-extremity ischemia. *J Vasc Surg* 1989; **10:** 57–67.
99. Seeger JM. Basic data related to laser angioplasty. *Ann Vasc Surg* 1990; **4:** 515–18.
100. Lammer J, Pilger E, Decrinis M, Quehenberger F, Klein GE, Stark G. Pulsed excimer versus continuous-wave Nd-YAG laser versus conventional angioplasty of peripheral arterial occlusions: prospective, controlled, randomised trial. *Lancet* 1992; **ii:** 1183–8.
101. Vroegindeweij D, Kemper FJ, Tielbeek AV, Buth J, Landman G. Recurrence of stenoses following balloon angioplasty and Simpson atherectomy of the femoro-popliteal segment: a randomised comparative 1-year follow-up study using colour flow duplex. *Eur J Vasc Surg* 1992; **6:** 164–71.
102. Ahn SS, Eton D, Yeatman LR, Deutsch LS, Moore WS. Intraoperative peripheral rotary atherectomy: early and late clinical results. *Ann Vasc Surg* 1992; **6:** 272–80.
103. Earnshaw JJ. Thrombolytic therapy in the management of acute limb ischaemia. *Br J Surg* 1991; **78:** 261–9.
104. Lammer J, Pilger E, Neumayer K, Schreyer H. Intra-arterial thrombolysis: long term results. *Radiology* 1986; **161:** 159–163.
105. Moran KT, Jewell ER, Persson AV. The role of thrombolytic therapy in surgical practice. *Br J Surg* 1989; **76:** 298–304.
106. Tonnesen KH, Holstein P, Andersen E. Femoropopliteal artery occlusions treated by percutaneous transluminal angioplasty and enclosed thrombolysis: results in 55 patients. *Eur J Vasc Surg* 1991; **5:** 429–34.
107. Seabrook GR, Mewissen MW, Schmitt DD, *et al.* Percutaneous intra-arterial thrombolysis in the treatment of thrombosis of lower extremity arterial reconstructions. *J Vasc Surg* 1991; **13:** 646–51.
108. Belkin M, Donaldson MC, Whittemore AD, *et al.* Observations on the use of thrombolytic agents for thrombotic occlusion of infrainguinal vein grafts. *J Vasc Surg* 1990; **11:** 289–94.
109. Hess H, Ingrisch H, Mietaschk A, Rath H. Local low dose thrombolytic therapy of peripheral arterial occlusions. *N Engl J Med* 1982; **307:** 1627–30.
110. Hess H, Mietaschk A, Bruckl R. Peripheral arterial occlusions: a six-year experience with local low dose thrombolytic therapy. *Radiology* 1987; **163:** 753–8.
111. Giddings AE, Walker WJ. Letter: Recombinant tissue-type plasminogen activator is superior to streptokinase for local intra-arterial thrombolysis. *Br J Surg* 1992; **79:** 976.
112. Johnson C. Specialisation in general surgery. *Br J Surg* 1991; **78:** 259–60.
113. Veith FJ, Goldsmith J, Leather RP, Hannan EL. The need for quality assurance in vascular surgery. *J Vasc Surg* 1991; **13:** 523–6.
114. Clason AE, Stonebridge PA, Duncan AJ, Nolan B, Jenkins AM, Ruckley CV. Acute ischaemia of the lower limb: the effect of centralizing vascular surgical services on morbidity and mortality. *Br J Surg* 1989; **76:** 592–3.
115. Darke SG. The provision of vascular services. *Eur J Vasc Surg* 1987; **1:** 217–18.
116. Michaels JA, Galland RB. Prospective audit of vascular surgical emergencies in a District General Hospital. *Br J Surg* 1991; **78:** 1271–2.
117. Ruckley CV. Mounting problems in vascular surgery. *Br Med J* 1988; **298:** 577–8.
118. Ruckley C. Report on questionnaire surveys 1988–89. Presented at the Annual General Meeting of the Vascular Surgical Society of Great Britain and Northern Ireland, 1989.
119. Roberts JP, Chant AC, Smallwood JA, Webster JHH. Local audit in vascular surgery. *Ann Roy Coll Surg Engl* 1990; **72:** 287–90.
120. Campbell WB, Souter RG, Collin J, Wood RFM, Kidson IG, Morris PJ. Auditing the vascular surgical audit. *Br J Surg* 1987; **74:** 98–100.

Index